THORACIC ONCOLOGY

Thoracic Oncology

Editors

Noah C. Choi, M.D.
Department of Radiation Therapy
Harvard Medical School, and
Department of Radiation Medicine
Massachusetts General Hospital
Boston, Massachusetts

Hermes C. Grillo, M.D.
Department of Surgery
Harvard Medical School, and
General Thoracic Surgical Unit
Massachusetts General Hospital
Boston, Massachusetts

Raven Press ■ New York

Raven Press, 1140 Avenue of the Americas, New York, New York 10036

Made in the United States of America

Library of Congress Cataloging in Publication Data
Main entry under title:

Thoracic oncology.

Includes index.
1. Chest—Cancer.   I. Choi, Noah C.   II. Grillo,
Hermes C., 1923–
RC280.C5T48   1983   616.99′494   79-63971
ISBN 0-89004-434-1

The material contained in this volume was submitted as previously unpublished material, except in the instances in which credit has been given to the source from which some of the illustrative material was derived.

Great care has been taken to maintain the accuracy of the information contained in the volume. However, Raven Press cannot be held responsible for errors or for any consequences arising from the use of the information contained herein.

Preface

We have drawn together in this book the opinions of the thoracic surgeon, medical oncologist, pulmonary radiologist, pathologist, radiation oncologist, and epidemiologist on the spectrum of thoracic neoplasms. Incidence, etiology, pathology, clinical behavior and treatment of tumors of the airways, lung, mediastinum, pleura and esophagus are presented by physicians in a variety of disciplines—physicians whose daily commitment is to treating patients with these diseases. The surgical management of each type of thoracic tumor is discussed, as are radiation therapy, immunotherapy and chemotherapy.

While our colleagues from the Massachusetts General Hospital provide the largest part of the authorship, we are pleased to be joined by several outstanding authorities from other institutions, each of whom presents a topic of his or her special interest.

We believe that this multidisciplinary focus on thoracic oncology in a single, comprehensive volume provides an unusually thorough perspective for physicians training in these areas and for all practitioners involved in the management of thoracic neoplasms.

Noah C. Choi, M.D.
Hermes C. Grillo, M.D.

v

Contents

Contributors

James A. Bennett, Ph.D. *Assistant Professor of Surgery, Department of Surgery and Physiology, Albany Medical College, Albany, New York 12208*

Robert W. Carey, M.D. *Associate Professor of Medicine, Department of Medicine, Harvard Medical School; Physician, Department of Medicine, Massachusetts General Hospital, Boston, Massachusetts 02114*

Noah C. Choi, M.D. *Assistant Professor of Radiation Therapy, Department of Radiation Therapy, Harvard Medical School; Associate Radiation Oncologist, Department of Radiation Medicine, Massachusetts General Hospital, Boston, Massachusetts 02114*

Reginald E. Greene, M.D. *Associate Professor of Radiology, Department of Radiology, Harvard Medical School; Radiologist, Department of Radiology, Massachusetts General Hospital, Boston, Massachusetts 02114*

Hermes C. Grillo, M.D. *Professor of Surgery, Department of Surgery, Harvard Medical School; Visiting Surgeon, Chief of General Thoracic Surgery, Massachusetts General Hospital, Boston, Massachusetts 02114*

John M. Head, M.D. *Clinical Professor of Surgery, Department of Surgery, Dartmouth Medical School; Chief of Surgery, Department of Surgery, Veterans Administration Hospital, White River Junction, Vermont*

David J. Kanarek, M.D. *Assistant Professor of Medicine, Department of Medicine, Harvard Medical School; Assistant Physician, Department of Medicine, Massachusetts General Hospital, Boston, Massachusetts 02114*

Mark R. Katlic, M.D. *Chief Resident in Thoracic Surgery, Department of Surgery, Massachusetts General Hospital, Boston, Massachusetts 02114*

Eleanor J. Macdonald, M.D. *Professor Emeritus of Epidemiology, Department of Cancer Prevention, The University of Texas System Cancer Center, M.D. Anderson Hospital and Tumor Institute, Houston, Texas 77030*

Eugene J. Mark, M.D. *Assistant Professor of Pathology, Department of Pathology, Harvard Medical School; Associate Pathologist, Department of Pathology, Massachusetts General Hospital, Boston, Massachusetts 02114*

Martin F. McKneally, M.D. *Associate Professor of Surgery, Department of Surgery, Albany Medical College; Attending Thoracic Surgeon, Albany Medical Center, Albany, New York 12208*

Donald L. Paulson, M.D. *Clinical Professor of Surgery, Department of Thoracic and Cardiovascular Surgery, University of Texas Health Science Center; Attending Surgeon, Department of Surgery, Baylor University Medical Center, Dallas, Texas 75246*

James G. Pearson, M.B., CH.B. *Professor of Radiotherapy and Oncology, Division of Radiation Oncology, University of Alberta Medical School; Director of Radiation Oncology, Dr. W.W. Cross Cancer Institute, Edmonton, Alberta, Canada*

Salvatore Saita, M.D. *Professor of Surgery, Institute of Surgical Pathology, University of Catania, Vittorio Emanuelle Hospital, Via Plebiscito, 95100 Catania, Italy*

J. Gordon Scannell, M.D. *Clinical Professor of Surgery, Department of Surgery, Harvard Medical School; Visiting Surgeon, Department of Surgery, Massachusetts General Hospital, Boston, Massachusetts 02114*

Herman D. Suit, M.D., D. Phil. *Professor of Radiation Therapy, Chairman of Department of Radiation Therapy, Harvard Medical School; Andres Soriano Director of Cancer Management, Chief of Department of Radiation Medicine, Massachusetts General Hospital, Boston, Massachusetts 02114*

Earle W. Wilkins, Jr., M.D. *Clinical Professor of Surgery, Department of Surgery, Harvard Medical School; Visiting Surgeon, Department of Surgery, Massachusetts General Hospital, Boston, Massachusetts 02114*

Thoracic Oncology, edited by N. C. Choi and
H. C. Grillo. Raven Press, New York © 1983.

Present Direction in the Epidemiology of Lung Cancer

Eleanor J. Macdonald

*Department of Cancer Prevention, The University of Texas System Cancer Center,
M. D. Anderson Hospital and Tumor Institute, Houston, Texas 77030*

Consideration of the epidemiology of cancer of the lung must start with an awareness of the present state of knowledge in many branches of scientific endeavor. The huge investment of cancer funds in basic research in all the sciences, especially in the last 35 years, has brought about a greater realization of the complexity and interrelationships of the factors that contribute to the etiology of this disease. The work of these scientists may be likened to that of the artisans in the Middle Ages who gave a whole life of effort to perfect one cornice of a beautiful edifice and considered the time well spent. Our scientific artisans, by explaining the mechanism of one fragment after another of genetic, biochemical, somatic, behavioral, environmental, epidemiological, nutritional, and carcinogen-related information, are building gradually the whole structure which upon completion will reveal for our use the mechanisms involved in the genesis of each of the conditions grouped under the term "cancer".

INCIDENCE

Knowledge of the population-based incidence of cancer is the baseline for measuring the size of the problem. Over time, incidence data enables a study of trends, which in turn provides clues to the populations at risk and the factors involved. The World Health Organization (WHO) has gathered together several yearly averages of incidence data from 69 population segments around the world (3). Among males, the variation in age-adjusted lung cancer incidence rates is from a high of 86.6 per 100,000 in Liverpool to a low of 13.3 per 100,000 in Bombay; among females, the variation is from 11.8 in Liverpool to 1.9 per 100,000 in Hungary. Among white males, the age-adjusted lung cancer incidence rates as percentages of total cancer incidence account for over one-fourth in every region in England, Scotland, Finland, and the German Democratic Republic. Rates for white females in the same regions fall in the same pattern (Table 1).

In Texas, an intensive, carefully controlled study (26), covering 23 consecutive years, examined the cancer incidence in a population of 4 million, in one-third of the state, comprising 56 contiguous counties and three major ethnic groups. Every known source of records was covered, including dermatologists' offices, clinics,

TABLE 1. *Incidence of total cancer and lung cancer for 23 countries, 69 population groups in 5 continents, average annual adjusted rates per 100,000*

	Latitude (degrees)	Total cancer				Cancer of the lung				Lung cancer as percentage of total cancer	
		Male		Female		Male		Female		Male	Female
		No. cases	Age-adjusted rates	No. cases	Age-adjusted rates	No. cases	Age-adjusted rates	No. cases	Age-adjusted rates		
Caucasians except Spanish-surnamed											
America											
United States											
Hawaii-Caucasian	18-22	843	265.1	808	235.4	131	43.8	34	10.2	16.5	4.3
Texas-Harlingen	26	1,648	458.3	1,355	354.6	131	36.3	27	6.8	7.9	1.9
Texas-Laredo	27-28	479	491.8	378	380.9	36	37.4	6	6.5	7.6	1.7
Texas-San Antonio	29-30	6,226	349.7	6,063	295.2	718	40.8	134	6.3	11.7	2.1
Texas-Houston	30	7,616	362.0	8,228	322.2	1,150	54.4	235	9.3	15.0	2.9
Texas-El Paso	31-32	1,200	330.9	1,289	306.2	95	28.3	25	6.3	8.6	2.1
Texas-Corpus Christi	27-28	3,547	577.6	3,015	442.9	298	48.5	58	8.9	8.4	2.0
Nevada	35-42	3,726	236.9	3,325	238.5	441	27.5	87	6.3	11.6	2.6
California-Alameda	38	5,573	254.1	6,090	226.0	1,032	47.8	198	7.4	18.8	3.3
Connecticut	41-42	12,229	257.8	11,935	220.0	2,062	44.0	423	7.8	17.1	3.5
Canada											
New Brunswick	45-48	1,725	275.5	1,760	286.5	156	27.0	24	4.2	9.8	1.5
Quebec	45-62	19,824	209.3	20,724	198.2	2,667	28.7	443	4.3	13.7	2.2
Newfoundland	46-60	2,148	265.2	1,607	207.2	182	23.5	24	3.1	8.9	1.5
Alberta	49-60	6,608	225.6	5,824	222.2	702	25.8	105	4.1	11.4	1.8
Manitoba	49-60	6,357	281.1	5,663	261.1	928	42.2	162	7.3	15.0	2.8
Saskatchewan	49-60	8,042	330.3	5,830	285.9	642	28.7	99	5.0	8.7	1.7
Asia											
India-Bombay	18-19	5,852	139.5	3,851	131.1	504	13.3	86	3.7	9.5	2.8
Israel											
All Jews	30-33	12,193	180.6	13,194	188.8	1,785	26.4	586	8.7	14.6	4.6
Jews born in Israel	30-33	880	138.6	902	144.7	55	17.3	28	7.0	12.5	4.8

Jews born in Africa or Asia	30-33	2,845	148.7	2,563	126.3	430	22.7	118	6.1	15.3	4.8
Jews born in Europe or America	30-33	8,468	203.7	9,729	225.0	1,300	29.6	440	9.8	14.5	4.4
Non-Jews	30-33	795	132.2	430	70.7	134	24.6	18	3.1	18.6	4.4
Europe											
Yugoslavia-Slovenia	45-46	8,070	204.1	8,645	165.6	1,537	38.5	238	4.4	18.9	2.7
Romania-Banat region	45	1,420	176.9	1,446	151.6	209	24.9	36	3.5	14.1	2.3
Hungary											
County Vas	46-47	1,599	174.7	1,606	157.9	216	22.8	58	5.4	13.1	3.4
Szabolcs-Szatmar	47-48	2,092	142.2	1,983	115.2	212	14.3	34	1.9	10.1	1.6
Miskolc	48	715	175.1	798	158.4	113	28.4	29	5.6	16.2	3.5
Poland											
Four rural areas	49	809	165.2	829	131.1	129	26.2	25	3.8	15.9	2.9
Warsaw city	49	2,383	214.9	3,691	204.7	522	46.9	160	8.4	21.8	4.1
Cracow city and district	49-50	3,540	154.8	3,592	122.2	654	27.9	118	3.9	18.0	3.2
Katowice district	49-50	4,236	136.3	5,038	122.2	919	29.4	116	2.7	21.6	2.2
German Democratic Republic (DDR)	50-54	74,783	211.7	88,572	190.0	17,617	48.8	2,230	4.3	23.1	2.3
England											
South-western region	45-52	20,849	245.1	21,064	198.0	5,059	60.3	953	8.7	24.6	4.4
Oxford region	51-52	10,777	234.2	10,317	175.8	2,920	63.1	575	9.8	26.9	5.6
Sheffield region	52-53	26,573	227.4	25,496	182.8	7,562	64.1	1,178	8.5	28.2	4.6
England and Wales-											
Liverpool region	52-54	19,655	288.7	18,536	199.9	5,982	86.6	1,109	11.8	30.0	5.9
England-Birmingham region	53	30,316	254.5	28,571	196.3	8,977	73.3	1,254	8.4	28.8	4.3
Denmark	55-57	33,112	221.1	35,842	223.3	4,609	31.4*	868	5.2*	14.2	2.3
Scotland	55-61	28,791	231.5	27,618	173.8	8,440	67.0	1,551	9.9	28.9	5.7
Sweden	55-69	45,582	199.4	48,168	203.2	4,363	19.2	1,142	4.4	9.6	2.2
Norway	57-71	13,763	174.8	14,023	164.9	1,263	16.5	279	3.1	9.4	1.9
Urban	57-71	6,397	207.1	6,966	181.8	784	25.2	168	4.2	12.2	2.3
Rural	57-71	7,366	153.7	7,057	151.2	479	10.5	111	2.2	6.8	1.5
Finland	60-70	21,591	259.7	21,247	182.8	5,980	70.0	530	4.4	27.0	2.4
Africa											
South Africa-Cape Province-white	33	2,012	371.2	1,934	276.7	237	44.7*	37	5.3*	12.0	1.9
Oceania											
New Zealand-European	34-47	15,734	242.1	14,261	200.0	2,865	45.1	428	6.1	18.6	3.1

TABLE 1. (continued)

	Latitude (degrees)	Total cancer				Cancer of the lung				Lung cancer as percentage of total cancer	
		Male		Female		Male		Female			
		No. cases	Age-adjusted rates	No. cases	Age-adjusted rates	No. cases	Age-adjusted rates	No. cases	Age-adjusted rates	Male	Female
Black											
America											
United States											
Texas-San Antonio	29-30	407	253.1	427	227.9	55	34.5	10	5.0	13.6	2.2
Texas-Houston	30	1,425	268.4	1,802	277.0	245	44.5	48	8.1	16.6	2.9
Texas-Corpus Christi	27-28	123	248.2	159	278.6	30	60.2	5	8.9	24.3	3.2
California-Alameda	38	545	251.1	552	195.7	106	43.8	22	9.0	17.4	4.6
Jamaica-Kingston and St. Andrew	7-18	713	212.3	1,079	200.2	83	24.6	35	7.5	11.6	3.7
Africa											
Nigeria-Ibadan	7-8	707	76.7	718	104.8	12	1.2	8	1.0	1.6	1.0
Rhodesia-Bulawayo	20	450	304.9	132	370.4	59	47.1	2	4.7	15.4	1.3
South Africa											
Natal-African	29-31	882	208.9	508	162.6	183	41.2	25	10.2	19.7	6.3
Natal-Indian	29-31	220	129.1	276	188.3	30	20.0	4	3.3	15.5	1.8
Cape Province											
Colored	33	728	217.0	777	164.5	129	42.8*	19	4.2*	19.7	2.6
Bantu	33	199	232.0	91	156.0	19	26.9*	2	4.9*	11.6	3.1

Spanish-surnamed											
America											
Colombia-Cali	3-4	1,698	245.9	2,441	260.3	107	17.5	31	3.8	7.1	1.5
Puerto Rico	17-18	6,100	205.0	5,457	180.1	392	13.6	149	5.0	6.6	2.8
United States											
Texas-Harlingen	26	819	216.5	1,107	258.4	106	28.8	31	7.6	13.3	2.9
Texas-Laredo	27-28	384	193.2	552	240.9	42	21.7	23	9.8	11.2	4.1
Texas-Corpus Christi	27-28	527	229.4	740	282.6	67	31.2	24	11.1	13.6	3.9
Texas-San Antonio	29-30	1,257	185.1	1,814	236.3	135	20.6	49	6.8	11.1	2.9
Texas-Houston	30	263	214.4	371	269.4	29	23.8	12	12.3	11.1	4.6
Texas-El Paso	31-32	404	186.3	702	248.1	45	22.8	27	10.7	12.2	4.3
Oriental											
America											
United States-Hawaii											
Hawaiian	18-20	376	313.6	362	264.8	82	70.3	28	22.3	22.4	8.4
Chinese	18-20	205	207.0	193	228.3	27	27.2	13	16.7	13.1	7.3
Filipino	18-20	325	131.0	96	180.9	43	17.1	8	17.4	13.1	9.6
Japanese	18-20	1,006	207.6	795	160.8	123	26.3	37	7.6	12.7	4.7
Asia											
Japan											
Okayama Prefecture	35	1,670	189.3	1,471	145.4	140	15.3	55	5.2	8.1	3.6
Miyagi Prefecture	37-39	4,082	196.0	3,623	142.8	321	15.6	151	6.0	8.0	4.2
Oceania											
New Zealand-Maori	34-47	512	259.3	560	276.8	124	70.1	60	37.7	27.0	13.6

*Not fully comparable.

Sources: Cancer Incidence in Five Continents (3); Texas data (1962-66, world standard), Macdonald, E. J., professor emeritus of epidemiology, Department of Cancer Prevention, The University of Texas System Cancer Center, M.D. Anderson Hospital and Tumor Institute, Houston, Texas.

laboratories, and group medical practices. Because of the unusual completeness and accuracy of the data, they are being cited as a microcosm of the cancer experiences in developed states and countries: these data represent varied degrees of urban density, industrial complexes, large seaports, rural agricultural communities, and altitudes and climates ranging from the temperate to the tropical, as well as genetic and sex differences. During this period of 23 consecutive years, there was a total of 9,551 cancers of the lung, of which 7,855 were in males, and 1,696 were in females.

The lung cancer rates for the entire period and for the last 5 years per 100,000 population in the six regions are given in Table 2, by ethnic group and sex. The age-adjusted rate for the six combined regions for males was 47.6 per 100,000. By

TABLE 2. *Cancer of the lung: number of cases and age-adjusted incidence rates per 100,000, six regions in Texas,[a] 1944–1966*

	White males	Nonwhite males	Spanish-surnamed males	White females	Nonwhite females	Spanish-surnamed females	Total population
All regions							
1944–1966	6,099	784	972	1,162	144	390	9,551
1944–1966	37.278	33.802	18.332	6.306	5.839	7.034	18.792
1962–1966	53.626	48.936	29.118	9.034	8.977	10.386	26.893
El Paso							
1944–1966	255	4	117	65	4	72	517
1944–1966	26.037	8.974	20.344	5.761	7.755	10.201	14.783
1962–1966	33.449	17.292	26.717	6.817	9.483	12.875	18.717
San Antonio							
1944–1966	1,782	155	321	347	25	118	2,748
1944–1966	30.706	29.072	15.987	5.158	4.006	5.630	15.258
1962–1966	47.438	40.855	24.854	7.339	5.897	8.123	22.578
Laredo							
1944–1966	130	2	118	25	0	56	331
1944–1966	42.662	26.058	19.289	8.401	.000	7.614	16.846
1962–1966	41.391	.000	26.325	7.123	.000	11.823	20.195
Harlingen							
1944–1966	336	2	195	66	2	62	663
1944–1966	28.688	8.687	17.077	5.464	13.298	5.567	13.882
1962–1966	42.563	.000	34.801	7.563	45.057	9.645	22.307
Corpus Christi							
1944–1966	725	59	138	112	17	50	1,101
1944–1966	38.767	38.597	20.470	5.555	10.057	8.110	19.903
1962–1966	56.417	68.946	37.966	9.734	10.807	13.104	30.182
Houston							
1944–1966	2,871	562	83	547	96	32	4,191
1944–1966	46.231	36.063	28.624	7.676	5.995	12.859	24.599
1962–1966	63.060	50.689	26.714	10.626	9.452	14.980	32.864

[a]1960 standard.
From Macdonald and Heinze (26).

ethnic groups, the rate per 100,000 for white males was 53.6, for nonwhite males, 48.9, and for Spanish-surnamed males, 29.1. The rate per 100,000 for white females was 9.0, for nonwhite females, 9.0, and for Spanish-surnamed females, 10.3. In all regions, the ratio between white and nonwhite males and females was approximately 6 to 1, and between Spanish-surnamed males and females, approximately 3 to 1. The other ethnic and regional differences are evident from these rates. The rates for Spanish-surnamed females were nearly double those for white females in El Paso and Laredo, and were also higher in every other region. The converse was true for Spanish-surnamed males and white males in the same regions.

MORTALITY

Public health measures in the United States have successively evolved a population that in 1980 is healthy beyond what anyone would have imagined 50 years ago. The mortality rate from all causes in the United States, in the most recent available year, 1977, was 8.9 per 1,000, an all-time low. The expected life span has risen from 59.7 years in 1930 to 72.5 years in 1975 (for males, 68.7 years, for females, 76.5 years) (45). Mortality from the greatest killers, the cardiovascular diseases, has dropped. Half of all people who develop cancer are over 65 at the time of diagnosis, and more than 10% of the total U. S. population is over 65—more than 23 million individuals. So there is a large number of people in the age groups in which cancer-susceptibles are clustered. A steady increase in the total cancer mortality rate has been observed. Despite all these potential reasons for a massive increase in cancer, total cancer, when adjusted for age, has increased only 2.5% in the 10-year period from 1968 through 1977, a very modest increase in percentage points, although it is large in numbers. This reflects the results of cancer programs in producing an increase in survivals, an increase in person-to-person education between concerned physicians and patients, and improvement in techniques for early diagnosis and treatment as well as supportive care.

Age-adjusted mortality rates for many kinds of cancer are either stabilizing or declining. The two exceptions are the rates for cancer of the digestive system and cancer of the respiratory system. The separation of true cancer of the respiratory system from other respiratory conditions is demonstrated in Fig. 1, which relates the advent of new antibiotics to the drop in communicable respiratory disease mortality. The gradual increase of reported lung cancer is inversely related to the drop in competing respiratory risks.

The steady decrease in mortality from tuberculosis has been almost exactly replaced by the increase in lung cancer. Wong (51) hypothesized that if people were susceptible to both tuberculosis and lung cancer, the deaths at earlier ages from tuberculosis would result in fewer deaths from lung cancer. But successful treatment has prevented much of the mortality from tuberculosis, with a consequent increase in lung cancer mortality. The association between these two causes of death is illustrated in a study by Ipsen (17), in which he observed that respiratory cancer occurred 5.3 times more often among those who had died of tuberculosis and that

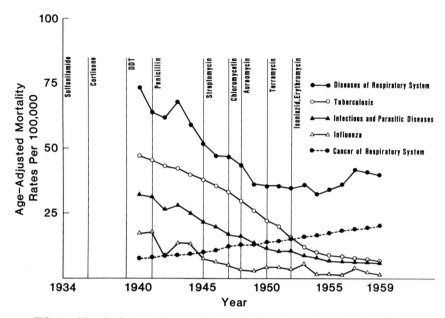

FIG. 1. Mortality from respiratory diseases by dates of introduction of antibiotics.

tuberculosis occurred 3.8 times more often among those who had died of respiratory cancer than among the general population.

Understanding the dynamics of change in the mortality rates for lung cancer among men and women can be aided by examining the rate of change over time in the death rates. This was done by approximating the first derivative of the empirical time function by a "moving slope, a linear slope calculated for consecutive overlapping time intervals of fixed length" (49). Analysis of the moving slope for the death rates from cancer of the bronchus, trachea, and lung from 1950 to 1975 showed an entirely different pattern for white males than for white females, as illustrated in Fig. 2. The moving slope for white male mortality indicates that until 1960 there was a gradually decreasing trend in the rate of increase, but that the rates accelerated sharply in the early 1960s and have been in a steady decline since then. For females, the corresponding graph shows a slowly increasing rate of increase until the late 1950s, when a sharp and steady acceleration began which lasted until almost 1970. Then a slight deceleration occurred, followed by a much more gradual acceleration than in the previous rise.

A 40-year interest in cancer mortality data culminated in a comprehensive study (50) published in 1979 on the relationship of environmental and ethnic factors to the mortality for each site of cancer for every state and region of the United States. A large number of factors, data for which were available for every state, were studied in depth, individually and in combination, to ascertain their influence on the geographic patterns of cancer of each site. In order to carry out a systematic analysis providing comparability across cancer sites, a pool of 12 variables was

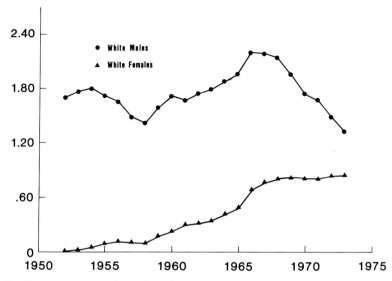

FIG. 2. Five-year moving slope of respiratory cancer mortality curve, United States, 1950–1975. Variation in the rate of increase (absolute net %) per 100,000 based on rates age-adjusted to 1970 U.S. population.

chosen for the derivation of the geographic models for each type of cancer mortality in the United States. The variables represented were smoking, consumption of different kinds of alcoholic beverages, ethnic background, pollution, income, temperature, and precipitation/elevation. Information on industrial employment risks was not available.

The male mortality models for cancer of the trachea, bronchus, and lung, specified as primary, indicate only one highly significant factor besides income (INCM), and that is the strongly positive effect of temperature (TEMP), a characteristic shared only by the corresponding female mortality models and by the skin cancer mortality models for both sexes. Pollution (POLLUT) also enters as a significant factor, but only when INCM is not in the model, indicating a possible interchange between the two effects. This appears to be even more the case in the models for the unspecified category, where an uninterpretable negative POLLUT effect alternates with a negative INCM effect. The correlation between these two variables is not large (.407), but the variation that they have in common could represent specifically those state differences that produce the varying quality in medical diagnosis and records.

Precipitation/elevation (PRELEV), a strong positive effect in most of the cancer mortality models, is notably weak in the models for primary lung cancer in males, and it does not even enter the female mortality models for this cancer category. A few of the consumption and ethnic factors enter these models positively but weakly: cigarettes (CIGS), wine, and Scandinavian ethnicity (SCAN).

It is clear that the variable pools do not contain all the factors needed to explain sufficiently the variation in lung cancer since only 44.26% is accounted for by the full 12-variable equation. The chosen models for lung cancer do explain a large proportion of this percentage however. In other sites of cancer, by contrast, the equations account for up to 90% of the variation in the rates.

CHEMICAL CARCINOGENESIS

The health hazards of cigarette smoking have been reported in too many investigations to need further amplification here (41). Those studies that have considered the fact of smoking and the presence of lung cancer have all reported an association. Many of these important studies have failed to examine adequately the relationship of occupation to cigarette smoking. Recent studies (42,44) have demonstrated that the smoking characteristics of males, and to some extent of females, are strongly associated with types of employment. The time has come to consider the epidemiologic evidence for factors other than smoking in the search for etiologic clues. Recognition of the carcinogenic implications in the workplace, in urban and even in home environments, suggests that the smoking connection should be considered in perspective as one of many etiologic factors in this complex disease.

The recognition of the importance of environmental (including nutritional) factors in causing cancer has been summarized recently by Sir Richard Doll (3): "That environmental factors contribute to the production of the majority of causes with which we have to contend is now obvious, and there is no need to review the evidence in detail. It rests on the great variation in the incidence of most cancers, both from place to place and almost certainly also from time to time; on the experience of migrants, among whom the risk of cancer changes to that of their adopted country in the course of one or two generations; on the recognition every year or so of a new occupational or iatrogenic hazard; and on the discovery that particular types of cancer can be related to specific types of behavior or correlated quantitatively with exposure to a known laboratory carcinogen."

Scientists who had previously reported urban pollution as an insignificant factor in lung cancer genesis have, after further research, reported a significant relationship between urbanization and lung cancer incidence and an even greater relationship between benzopyrene exposure and lung cancer incidence (4). These relationships held when standardization for cigarette smoking was done, which confirmed the fact that air pollution itself is a significant factor in the etiology of lung cancer.

Asbestos exposure is a similar case in point. In the early reports (12) it was hypothesized that asbestos exposure and cigarette smoking were synergistic. Later reports on the same data showed that the relative mortality risk for lung cancer among asbestos workers was the same for nonsmokers as for smokers. A mounting increase in the identification of one industrial lung cancer carcinogen after another has opened many avenues of study and emphasized the importance of the industrial environment. Control of these carcinogens at their source offers a positive potential for prevention.

While man has proved himself over the ages to be remarkably adaptable in his biological responses to the evolution from a primitive to an agricultural to an industrial environment, the change in the last 100 years to a near-artificial man-made environment, through the introduction of new physical and chemical agents (pesticides, plastics, herbicides, artificial colors, food additives, among others), has been too fast to allow a natural defense mechanism to develop. Whereas this generation has the advantages of longevity, leisure, and control of communicable diseases, it also has, as a by-product of material progress, the new type of health hazard represented by exposure to chemical and physical agents possessing carcinogenic properties.

An estimate by the Environmental Protection Agency (EPA) that 60,000 chemicals are in commercial use and that new ones are being introduced at the rate of 1,000 a year may be a modest estimate. Many of these chemicals have been recognized as carcinogenic, and some have been banned. Because it takes so long to identify carcinogens, and because the latent period to carcinogenesis after exposure often is so long, many people who have been exposed to carcinogens will develop cancer before these chemicals are recognized as carcinogens. That many chemicals become carcinogenic only in combination with other chemicals enlarges the pool of agents to be studied. Many chemicals that in themselves are only weakly carcinogenic are present in such large quantities in our environment that their total cancer-producing effect may be greater than that of known strong carcinogens (2).

Most known carcinogenic agents were first identified by clinical physicians examining humans who had been subjected to occupational exposure. Notable examples of this are provided by Percival Pott (15), who in 1775 identified chimney-sweeps' cancer; Creech and Johnson (7), who identified angiosarcoma in vinyl chloride workers; and Rehn (40), who identified bladder cancer in aniline dye workers. Often the specific cause-and-effect relationship has been obscured by the long latent period between biological insult and onset of disease and because until recently it was not realized that the exposure does not have to be continuous.

The tremendous variety of toxic and carcinogenic airborne chemicals produced by modern society and released into our indoor and outdoor environment, in our homes and in our workplaces, places a heavy burden on each of us physically from repeated and cumulative exposures.

Research toward identification of carcinogens is more effective and potentially more productive in controlled populations in the workplace than in studies of the general population. In such studies it is recognized that the physical requirements of good health at the time of first employment, followed by regular health checkups, make the work force healthier than the population at large. The employed population may be considered a "healthy survivor" group. In contrast, the general population includes large numbers of individuals unemployed because of sickness, disability, or previous occupational injury or disease, as well as the institutionalized population. As a result, in such studies the expected cancer rate derived from the general population for a particular type of cancer will be high, which tends to lessen the difference between the observed rates in industry and the expected rates. This dilutes the true magnitude of the work-related risk.

Governmental and nongovernmental organizations are at work trying to determine the increased risk for each suspected carcinogen, together with its impact on the industrial population and on society as a whole. The underlying objective is to institute measures for prevention and control. The Occupational Safety and Health Administration (OSHA) has officially listed 17 carcinogens, 6 of which are etiological factors in the induction of lung cancer (28). These are asbestos fibers, coke-oven emissions, 3,3'-dichlorobenzidine (and its salts), vinyl chloride, chloromethyl methyl ether (CMME), and bis-chloromethyl ether (BCME). The International Agency for Research on Cancer (IARC) of the WHO has published a series of monographs (18) on industrial carcinogens, in the summary of which nine are listed as carcinogenic for lung cancer: arsenic and certain arsenic compounds, asbestos, BCME and CMME, chromium and certain chromium compounds, underground mining of hematite, mustard gas, nickel refining, soots, tars, mineral oils, and vinyl chloride. The IARC also lists 12 other chemicals as suspected lung cancer carcinogens: acrylonitrile, beryllium and certain beryllium compounds, cadmium and certain cadmium compounds, dimethyl sulfates, epichlorohydrin, hematite (ferric oxide), hexachlorocyclohexane, isoniazid, lead and certain lead compounds, nickel and certain nickel compounds, 2,3,7,8-tetrachlorodibenzo-p-dioxin, and vinylidene chloride.

In a recent communication, reevaluation by Kang, Infante, and Carra (20) of the data previously interpreted as supporting noncarcinogenicity of lead in humans showed a significant excess of mortality from two categories of cancer, digestive and respiratory, among workers exposed to lead. Cancer of the respiratory system in lead-smelter workers and battery-plant workers was demonstrated to be statistically significant regardless of the type of statistical analysis employed. The magnitude of the risk among the lead-exposed workers in the study by Cooper and Gaffey may still be underestimated, because the latency period for 59% of the smelter workers and 36% of the battery-plant workers was less than 20 years. The IARC has issued two caveats for research into the identification of carcinogenic risks by epidemiologic means: (a) failure to analyze data by latency categories presumably will result in a dilution of findings in studies of any disease characterized by long latency; (b) such studies must emphasize the need for use of appropriate epidemiologic methodology and statistical analysis and for full presentation of data in a format that permits an assessment of latency.

Ionizing radiation has long been recognized as a carcinogen for cancer of the lung and even other sites (15). The Joachimsthal and Schneeberg miners in Europe and uranium miners of the United States have demonstrated on a large scale the excess lung cancer risk.

The carcinogenic potential of chemicals extends to the neighborhood surrounding an industry as well as the workplace itself. Examples of this include beryllium, coal-tar fumes, asbestos, isopropol oil, ionizing radiation, and arsenic (copper smelters).

A recent publication by Hoover and Fraumeni (14) showed that in a county by county mortality study of the general population of the United States there was a

10% excess of cancer of the lung, liver, and bladder among males in the 139 counties where the chemical industry is most highly concentrated. The authors state that if this excess is due to occupational exposure, then the risk of these cancers would be two to three times the risk for the general population. This study suggests fresh leads to chemical exposure that may be carcinogenic and states that of particular note are elevated risks of lung cancer in counties producing pharmaceutical preparations, soaps and detergents, paints, inorganic pigments, and synthetic rubber.

In the evaluation of epidemiologic data relative to the effects of exposure to industrial carcinogens, results are more acceptable when the comparisons by different lengths of exposure are made using cohorts of exposed workers and control cohorts in the same industry and in other industries not exposed to the carcinogen being studied, but for the same age groups and years of observation. There are limitations to estimation of risk when studies of industrial hazards compare the morbidity and mortality of the general population with that of the industrial population. The differing latent periods between internal exposure and onset of cancer for different carcinogens make interpretation more difficult.

The cohort study (48) of workers exposed to vinyl chloride demonstrates the importance of considering duration of exposure. When a comparison was made between the risk for a cohort of workers with 10 years of exposure and the risk for a cohort of workers with 15 years of exposure, the excess risk of each site-specific cancer was increased. Although it was angiosarcoma of the liver, occurring in a cluster of surgical patients, that brought the danger of vinyl chloride to public attention, it was found that the respiratory system, the brain, and the hematopoietic system also experienced increased risk among exposed workers. Vinyl chloride also causes chromosomal aberrations in male workers and an excess of miscarriages in their wives.

Investigations of cancer in the rubber industry have emphasized the complexity of the epidemiologic aspects in the recognition of occupational cancers, not only in the rubber industry but in every industry. Because different chemicals are introduced at different times by companies engaged in the manufacture and processing of various products, this results in the appearance of biological effects during different periods of time. The detection of cancer risk is enhanced by studying cohorts of employees in a departmental comparison, with periods of observation of 20 to 30 years or more. For example, all deaths from lung cancer in a curing department were from a cohort of employees over 30 years of age (31).

Exposure to all types of commercial asbestos fibers results in a high incidence of lung cancer in humans, not only in the workplace but also in the neighborhood of asbestos factories and in asbestos mines, as well as among persons living with asbestos workers.

One of the important leads found by Fraumeni et al., in their U.S. county-by-county study (1,9) suggests exploration of the shipbuilding industry, in which asbestos and other shipyard exposures occurring during wartime employment accounted for part of the excess lung cancer mortality reported later in certain coastal areas of the United States.

An increased risk of lung cancer, particularly oat cell cancer, has been demonstrated (23,38) in workers exposed to chloromethyl ethers and to BCME which was directly related to intensity and duration of exposure and was not cigarette-related.

There is an increased incidence of lung cancer (29) among workers in the chromate industry and among those working with chromium plating and chrome pigment, which has raised the question of whether or not all forms of chromium may be carcinogenic. Lung cancer mortality among chromate workers clusters at 27 to 36 years from exposure, which demonstrates how long the latent period can be from cause to effect and how long a follow-up period of observation is required.

Exposure to mustard gas causes lung cancer, especially among those who have experienced chronic industrial exposure. The incidence of lung cancer is higher than was expected among workers in nickel refineries. Soots, tars, and mineral oils have long been recognized as causes of lung cancer, and many recent studies support this finding. Underground hematite miners have a high incidence of lung cancer (18). Whether this is caused by radon or inhalation of ferric oxide or by a combination of these and other factors is not known.

The case for beryllium as a lung carcinogen has been demonstrated in recent reports (30). Mancuso's study, reported in 1980, showed that the amount of exposure necessary to establish a biologically effective dose for the induction of lung cancer can occur within a few months of exposure regardless of whether the individual is employed for less than 1 year or for 10 years or more. The latent period from exposure to carcinogenesis was from 20 to 30 years. Once inhaled, this substance is retained in the body for a long time, and it has been detected in the urine 10 years after exposure. Once the biologically effective carcinogenic dose has been received, additional exposure to beryllium may not be required.

The long-term mortality findings of increased lung cancer for cohorts of coke-oven workers at 12 North American steel plants, found to be 2.85 times greater than for workers in other parts of the plant, showed a dose–response relationship between some carcinogenic element or elements in the coke-oven effluents and the development of lung cancer (24,39).

Excessive liability to lung cancer among American uranium-ore miners has been established by a series of studies. It has been ascertained that the cumulative dose of airborne radiation contained within uranium-ore mines was responsible for the excess of lung cancer among the miners (33,47).

It was found that inhalation of high concentrations of arsenic trioxide increased the risk of lung cancer as much as 4 to 12 times among copper-smelter workers; other potential carcinogens were present, the effect of which could not be excluded (22). More recent studies (35) have demonstrated the increased risk to individuals living in communities around copper smelters. Follow-up of the exposed populations, particularly the children, is imperative. As an indication of carcinogenic exposure, the urinary arsenic levels for men working at the smelter were similar to those found in people living near it. The urinary arsenic levels showed an inverse relationship to age, with younger children showing consistently higher concentrations.

The part played in lung carcinogenesis by the petrochemical industries is not yet completely documented, but the county-by-county study of Mason and McKay (34) gives some thought-provoking leads by pinpointing counties with high incidences of lung cancer in those areas with great petrochemical exposure. Half the petrochemical industry of the United States is located in Houston, Texas, and most of the plants are on the Houston Ship Channel. A study (25) was made in Houston of age-adjusted mortality rates for each cause of death for a 30-year period which grouped the data by the census tracts surrounding the 15 air-pollution sampling stations. It revealed high mortality from lung cancer, heart diseases, and all other respiratory diseases from the ship channel in the southeast to the northwest in the pathway of the winds prevailing 11 months of the year. In the last 15 years of the study, deaths from respiratory cancer and other respiratory diseases and heart diseases had doubled, whereas the 30-year rates outside this pathway had remained relatively stable. A similar finding was reported by Clemmesen (6) in Fredericia, an industrial town in Denmark. These epidemiologic findings are suggestive of the multiple factors underlying the etiology of lung cancer.

Preliminary epidemiologic studies in Virginia, Maryland, North and South Carolina, Georgia, and Texas were performed by Hitchcock (13) in which comparisons were made between lung cancer mortality rates in counties graded for urbanization, employment in higher-risk industries, and surrogate measures of natural biogenic sulfide production. The surrogate measures were mean annual precipitation, drainage, and landform features. Her field studies in salt marshes and other coastal sites confirmed that hydrogen sulfide produced by bacteria in flood sediments is rapidly converted in the atmosphere to respirable particulate sulfate. She suggested that the high rates of lung cancer among oil- and gas-field workers in Texas and Louisiana are related to such sulfate production and that other mining and manufacturing operations that involve release of this gas may also carry the added pulmonary hazard. In another study (46), the authors related respiratory cancer to wetlands residency in Louisiana.

These studies may explain the strength of the precipitation/elevation factor in the models of the geographic distribution of cancer in the United States (50). Even after correction for most of the factors that come under the urban umbrella, areas of high precipitation and low elevation were found to have high rates for almost every type of cancer mortality, including the respiratory group, and areas of low precipitation and high elevation experienced very low cancer mortality.

The response to potentially carcinogenic industrial insults varies in individuals, not only in terms of genetic makeup but perhaps more important in terms of general nutritional and basic health and environmental background. A study of cancer among migrants has been a very productive form of research. In the past, the focus on migrants was on individuals from foreign countries. Mancuso et al. (32) found differences among migrants from different parts of the United States. An important consideration in the development of cancer among migrants is their background, especially among blacks, of general malnutrition and related diseases as a result of decades of poverty, with associated physiological impairments affecting the susceptibility and adaptability of the individual in subsequent years of life. The direct bearing on cancer development of malnutrition in combination with subsequent environmental factors is virtually an unexplored area. The migrant study within the United States revealed that the high incidence of lung cancer among blacks in Ohio was among migrant blacks. Ohio-born blacks had the same lung cancer death rates as Ohio-born whites. The indications are that this was related to the fact that the migrant blacks who were born in the south and migrated to Ohio were employed in the lowest jobs with the greatest industrial exposures.

An interesting further potential study (28) may show a reverse migration of blacks caused by major employment dislocations in northern cities. Often blacks who spend their working lives in the industrial north return to their original communities in the south. The long latent period between exposure and onset of lung cancer means that in time there will be an upward death rate in the southern communities to which these exposed workers have returned. It would be a major contribution to our understanding of cancer development to establish a mechanism for identifying and following these workers so that the prior work-industry exposure could be properly documented for subsequent evaluation of the future lung cancer patterns in these areas of the south.

A relatively recent avenue of research is opening up because of awareness of the part played in lung cancer by indoor air pollution. In our own study (27) in El Paso an attempt was made to determine why Mexican-American women had an incidence of lung cancer twice as high as that for other white women in the same community. About 60% of both the Mexican-American women and other white women smoked cigarettes, so this was not the major causative factor. El Paso has had a total registry since 1950 cooperated in by all the medical profession. Interviews with the women with cancer and their relatives were carried out prospectively. Each patient was asked for her thoughts as to what might have caused her disease. They all mentioned the stifling environment when heating braziers were used in the airtight adobe houses in which they had all spent at least 20 years, and this was found to be a significant causative factor. Analysis of wall scrapings of the Mexican-American women's houses demonstrated the presence of benzopyrene and DDT. No unusual radiation levels were detected.

Because of a recent review of the current status of a number of studies (10,43) on the subject, insights into the extent of indoor pollution and its sources are coming into focus. Because people spend an estimated 70% of their time in their homes, this may be an important consideration. A demonstration energy-saving house built in Mount Airy, Maryland, was described as a "veritable fortress against the loss of energy." When the conservation-minded designers studied the results of their airtight house, they found that without the drafts of outside fresh air typical of most homes the indoor air went bad. High concentrations of formaldehyde gas were found, as was 100 times the natural background level of radioactivity. These pollutants originated in the home itself. Formaldehyde, a bonding agent in foam insulation and in furniture made of plywood and particle board, and a common ingredient of adhesives in carpeting, escapes into the inside air.

The most alarming pollutant discovered in these studies is radon, a radioactive gas. Radon's charged decay products cling to dust particles that often lodge in the lungs and result in short-range radiation. In regions of the country with large deposits of radioactive minerals, indoor levels of radon can become high. Assuming that most American homes contain several times the normal radiation background, as the limited data suggest, the Lawrence Berkeley researchers (10) have estimated that this might be responsible for thousands of lung cancer cases per year. The EPA has suggested that if ventilation in all U. S. homes were cut in half, the increased exposure to radon alone might increase lung cancer cases by as much as 20,000 per year.

The National Academy of Sciences has recognized the importance of indoor air pollution in the development of cancer and other biological effects. Recently, the WHO recommended that governments that reduce ventilation requirements in the interest of energy conservation be mindful of the impact on the quality of air that will result (10).

GENETICS

The expanding knowledge of genetics and its relationships to disease processes gives rise to ideas that are "speculative, but represent reasonable extensions of our knowledge of genetics and lung disease" (21). An individual is born with his own immutable set of genes. The interaction of the individual genotypes with factors in the environment, in the diet, and in individual behavior determine the health or illness of the individual. Different sets of genes condition an individual to different responses to environmental factors. When limits of tolerance are reached, illness results. It follows naturally that sets of genes differ from person to person. The limits of tolerance to environmental insults also differ.

Genetic factors are characterized as predominantly single-gene factors or multigenic, due to one or more genes acting together. The search of clinical geneticists for susceptibles in the population with single-gene disorders or inborn errors in metabolism has been diverted to the more productive study of hereditary factors predisposing individuals to common disorders. The aim is prevention. Single-gene disorders are rarely causes of disease. In lung cancer the etiology of the disease seems to be a result of a combination of environmental and genetic factors. These environmental factors have been set forth broadly as pathogens (bacteria and viruses), irritants, pollutants (cigarette smoke and coal dusts), drugs, and nutrition.

In the more prevalent histological type of lung cancer, squamous cell, as in most human diseases, pathological heterogeneity seems to underlie important influences, and little evidence exists for inherited influences.

In the rarer types of lung cancer histology, the relationship is more apparent between genetic factors and onset of disease. Mulvihill (37), in 50 reported cases, listed scleroderma or progressive systemic sclerosis as a forerunner of alveolar cell adenocarcinoma of the lung, with the unusual ratio of 7 females to 1 male, whereas the ratio in scleroderma is usually 3:1. Also reported is a direct relationship between the level of the enzyme aryl hydrocarbon hydroxylase and the induction of lung cancer and fibrocystic pulmonary dysplasia.

Geneticists are recognizing hereditary traits or syndromes in families which pre-dispose to certain types of cancer. Mulvihill (36) states that the clinician who diagnoses the cancer, but not the syndrome of which it is a manifestation, makes an incomplete diagnosis.

The genetic and hereditary factors that are coming into focus give a means of screening persons at high risk, with the anticipation of interrupting the process and preventing the development of cancer.

As of 1980, the multistage or two-stage theory of carcinogenesis, initiation and promotion, is the working hypothesis of many scientists (5). Elucidation of the roles of DNA damage and repair mechanisms in the carcinogenic process and of the relationship of the wide range of individual genetic variations to carcinogenic susceptibility has broadened the base for continuing the exploration of this complex subject. An important avenue of great potential involves attempts to identify and exploit agents capable of inhibiting or reversing the biological mechanism involved in initiation and promotion of carcinogenesis. The increasing sociological impact of environmental carcinogens is clearly shown in national and international incidence and mortality studies. It appears that most cancers are initiated by external agents. Intrinsic to that observation is the idea that cancer may be a preventable disease. The difficulty of translating this to a reality lies not only in individual responsibility for health protection but also in a more careful awareness and regulation of the by-products of our technological development.

NUTRIENTS AND ANTINUTRIENTS

There is a convergence of scientific interest in 1980 on the relationship between nutrition and disease. In a recent article, Dubos (8) observed that many people in the Western world, especially the United States, are intensely worried about their nutritional status, not necessarily because they are suffering from malnutrition but because they are constantly hearing and reading about the dangers of bad diets and of food contaminated with additives and other chemicals. Any departure from a hypothetical "ideal natural diet" is publicized by the media, thus contributing to the prevalent social neuroses about the general state of the world. Dubos goes on to say that if some, and perhaps many of us, are in a state of malnutrition it is because our dietary regimen is ill-adapted to modern conditions: "It would be surprising if the nutritional regimens designed for the old ways of life were the right ones for the conditions prevailing in today's wheel-borne, well-heated, air-conditioned societies." A relatively new departure in nutritional research is the study of individual differences in nutritional requirements. The scientific evidence is increasing that a diet suitable for one individual may be dangerously deficient for another. Dubos reports as an example of the trend in this type of research, a recent study of 19 healthy men in which an almost fivefold difference was found in their daily requirements for calcium (from 220 to 1,018 mg), and twofold to sevenfold differences in their needs for the various essential amino acids that maintain nitrogen balance. Examinations of many population groups under widely different circumstances have demonstrated that the nutritional needs of an individual undergo profound changes as a result of adaptations to shortages or abundance of certain nutrients.

Basic laboratory research is continuing in physiological, biochemical, cellular, and molecular areas. The time is at hand to identify individual dietary requirements, taking into account the different genetic, somatic, behavioral, and environmental situations of individuals (11). In expert hands, assays for trace mineral contents can provide a satisfactory method of determining the balance or imbalance existing in a given individual. Mineral rebalancing by nutritional or pharmacological manipulations should increase the well-being of the individual by balancing his personal equation and may prove to affect the probability of a favorable prognosis, even in early clinically observable stages in the malignant progression.

Delineation of the epidemiology of cancer of the lung emphasizes again that awareness of the whole person, his work history and his environment, not only his cancer, must be considered to effect improvement in the present picture.

In an adequate detailed history, carefully elicited from the patient in the clinician's office, covering the entire lifetime work experience, family medical history, and residential and other usual environments, may lie the clues to identification of the causes of lung cancer. As in the El Paso lung cancer study, the patients themselves give the most important clues, but they must be listened to and encouraged by careful questioning. Minimum-form registry data, although it allows a head count, defeats the epidemiologist by its omissions in the search for etiological clues. A retrogressive step was taken recently when the known primary lung cancer deaths were combined with lung cancer deaths not specified as primary or secondary in the International Classification of Diseases, 1965 revision (19). Scientific evaluation has shown these two categories to be clearly different (50).

Epidemiologists must work toward amending the official reporting of lung cancer by separating histological types, because different cell types often have different natural histories and causes.

It is in the best interest of science to take a comprehensive approach and to avoid the fatal fixed idea in considering the epidemiology, etiology, and eventual prevention of lung cancer. Obviously there are causative factors or combinations of factors that science has not yet pinpointed. As we strive for objectivity in the face of numerous pressures, we might consider the wry comment of one of our contemporary philosophers that "the great tragedy of science is the slaying of a beautiful hypothesis by an ugly fact" (16) and, after disappointments, go on with courage to try again.

It is vital that research continue in an unbiased, open-minded atmosphere with a broad perspective as a basis, so that potential or proved environmental, nonenvironmental, social, and economic carcinogenic factors will fall into their proper places for the eventual solution of the lung cancer problem. It may be that action by the upcoming health-conscious generation will lead us to realize that there are many carcinogen-producing luxuries to which we have become accustomed and without which we can learn to live.

Epidemiologists must continue to work closely with clinicians and scientists from every field and maintain an essential objectivity in the common goal, the prevention and control of lung cancer.

REFERENCES

1. Blot, W. J., and Fraumeni, J. F., Jr. (1979): Studies of respiratory cancer in high risk communities. *J. Occup. Med.*, 21:276–278.
2. Cameron, E., and Pauling, L. (1979): *Cancer and Vitamin C*. Linus Pauling Institute of Science and Medicine, Menlo Park, Calif.; Distributed by W. W. Norton, New York.
3. Doll, R., Muir, C., and Waterhouse, J., editors (1970): *Cancer Incidence in Five Continents, Vol. II*. Distributed for UICC by Springer-Verlag, New York.
4. Carnow, B. W. (1978): The "urban factor" and lung cancer: Cigarette smoking or air pollution? *Environ. Health Perspect.*, 22:17–21.
5. Clark, R. L. (1979): Introduction to the 31st annual symposium on fundamental cancer research. In: *Carcinogens: Identification and Mechanisms of Action*, edited by A. C. Griffin and C. R. Shaw, pp. 1–2. Raven Press, New York.
6. Clemmesen, J. (1977): Is lung cancer associated with air pollution? A tale of two towns: Houston and Fredericia. *Acta. Pathol. Microbiol. Scand. [A] [Suppl. 261]*, 5:56–64.
7. Creech, J. L., and Johnson, M. N. (1974): Angiosarcoma of liver in the manufacture of polyvinyl chloride. *J. Occup. Med.*, 16:150.
8. Dubos, R. (1980): Nutritional ambiguities. *Natural History*, 89:14–21.
9. Fraumeni, J. F., Jr. (1979): Epidemiological studies of cancer. In: *Carcinogens: Identification and Mechanisms of Action*, edited by A. C. Griffin and C. R. Shaw, pp. 51–63. Raven Press, New York.
10. Gold, M. (1980): Indoor air pollution. *Science*, 80:30–33.
11. Gori, G. B. (1978): Diet and nutrition in cancer causation. *Nutrition and Cancer*, 1:5–8.
12. Hammond, C. E., Selikoff, I. J., and Seidman, H. (1979): Asbestos exposure, cigarette smoking and death rates. *Ann. N.Y. Acad. Sci.*, 330:473–490.
13. Hitchcock, D. R. (1981): Lung cancer, wetlands and hydrogen sulfide. In: *Trace Substances in Environmental Health, XIV*, edited by D. Hemphill, pp. 43–50. University of Missouri, Columbia.
14. Hoover, R., and Fraumeni, J. F., Jr. (1975): Cancer mortality in U.S. counties with chemical industries. *Environ. Res.*, 9:196–207.
15. Hueper, W. C. (1966): *Occupational and Environmental Cancers of the Respiratory System. Recent Results in Cancer Research, No. 3*. Springer-Verlag, New York.
16. Huxley, T. H. (1879): Biogenesis and abiogenesis. Presidential address, 1870, British Association for the Advancement of Science. In: *Discourses, Biological and Geological. Collected Essays. Vol. 8*. D. Appleton, New York.
17. Ipsen, J. (1966): The epidemiology of lung cancer in relation to pulmonary tuberculosis. Special Lecture, University of Pennsylvania.
18. International Agency for Research on Cancer (1979): *Evaluation of the Carcinogenic Risk of Chemicals to Humans. IARC Monographs, Vols. 1–20, Suppl. 1*. IARC, Lyons.
19. WHO (1967): *International Classification of Diseases, Vols. 1 and 2*. 1965 revision. WHO, Geneva.
20. Kang, H. K., Infante, P. F., and Carra, J. S. (1980): Occupational lead exposure and cancer. *Science*, 207:935–936.
21. Kazazian, H. H. (1976): A geneticist's view of lung disease. *Am. Rev. Respir. Dis.*, 113:261–266.
22. Lee, A. M., and Fraumeni, J. F., Jr. (1969): Arsenic and respiratory cancer in man: An occupational study. *J. Natl. Cancer Inst.*, 42:1045–1052.
23. Lemen, R. A., Johnson, W. M., Wagoner, J. K., Archer, V. E., and Saccomanno, G. (1976): Cytologic observations and cancer incidence following exposure to BCME. *Ann. N.Y. Acad. Sci.*, 271:71–80.

24. Lloyd, J. W. (1971): Long-term mortality study of steelworkers. V. Respiratory cancer in coke plant workers. *J. Occup. Med.*, 13:53–68.
25. Macdonald, E. J. (1976): Demographic variation in cancer in relation to industrial and environmental influence. *Environ. Health Perspect.*, 17:153–166.
26. Macdonald, E. J., and Heinze, E. B. (1978): *Epidemiology of Cancer in Texas: Incidence Analyzed by Type, Ethnic Group and Geographic Location.* Raven Press, New York.
27. Macdonald, E. J., Lichenstein, H., Nooner, D., Flory, D., Wikstrom, S., and Oro, J. (1973): Epidemiologic factors in lung cancer among women in El Paso County, Texas, 1944–69. *J. Am. Med. Wom. Assoc.*, 28:459–467.
28. Mancuso, T. F. (1979): *Cancer in the Workplace: An Overview.* Proceedings of a seminar for news media on lost in the workplace: Is there an occupational disease epidemic? Sept. 13–14, 1979. U.S. Department of Labor, Occupational Safety and Health Administration, Chicago.
29. Mancuso, T. F. (1975): Consideration of chromium as an industrial carcinogen. In: *Proceedings of the International Conference on Heavy Metals in the Environment*, Toronto, Ontario, October, 1975, pp. 343–356.
30. Mancuso, T. F. (1980): Mortality study of beryllium industry workers' occupational lung cancer. *Environ. Res.*, 21:48–55.
31. Mancuso, T. F. (1976): Problems and perspective in epidemiological study of occupational health hazards in the rubber industry. *Environ. Health Perspect.*, 17:21–30.
32. Mancuso, T. F., Coulter, E. J., and Macdonald, E. J. (1973): Migration and cancer mortality experience: A study of native and southern born nonwhite Ohio residents. *Trace Substances in Environ. Health.*, 6:49–56.
33. Mason, T. J., Fraumeni, J. F., Jr., and McKay, F. W. (1972): Uranium mill tailings and cancer mortality in Colorado. *J. Natl. Cancer Inst.*, 49:661–664.
34. Mason, T. J., and McKay, F. W. (1974): *U.S. Cancer Mortality by County: 1950–1969.* DHEW publication no. (NIH) 74–615. U.S. Government Printing Office, Washington, D.C.
35. Milham, S., Jr., and Strong, T. (1974): Human arsenic exposure in relation to a copper smelter. *Environ. Res.*, 7:176–182.
36. Mulvihill, J. J. (1975): Congenital and genetic disease. In: *Persons at High Risk of Cancer. An Approach to Cancer Etiology and Control*, edited by J. F. Fraumeni, Jr., pp. 3–35. Academic Press, New York.
37. Mulvihill, J. J. (1976): Genetic factors in pulmonary neoplasms. *Birth Defects*, 12:99–111.
38. Nelson, N. (1976): The chloroethers—occupational carcinogens: A summary of laboratory and epidemiology studies. *Ann. N.Y. Acad. Sci.*, 271:81–90.
39. Redmon, C. K., Ciocco, A., Lloyd, J. W., and Rush, H. W. (1972): Long-term mortality study of steelworkers: VI. Mortality from malignant neoplasms among coke oven workers. *J. Occup. Med.*, 14:621–629.
40. Rehn, L. (1906): Über Blasenerkrankungen die Anilinarbeitern. *Verh. Dtsch. Ger. Chir.*, 35:313–314.
41. DHEW (1979): *Smoking and Health, A Report of the Surgeon General.* DHEW publication no. (PHS) 79–50066. U. S. Government Printing Office, Washington, D. C.
42. Sterling, T. D. (1980): Smoking, occupation and respiratory disease. Presented at the American Lung Association Occupational Health Task Force Meeting, Clearwater, Florida *(in press)*.
43. Sterling, T. D., and Kobayashi, D. M. (1977): Exposure to pollutants in enclosed "living spaces." *Environ. Res.*, 13:1–35.
44. Sterling, T. D., and Weinkam, J. J. (1976): Smoking characteristics by type of employment. *J. Occup. Med.*, 18:743–754.
45. U.S. Bureau of the Census (1978): *Statistical Abstract of the United States, 1978*, ed. 99. Washington, D.C.
46. Voors, A. W., Johnson, W. D., Steele, S. H., and Rothschild, H. (1978): Relationship between respiratory cancer and wetlands residency in Louisiana. *Arch. Environ. Health*, 33:124–129.
47. Wagoner, J. K., Archer, V. E., Lundin, F. E., Jr., Holaday, D. A., and Lloyd, J. W. (1965): Radiation as the cause of lung cancer among uranium miners. *N. Engl. J. Med.*, 273:181–188.
48. Wagoner, J. K., and Infante, P. F. (1977): Vinyl chloride: A case for the use of laboratory bioassay in the regulatory control procedure. In: *Origins of Human Cancer*, edited by H. H. Hiatt, J. D. Watson, and J. A. Winsten, pp. 1797–1805. Cold Spring Harbor Laboratory, New York.

49. Wellington, D. G. (1980): Time characteristics of U.S. lung cancer mortality. In: *Time Series Analysis*, edited by O. D. Anderson and M. R. Perryman, pp. 617–631. North-Holland Publishing Co., Amsterdam.
50. Wellington, D. G., Macdonald, E. J., and Wolf, P. F. (1979): *Cancer Mortality: Environmental and Ethnic Factors*. Academic Press, New York.
51. Wong, O. (1977): A competing-risk model based on the life table procedure in epidemiological studies. *Int. J. Epidemiol.*, 6:153–159.

Thoracic Oncology, edited by N. C. Choi and
H. C. Grillo. Raven Press, New York © 1983.

Pathology of Bronchopulmonary Neoplasms

Eugene J. Mark

Department of Pathology, Massachusetts General Hospital, Boston, Massachusetts 02114

Pathologic categorization of lung neoplasms can be as simple or as complex as one desires. In the early part of the twentieth century, when lung tumors were rare and therapy was supportive, a pathologic diagnosis of bronchogenic carcinoma was considered sufficient and specific. As lung tumors became more prevalent and therapy became more aggressive, pathologists refined their diagnosis. Histologic subdivision of lung tumors can sometimes exceed its epidemiologic or clinical relevance. Although elaborate diagnostic labels are useful to pathologists in communicating their findings, and although an occasional subtype of a tumor may later prove to be a clinicopathologic entity in its own right, excessively detailed diagnoses do not necessarily serve the best interests of the patient or his attending physician. This chapter discusses histologic typing of tumors as far as it is useful either to the understanding of the histogenesis and growth patterns of lung tumors or to their surgical and medical therapy.

The classification of bronchopulmonary neoplasms used here appears in Table 1. Neoplasms which are usually primary in organs other than the lung but rarely originate in the lung, e.g., Kaposi's sarcoma or granular cell tumor, are not included. The pathologic description of each tumor lists the histologic features essential for its diagnosis. It emphasizes histologic parameters that have been proven to possess or to lack prognostic value. Each description is intended to provide the information about pathology of a lung tumor that an oncologist would find valuable before sitting down with the pathologist to examine the slide of his patient's biopsy.

In addition to classifying and histologically staging a lung tumor, the pathologist can contribute to a better understanding of pulmonary oncology by recording three other facts in his report: (i) inflammation directly associated with the tumor, (ii) concurrent pulmonary disease, and (iii) arteriopathy associated with the tumor. Carcinomas elicit a local cellular immune response. Lymphocytic and plasmacytic infiltration is greatest in squamous cell carcinoma and least in small cell carcinoma (66). The amount of inflammation correlates positively with the degree of differentiation, and it is not related to necrosis. Granulomatous inflammation and granulomas occur in hilar and mediastinal lymph nodes draining a carcinoma and do not necessarily indicate concominant tubercular or fungal disease or sarcoidosis (135). Concurrent diseases very commonly found in excisions of lung tumors include chronic bronchitis, emphysema, and pneumoconioses. Chronic bronchitis can be evaluated morphologically from bronchi proximal to the tumor, including the section

TABLE 1. *Bronchopulmonary neoplasms*

Epithelial tumors with squamous differentiation
 Squamous cell carcinoma
 Verrucous squamous cell carcinoma
 Squamous papillomatosis

Epithelial tumors with glandular differentiation
 Adenocarcinoma
 Bronchoalveolar carcinoma
 Mucoepidermoid tumor
 Adenoid cystic tumor
 Bronchial cystadenoma

Epithelial tumors with neurosecretory differentiation
 Oat cell carcinoma
 Carcinoid tumor
 Benign clear cell tumor

Epithelial tumors without differentiation
 Small cell carcinoma
 Large cell carcinoma
 Giant cell carcinoma

Mixed-pattern carcinoma

Metastases in the lung

Mesenchymal tumors
 Carcinosarcoma
 Blastoma
 Leiomyosarcoma
 Fibrosarcoma
 Bronchial hamartoma

Vascular tumors
 Sclerosing epithelioid angiosarcoma
 Intimal sarcoma
 Hemangioendotheliomatosis
 Sclerosing hemangioma

Lymphoproliferative tumors
 Lymphoma of small cell or large cell type
 Hodgkin's disease
 Lymphoma of lymphomatoid granulomatosis type
 Eosinophilic granuloma
 Plasmacytoma
 Plasma cell granuloma

Leukemia

---

taken as documentation of the bronchial resection margin. Emphysema should be evaluated in the gross specimen. Emphysema noted histologically only adjacent to the tumor probably represents scar emphysema and, as such, is a secondary phenomenon with little epidemiological or clinical importance. Asbestosis, silicosis, berylliosis and other pneumoconioses should be excluded if interstitial or pleural fibrosis, nodular scars, or extensive interstitial or intra-alveolar inflammation are found at a distance from the tumor. At least one slide of the lung should be examined with polarized light to quantitate any silica, talc, or other birefringent material which may be present but inconspicuous or invisible on the routine hematoxylin-eosin stain. Pulmonary and bronchial arteries adjacent to tumor are usually hypertrophic and may have medial and intimal thickening. Elastic tissue stain facilitates quantitation of these vascular changes. Patients with lung tumors sometimes have unexpectedly large perfusion defects on scintillation scans or arteriograms, and thus quantitation of the pathologic changes in the blood vessels may prove valuable for future studies.

EPITHELIAL TUMORS WITH SQUAMOUS DIFFERENTIATION

Squamous Cell Carcinoma

Squamous cell carcinoma accounts for one-half of all lung carcinomas (131,150). Usually located in the central zone of the lung, it may be at the periphery when associated with a scar or with Pancoast's syndrome, which is most commonly caused by squamous cell carcinoma. It is the pulmonary neoplasm with the best documented pathologic progression of hyperplasia, metaplasia, dysplasia, carcinoma *in situ*, and invasive carcinoma (8). The bronchial epithelium is normally columnar, pseudostratified, and ciliated. Hyperplasia is the conversion of columnar and ciliated cells to flattened and keratinizing cells, and dysplasia is the enlargement, hyperchromaticity, and pleomorphism of the epithelial nuclei. Carcinoma *in situ* is defined as an epithelial lesion composed entirely of cells with highly atypical nuclei, and loss of cellular stratification and of ciliated surface epithelium, but an intact basement membrane (8). It includes tumors in which malignant cells fill or even distend bronchial mucus glands but do not disrupt or permeate them. Invasive carcinoma is defined as an epithelial lesion in which malignant cells penetrate through the subepithelial basement membrane into either stroma, vessels, or lymph nodes. The premalignant changes, as observed in smokers and uranium miners, generally involve more of the surface of the bronchial mucosa than just the area adjacent to the tumor and generally are multifocal. If invasive squamous cell carcinoma is associated with *in situ* carcinoma, the *in situ* carcinoma generally extends proximal to the invasive lesion (28). Frozen section examination of bronchial resection margin at the time of definitive surgery can prevent an unpleasant, unexpected finding on permanent sections of carcinoma *in situ*. Multiple, primary, invasve carcinomas have been found in up to 15% of patients when deliberately sought at autopsy (9). Mediastinal lymph node metastases from squamous cell carcinoma do not necessarily contraindicate resection for cure (118).

The essential histologic features of squamous cell carcinoma are keratin pearls, intercellular bridges, or both, on light microscopy (78) (Fig. 1), and desmosomes and tonofilaments on electron microscopy. Squamous cell carcinoma is classically subdivided according to the degree of differentiation, which in turn depends upon the degree of keratinization. Early invasive squamous cell carcinoma associated

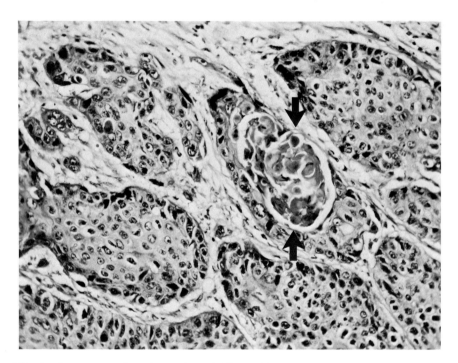

FIG. 1. Squamous cell carcinoma (×256). Nests of large cells with pleomorphic nuclei and sharply outlined cytoplasm invade fibrous tissue. A keratin pearl *(arrows)* has whorled cells with darkly staining cytoplasm and pyknotic nuclei.

with *in situ* squamous cell carcinoma is particularly well differentiated and curable by surgery (92,149). Invasive carcinoma which is well or moderately differentiated has a better prognosis than that which is poorly differentiated (110). The latter is often difficult to separate from either large or small cell undifferentiated carcinoma and shares the bad prognosis of these types (110).

Squamous cell carcinoma can be composed predominantly of spindle cells, clear cells with abundant glycogen, malignant multinucleated giant cells, or small cells. As anaplasia worsens, the distinction between a squamous cell carcinoma with small cells and a small cell undifferentiated carcinoma becomes tenuous, particularly when evaluating a small bronchoscopic or needle biopsy of lung or a metastasis in a hilar or mediastinal lymph node. Furthermore, squamous cell carcinoma is frequently associated with small cell undifferentiated carcinoma. A prevalence of 24% of this association was found in one autopsy series (22). When the two cell types are intermixed in the same mass, it is unlikely that they represent two different primary tumors. Rather, they probably reflect variable degrees of differentiation from a common cell of origin. The squamous cell carcinoma commonly manifests itself after treatment of the small cell carcinoma. Radiation and chemotherapy may cause differentiation of the anaplastic small cells to squamous cells. Alternatively, treatment may preferentially destroy primitive, undifferentiated, small cells and give more differentiated and more resistant cells time to assert themselves. The natural history of coexistent squamous cell carcinoma and small cell carcinoma is unknown. This poses a dilemma for therapy.

Verrucous Squamous Cell Carcinoma

Verrucous squamous cell carcinoma is a papillary neoplasm composed of highly differentiated and only slightly atypical keratinizing epithelium (Fig. 2). A solitary lesion typically obstructs a bronchus but invades for only a short distance into the bronchial wall (125). Prognosis is excellent. Histologic diagnosis of malignancy may be difficult in a biopsy taken from the surface of the exophytic tumor, because dysplasia is slight and invasion will not be seen.

Squamous Papillomatosis

Squamous papillomas of the lower respiratory tract may be single or multiple. Solitary squamous papilloma may be difficult or impossible to distinguish from a verrucous squamous cell carcinoma *in situ* (80). Squamous papillomatosis constitutes a clearer clinicopathologic entity (82). Multiple squamous papillomas in this condition may carpet the larynx, trachea, and bronchi. Viral ctiology has been

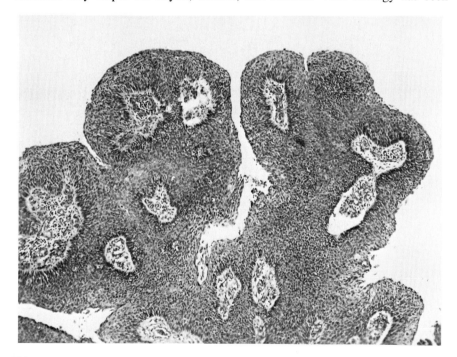

FIG. 2. Verrucous squamous cell carcinoma (×100). Papillae with fibrovascular cores are covered by squamous epithelium which is 5 to 10 cells in thickness. Cells mature and flatten toward the surface. Nuclear pleomorphism is absent.

suspected but not proven. Bronchial papillomatosis in children is self-limited. Bronchial papillomatosis in adults may run a protracted course, behaving as a low grade malignancy which disseminates within the major airways and sometimes invades lung parenchyma and metastasizes to hilar lymph nodes. Laryngeal involvement is frequent in children and rare in adults. Slight cellular dysplasia and rare mitoses have no prognostic import, but loss of polarity, marked pleomorphism, and extensive dyskeratosis increase the likelihood that the lesion is or will become an invasive carcinoma (4).

EPITHELIAL TUMORS WITH GLANDULAR DIFFERENTIATION

Adenocarcinoma

Adenocarcinoma classically arises in the peripheral zone of the lung distal to a segmental bronchus. It originates from bronchial or bronchiolar mucosa, but adenocarcinoma *in situ* confined to the mucosa is rarely encountered. The essential histologic features of adenocarcinoma are tubular or glandular formations (78) and/or abudant intracellular mucin on light microscopy (Fig. 3), and secretory granules and microvilli on electron microscopy (76). Ultrastructurally the cells may have features of goblet cells of the bronchial surface epithelium, mucus cells of bronchial

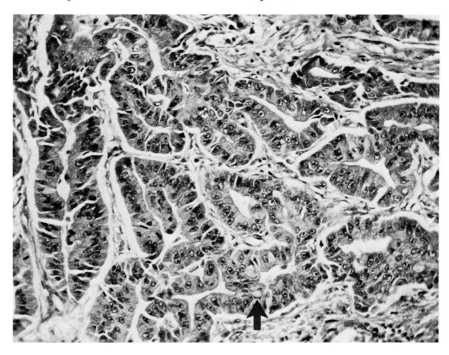

FIG. 3. Adenocarcinoma (×256). Serpentine glands with well developed lumens are lined by columnar epithelial cells. Nuclei are pleomorphic and have prominent nucleoli. Cytoplasm of a few cells contains a vacuole *(arrow)*.

mucus glands, nonciliated columnar cells of the bronchiole, or type II alveolar lining cells (76). A precursor lesion is the dysplastic epithelial proliferation commonly seen within diffuse interstitial pneumonitis and fibrosis or around focal scars (34,94). Atypical epithelial hyperplasia in a pseudocarcinomatous pattern can closely mimic carcinoma, particularly on frozen section diagnosis in cases of cholesterol pneumonitis, and is a pitfall which must be avoided. Pulmonary fibrosis from any cause and in any pattern predisposes to carcinoma in general and to adenocarcinoma in particular (7). Adenocarcinoma constitutes about one-third of all primary lung carcinomas, almost three-fourths of all carcinomas associated with a scar (7), and is increasing in prevalence relative to other types of lung cancer (142). Scar carcinomas are more frequently associated with a focal scar than with diffuse fibrosis, probably because the diffuse fibrosis causes death due to respiratory failure before malignancy has time to develop. Multiple areas of scarring with attendant epithelial atypicality may be the source of multiple primary adenocarcinomas, and thus multiple foci of adenocarcinoma in one or both lungs does not necessarily mean that metastasis has occurred (20).

Surgical staging influences prognosis but histologic grading of adenocarcinoma does not. Largeness of the primary tumor and occult metastases in hilar lymph nodes worsen prognosis. Well-differentiated adenocarcinomas may be papillary and have psammoma bodies. Poorly differentiated adenocarcinomas may be predominantly solid with extensive necrosis. Neither the degree of differentiation nor the presence of vascular or pleural invasion has prognostic value (20). Surgical extirpation of adenocarcinoma is infrequently curative, despite the common peripheral location, probably because vascular and pleural invasion occur so early and so often.

Clear cell carcinoma is a subtype of poorly differentiated adenocarcinoma, composed of broad sheets or solid nests of cells with small central nuclei and copious clear cytoplasm. When present, glands form poorly and infrequently. The reason for distinguishing this particular subtype of adenocarcinoma is so as not to confuse it pathologically with metastatic renal cell carcinoma, which it resembles. In primary clear cell carcinoma of the lung the clarity on hematoxylin-eosin stain is due to abundant intracellular mucin, whereas in metastatic renal cell carcinoma the clarity is due to intracellular lipid. Clear cell variant of adenocarcinoma has the same prognosis as adenocarcinomas of the lung in general.

Bronchoalveolar Carcinoma

Bronchoalveolar carcinoma is a distinct clinicopathologic entity with four characteristic histologic features: (i) well differentiated cytology, (ii) peripheral origin distal to a grossly recognizable bronchus, (iii) growth along walls of distal air spaces, and (iv) dissemination via airways and lymphatics (83) (Fig. 4). The cell of origin of bronchoalveolar carcinoma has been variously purported to be a bronchiolar mucinous epithelial cell, a bronchiolar nonmucinous epithelial cell, or a type II alveolar lining cell (18). An animal model of a precursor lesion of bron-

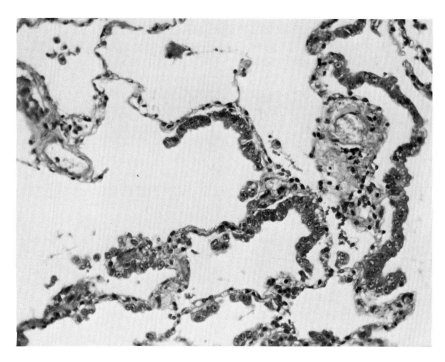

FIG. 4. Bronchoalveolar carcinoma (×256). A single layer of malignant, cuboidal, epithelial cells lines alveolar duct *(right)* and portions of two alveoli *(center)*. Tumor terminates abruptly. Alveolar architecture is delicate and preserved.

choalveolar carcinoma is pulmonary adenomatosis of sheep (104). A similar lesion with diffuse proliferation of cytologically innocuous cells rarely is seen in humans. Because highly atypical alveolar lining cells are seen in various settings that include pulmonary fibrosis, bronchoalveolar carcinoma has been associated causally with idiopathic diffuse interstitial fibrosis, with interstitial fibrosis of rheumatoid disease (60), and with honeycomb lung of scleroderma (25). The salient feature of bronchoalveolar carcinoma is not its histogenesis, however, but its propensity to aerogenous spread.

Bronchoalveolar carcinoma sometimes has been categorized as a well-differentiated adenocarcinoma since it may contain glandular structures and/or mucin. Many an adenocarcinoma which has poorly differentiated cytology in its center will merge gradually at its advancing edge into the pattern of a bronchoalveolar carcinoma. Conversely, an occasional bronchoalveolar carcinoma will have areas of solid tumor and poor cellular differentiation, lending a worse prognosis than bronchoalveolar carcinoma lacking these features (37). Prognosis also correlates with radiographic and gross features. A solitary nodule has a better prognosis than segmental consolidation by tumor or diffuse reticular infiltration. The latter reflect later stages of disease where aerogenous or lymphangitic metastasis, respectively, have already occurred (87,100).

Bronchoalveolar carcinoma can induce sclerosis of the interalveolar septa along which it grows, although in its most characteristic phase it uses the septa of distal airways as scaffolding without altering them. Bronchoalveolar carcinoma can produce voluminous mucoid fluid which, when coughed up by the patient, may cause electrolyte depletion (65). Abundant intra-alveolar mucin may spill into pulmonary lobules, unaccompanied by malignant cells, and thereby mimic colloid carcinoma metastatic from the colon on frozen section diagnosis. Nuclei of bronchoalveolar often contain glassy eosinophilic inclusions. Ultrastructurally these intranuclear inclusions are composed of membranous tubules which might result from virus infection but are not themselves virions (138). Such intranuclear inclusions are seen rarely in alveolar lining cells in asbestosis and in few other pulmonary conditions, and their recognition is therefore most useful.

Mucoepidermoid Tumor

Mucoepidermoid tumor is a rare neoplasm which arises from mucus glands of the major bronchi, generally grows as a sessile intrabronchial mass, may obstruct the lumen, and invades locally. In histologic appearance and clinical behavior it generally resembles the better known mucoepidermoid tumor of salivary gland origin. The essential histologic features are the presence of two types of cells, one keratinizing and the other producing glands and mucin. Some examples are composed in large part of an intermediate or transitional cell type. Low grade and high grade tumors have different prognoses and should be distinguished pathologically. The low grade tumor is more common, well circumscribed, exophytic, and composed of cells with small and regular nuclei, abundant cytoplasm and no mitoses. The high grade tumor is less common, poorly circumscribed, endophytic, focally necrotic, and composed of cells with large and pleomorphic nuclei, scant cytoplasm, and mitoses (32). However, the relative proportions of keratinizing cells, mucin-producing cells, and transitional cells are not useful in grading mucoepidermoid tumors of the bronchi. All reported cases of mucoepidermoid tumor in childhood have been low grade and acted in a benign fashion (98).

Adenoid Cystic Tumor

Adenoid cystic tumor is a locally aggressive tumor originating in mucus glands of major bronchi. The essential histologic features are solid or lobulated nests and cords composed of small, basaloid, epithelial cells with dark and regular nuclei, scant cytoplasm, and deposition of hyaline stroma within and around the cords. The corded pattern accounts for the alternative name of cylindroma. The cells may form glands and produce mucin. The tumor cells characteristically array themselves as packets of cells interrupted by spaces like perforations in a sieve. Adenoid cystic tumor occurs in many organs of the body, and in all locations this cribiform pattern is its histologic *sine qua non*. Bronchial adenoid cystic tumor usually has extended beyond the external perichondrium of the bronchial cartilage by the time of surgery. Adenoid cystic tumor has a predilection for perineural and intraneural invasion.

Mucosal infiltration proximal, distal and circumferential to the grossly obvious tumor is common, and frozen section examination of bronchial resection margin is advisable. Adenoid cystic tumor is always potentially malignant. Its permeative character accounts for its ill-defined borders grossly and its potential for local recurrence (19). The degree of histologic differentiation of the tumor, in contradistinction to mucoepidermoid tumor, does not have prognostic value (90). Metastasis in hilar lymph nodes removed en bloc at the time of original excision does not alter prognosis (32). Death due to tumor usually results from bronchial and mediastinal recurrences, but distant metastases occur in some cases.

Bronchial Cystadenoma

Bronchial cystadenoma is the only truly benign bronchopulmonary neoplasm with glandular differentiation and therefore the only one for which the term "adenoma" is appropriate. It arises from and recapitulates the mucus glands of the bronchus and remains confined to the bronchial mucosa internal to the cartilage. The essential histologic features are glands which are dilated, filled with mucin, and lined by benign columnar epithelial and goblet cells. The dilated glands may coalesce into microcysts. Papillary infolding of the epithelium is common. Local resection is curative (79,108).

EPITHELIAL TUMORS WITH NEUROSECRETORY DIFFERENTIATION

Oat Cell Carcinoma

Oat cell carcinoma is so highly malignant for three reasons: (i) it usually occurs in the central zone of the lung, (ii) it infiltrates facilely through the bronchial mucosa and between cartilage plates into mediastinal lymph nodes, and (iii) it has already metastasized to the bone marrow at the moment of diagnosis in 20% of patients (62). The essential histologic features are malignant epithelial cells with hyperchromatic nuclei, scant cytoplasm with indistinct cell borders, and absence of keratinization and glands (Fig. 5). Other features include solid mass with extensive necrosis, cells arrayed in ribbons and rosettes, diffuse permeation of lung and lymph nodes by tumor cells that are not aggregated like epithelial cells but are dispersed individually like lymphocytes, nuclei that appear squeezed and smudged in small biopsies, and encrustation of walls of blood vessels by hematoxylinophilic nuclear material released from disintegrated tumor cells (10).

Historically, Barnard (1926) introduced the terminology for oat cell carcinoma (12), emphasizing that such small cell tumors of the central lung and mediastinum were carcinomas and not lymphomas or sarcomas, a belief commonly held at the time. His original paper included illustrations of cells of polygonal and fusiform cell types as well as smaller cells of oat cell type. The classification (78) of the World Health Organization (1981) recognized three histologic subtypes of small cell carcinoma: oat cell, intermediate (polygonal and fusiform) and combined.

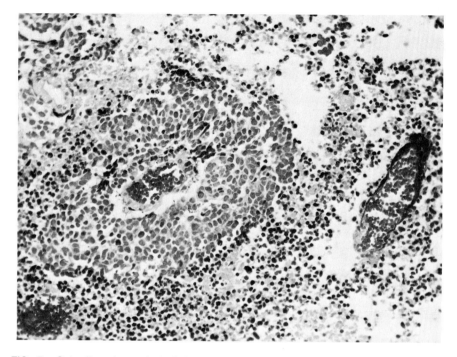

FIG. 5. Oat cell carcinoma (×256). Intact nuclei *(left)* surround a blood vessel. They are oval, uniform in size, and slightly larger than the red blood cells within the vessel. Necrotic and disintegrating tumor *(right)* has smaller, pyknotic nuclei. Wall of another blood vessel *(right)* is darkly outlined due to encrustation by nucleoplasm.

Although classic examples of intermediate cell and oat cell types are separable, they have overlapping features, and more than one subtype may be seen in a single tumor. However, prior to the classification of the World Health Organization, the term oat cell carcinoma had come to be used, imprecisely, as a synonym for small cell undifferentiated carcinoma of any subtype and continues to be used today. Whether or not these three morphologic subtypes have histogenetic relevance or clinical importance is unknown. Reports conflict as to which, if any, subtype has a better prognosis (103,110). All three subtypes have the same prevalence of bone marrow metastases at initial diagnosis.

Neurosecretory granules of Kultschitzky cells of the normal bronchial epithelium in bronchial carcinoid tumors and in oat cell carcinomas have similar histochemistry and ultrastructure. Oat cell carcinoma has been assumed to be derived from cells of the neuroendocrine system (21). Argyrophilic granules and neurosecretory granules have been found on light and electron microscopic examination in some examples of each of the subtypes (46,136) of small cell carcinoma (46,136) but are reported most frequently in oat cell carcinoma (21,55). As used here, oat cell carcinoma signifies a small cell carcinoma with oval nuclei about the size of the nucleus of a small lymphocyte (approximately 10–20 microns), so dense as to obscure the nucleolus, minimal cytoplasm, and proven or suspected neurosecretory differentiation.

Oat cell carcinoma is the bronchopulmonary neoplasm which is most commonly associated with various paraneoplastic syndromes and with ectopic production of hormones. It can cause Cushing's syndrome, carcinoid syndrome, or diabetes insipidus. Ectopic production of other hormones may be due to other types of tumors. Squamous cell carcinoma may produce parathormone with hypercalcemia; large cell carcinoma or giant cell carcinoma may produce gonadotrophin with acromegaly; and large cell carcinoma or adenocarcinoma may produce somatomammotrophin with acromegaly.

Carcinoid Tumor

Carcinoid tumors are slowly growing neoplasms derived from the neuroendocrine Kultschitzky cell of the bronchial epithelium. Two types exist: central and peripheral. They differ in clinical presentation, radiologic and gross appearance, histology and behavior. Central carcinoids outnumber peripheral carcinoids by four to one.

Central carcinoids come to medical attention by causing hemoptysis or signs and symptoms of bronchial narrowing. They are distributed along the tracheobronchial tree in a frequency which parallels the normal frequency of distribution of Kultschitzky cells, i.e., their concentration is highest in lobar bronchi and decreases both proximally and distally. Central carcinoids can be exophytic, endophytic, or both. Even when locally invasive in the lung, carcinoid tumors retain a discrete gross border. Histologically, central carcinoids are composed of monotonous cells of medium size with granular eosinophilic cytoplasm and regular nuclei arranged in either islands or trabeculae. Histologic variations include sheets of clear cells imitating metastatic renal cell carcinoma, papillae imitating papillary adenocarcinoma, and mucin production in carcinoids of goblet cell type (134).

Peripheral carcinoids are usually detected as solitary discrete nodules on chest radiographs of patients who do not have symptoms attributive to the tumor. Grossly, they are firm and encapsulated. They are rarely attached to the pleura. Histologically, peripheral carcinoids are composed of interlacing fascicles of spindle-shaped cells, which are reminiscent of neurofibroma on frozen section examination (121,126). Neurosecretory granules can be demonstrated by argyrophilic or argentaffinic staining in more than one-half of cases and can always be visualized by electron microscopy in both central and peripheral carcinoids.

The neuroendocrine cell of origin of carcinoid tumors increases in number in inflammatory diseases such as chronic bronchitis (39) and in experimental animal models such as challenge with nitrosamines (112). Small nodular proliferations of these cells are frequently found in surgical or autopsy specimens, particularly as associated with bronchiectasis, old infarcts, and scars of diverse etiology. These tumorlets of carcinoid type represent a precursor lesion of carcinoid tumors (31,109). Tumorlets of carcinoid type may be multiple, scattered diffusely through the lungs, and associated with restrictive lung disease (95).

Most central carcinoids have cells which appear innocuous, and surgical resection usually cures the patient. Occult metastasis to regional lymph nodes has already occurred by the time of primary resection in 5% of cases and decreases (105,121) the five year survival from 94% to 71%. All carcinoid tumors are potentially malignant, but 1 in 10 has histologic features which should alert one to an increased likelihood of both local and distant metastases. These atypical features are (i) increased cellularity, (ii) disorganization of insular or trabecular pattern, (iii) nuclear pleomorphism, (iv) necrosis, and (v) mitoses. Size of tumor and invasion of contiguous lymphatic vessels are not of prognostic value. Metastasis occurs in 66% of atypical carcinoids and the five year survival is 57% (105). Recurrent tumor in bronchus or mediastinum is more commonly lethal than is distant metastasis to liver and bone. Cellular atypicality, metastasis, and death due to tumor ensue less commonly with peripheral carcinoids than with central carcinoids. Typical histology dictates a diagnosis of carcinoid tumor, while the presence of cellularity, disorganization, necrosis, and mitosis dictate a diagnosis of carcinoid tumor with slight, moderate, or marked atypicality (6,45).

Further histologic dedifferentiation leads to a difficult problem for the pathologist—distinguishing markedly atypical carcinoid tumor from oat cell carcinoma. Both derive from the Kultschitzky cell, both have neurosecretory granules, and both may cause the carcinoid syndrome (123), although their epidemiologies differ (43). The pathologist must exercise caution, particularly before making a diagnosis of oat cell carcinoma based on a biopsy of a solitary peripheral lesion. Some long-term survivors with a diagnosis of oat cell carcinoma may actually have had atypical carcinoid tumors. Oat cell carcinoma becomes the diagnosis when the cellularity becomes solid and dense, necrosis becomes extensive, nuclei become shrunken and so hyperchromatic that they lose visible internal structure, and invasion by individual cells occurs.

Benign Clear Cell Tumor

Benign clear cell tumor is a classic coin lesion: peripheral, solitary, well circumscribed, and asymptomatic. It lies unencapsulated in the parenchyma without connection to bronchi or pleura. The essential histologic features are masses of rounded or polygonal cells with abundant clear cytoplasm, well-defined cell membranes, and small regular nuclei (85). The clarity of the cytoplasm is due to a high content of glycogen, from which stems the alternate name of sugar tumor. Benign clear cell tumors are served by a rich network of sinusoidal blood vessels. Necrosis may occur. Electron microscopic studies have shown neurosecretory granules in some cases (17,54), although an origin from pericytes has also been suggested (63). Benign clear cell tumor may histologically imitate exquisitely a metastasis from renal cell carcinoma, and therein lies its claim to fame.

EPITHELIAL TUMORS WITHOUT DIFFERENTIATION

Small Cell Carcinoma

Small cell carcinoma designates a tumor composed of epithelial cells which lack squamous, glandular, or neurosecretory differentiation and whose nuclei measure 25 microns or less in greatest diameter in slides of paraffin-embedded tissue (103). Four facts support the classification of the World Health Organization, which segregates oat cell carcinoma from other small cell carcinomas on purely morphologic grounds. First, foci of squamous cell carcinoma or adenocarcinoma are found in 10–20% of cases of small cell carcinoma (122). Second, after chemotherapy or radiotherapy the small cell carcinoma may disappear entirely, but one finds a residue of squamous cell carcinoma, adenocarcinoma, or large cell carcinoma at autopsy (1,22). This sequel seems to occur particularly with the intermediate cell subtype of small cell carcinoma (1). Third, some but not all small cell carcinomas contain neurosecretory granules on electron microscopy (46,49), and small cell carcinomas often lack argyrophilic or argentaffinic granules even when a large volume of tissue is thoroughly sampled. Fourth, a plasma-membrane antigen demonstrated by immunostaining and associated with the presence of neurosecretory granules has been found in only two-thirds of small cell carcinomas, indicating heterogeneity of the group.

These facts suggest that small cell carcinomas do not all have the same histogenesis. Those which have neuroendocrine features, and presumably derive from the Kultschitzky cell, are commonly diagnosed as oat cell carcinoma. Those which lack any differentiation at all, and presumably arise from the small, primitive, reserve cell normally present in the basal layer of the bronchial epithelium, can be properly diagnosed as small cell carcinoma. Tumors derived from this undifferentiated epithelial cell could be expected to show squamous or glandular differentiation under certain conditions. Unless neurosecretory differentiation is demonstrated, a diagnosis of undifferentiated small cell carcinoma is more accurate than oat cell carcinoma, particularly when the biopsy is small, distorted, or from a peripheral lesion. It leaves open the possibility of a concomitant or subsequent carcinoma of other cell type. Unanswered is whether or not undifferentiated small cell carcinoma has a natural history different from neurosecretory oat cell carcinoma, and whether or not the treatment of the two should differ.

Large Cell Carcinoma

The essential histologic features of large cell carcinoma are undifferentiated malignant epithelial cells, nuclei measuring more than 25 microns in greatest diameter in sections of paraffin-embedded tissue, and the absence of intercellular bridges, keratin pearls, gland formation, or extensive mucin by optical microscopy. Ultrastructural analysis can usually identify some keratinocytic or glandular differentiation (30). Since no large, undifferentiated, reserve cell normally exists in the bronchopulmonary epithelium that might represent a cell of origin for large cell carcinoma, one assumes that large cell carcinoma is a tumor which has dedifferentiated from some other cell type.

The diagnosis of large cell carcinoma is primarily one of exclusion and is associated with great observers' variability in diagnosis. Therefore, histochemical and ultrastructural examination should be rigorous to minimize the number of cases falling into this generic category. Undifferentiated large cell carcinoma has received little specific investigative attention.

Giant Cell Carcinoma

Giant cell carcinoma is giant at both the macroscopic and microscopic level. Grossly, it has usually attained massive proportions by the time it is detected on chest radiograph (50). It is highly prone to invade the pleura and chest wall. After squamous cell carcinoma, it is the second most common tumor to cause the Pancoast syndrome. The essential histologic features are four: (i) giant, anaplastic multinucleate, tumor cells, (ii) abundant, glassy, eosinophilic cytoplasm with microvacuoles, (iii) extensive phagocytosis of inflammatory cells by tumor cells, and (iv) cannibalism of one tumor cell by another (59,101). The giant cells measure 50 to 120 microns in minimal diameter in sections of paraffin-embedded tissue and should comprise the predominant cell type either in the entire mass of tumor or in several large foci (50,57). The giant cells each contain from 2 up to 50 malignant nuclei. Nucleoli are large and often gigantic. Ultrastructurally, some giant cell carcinomas contain characteristic concentric whorls of tonofilament-like fibrils in the cytoplasm (145).

Most giant cell carcinomas contain a small amount of intracytoplasmic mucin and probably represent dedifferentiated adenocarcinomas (59). Small foci of keratinization are also found occasionally (50). Fulminant behavior characterizes giant cell carcinoma. Overall survival is worse than that for adenocarcinoma (57,75).

MIXED-PATTERN CARCINOMA

Mixed-pattern carcinoma designates two or more distinct, synchronous, histologic types of carcinoma in a single tumor. It excludes multiple primary carcinomas, carcinoma metastatic to carcinoma, and carcinoma which changes morphology over time, with or without therapy. The best recognized mixed-pattern carcinoma is combined squamous cell carcinoma and adenocarcinoma, also known as adenosquamous carcinoma. Data is insufficient to determine whether the relative proportions of squamous cell carcinoma and adenocarcinoma influence prognosis. Mixed-pattern carcinomas account for approximately 1% of all carcinomas (142).

METASTASES IN THE LUNG

Metastatic carcinoma in the lung may be difficult to distinguish from primary bronchopulmonary carcinoma. Particularly perplexing is the evaluation of a solitary nodule of adenocarcinoma. Central fibrosis within an adenocarcinoma might suggest that it is a primary lung tumor arising in a scar, but metastases can become centrally necrotic and then fibrotic. A scar can also alter lymphatic drainage and thereby act as a nidus toward which metastases will drain. Signet-ring cells in adenococarcinoma are characteristic of gastrointestinal primaries but do occur occasionally in bronchopulmonary primaries. Heterotopic ossification occurs in pulmonary metastases from primary carcinoma of the stomach, colon, gallbladder, breast, ovary and prostate (113), as well as in primary bronchogenic carcinoma (106).

As a general rule, an adenocarcinoma in the lung removed at thoracotomy from a patient without a history of previous malignancy is ten times more likely to be primary than metastatic (61,81). How thoroughly such a patient should be investigated for an improbable primary adenocarcinoma is an open question (61) that arises frequently. If a patient with a known carcinoma of the colon develops a solitary lung shadow, the likelihood that this is a primary carcinoma of the lung is about equal to the likelihood that it is a metastasis from the colon (25).

Metastases from an occult renal cell carcinoma are sufficiently distinctive to prompt an intravenous pyelogram. If a primary renal cell carcinoma is thereby discovered and the pulmonary metastases are unilateral, nephrectomy will improve survival (73).

Pulmonary metastases from an extrathoracic squamous cell carcinoma usually show a greater degree of keratinization and pearl formation than primary squamous cell carcinoma of the lung (114). Squamous cell carcinoma *in situ* should always be sought in near bronchi when trying to distinguish primary and metastatic squamous cell carcinoma.

Microscopic tumor embolization in small pulmonary arteries and arterioles may cause dyspnea and cor pulmonale. This occurs particularly with metastases from primary adenocarcinoma of the breast, prostate, liver, and stomach (70). The primaries in breast or prostate are usually clinically known whereas those in liver or stomach are often occult. Pulmonary tumor emboli have also been reported in 17% of patients dying with primary adenocarcinoma of the lung and in 6% dying with primary squamous cell carcinoma of the lung (44). Arterial occlusion can result from plugs of tumor, associated thrombosis by fibrin and platelets, or intimal proliferation. Concentric, cellular, intimal proliferation in embolic carcinomatosis differs from the fibrous organization of thromboemboli and has been called carcinomatous vasculitis.

Lymphangitic carcinomatosis can be diagnosed by transbronchial lung biopsy (5). This pattern of metastasis does not favor either pulmonary or extrapulmonary primary. Apart from lymphatic spread, intrabronchial extension of tumor has been found in 18% of patients dying from metastatic disease from a primary extrapulmonary malignancy (77).

Extrathoracic sarcomas are rarely occult when thoracotomy discloses a nodule of sarcoma. Even if the histology of the nodule of sarcoma resected from the lung differs markedly from that of a known primary sarcoma, it is still almost surely a metastasis. Metastatic sarcoma generally appears worse differentiated than the primary, but after chemotherapy the metastasis may appear better differentiated. Two-thirds of nodules of metastatic osteogenic sarcoma exhibit histology mirroring the primary tumor, but neither the type nor the degree of differentiation of the mesenchymal elements is useful in prognosis (38).

MESENCHYMAL TUMORS

Carcinosarcoma

Carcinosarcoma is a highly unusual and highly malignant neoplasm which occurs in the central zone of the lung. In an early phase it may grow principally by endobronchial extension. The essential histologic feature is bimorphism, consisting of an admixture of malignant epithelial and malignant mesenchymal elements. The carcinoma is usually squamous cell carcinoma. The sarcoma is usually fibrosarcoma, sometimes combined with osteogenic sarcoma or chondrosarcoma. Metastases are present in regional lymph nodes at the time of resection in one-half of cases. The metastases are generally carcinomatous only but may be sarcomatous only or bimorphic (29,36,130).

Blastoma

Pulmonary blastoma is a malignant tumor that grows typically as a solitary, discrete mass in the peripheral zone of the lung. Males are affected more than females. Grossly, the tumor is usually solid, circumscribed, and unrelated to a bronchus. The essential histologic features are a primitive mesenchyme surrounding embryonic tubules lined by immature, nonciliated, columnar cells. Cartilage and bone may exist within the malignant stroma. The columnar cells often contain distinctive basal vacuoles filled with glycogen. The histology is reminiscent of peripheral lung tissue during the first trimester of embryogenesis (14,127). The name blastoma stems from the presumption that the tumor derives from a single germ cell layer or blastema. Pulmonary blastoma would thus be analogous to Wilms' tumor (renal blastoma). However, pulmonary blastoma is a neoplasm of adults, and is rare, whereas Wilms' tumor is a neoplasm of children and relatively common. In addition, ultrastructural evidence suggests that two germ cell layers are present, mesoderm and endoderm (41,93). Approximately one-third of patients have survived for one or more years after surgical excision. One-half of patients develop distant metastases (71). The mean diameter of the tumor influences prognosis, greater diameter indicating lesser survival. Neither the character nor the degree of histologic differentiation of the tumor affects prognosis, however. Pulmonary blastoma has a more peripheral location and better prognosis than pulmonary carcinosarcoma and should be distinguished from it (130).

Leiomyosarcoma

Bronchopulmonary leiomyosarcoma arises from smooth muscle cells, which normally are found in the bronchial tree as far distally as the alveolar duct, in the interstitium of interlobular septa, and in the walls of blood vessels. This rare tumor occurs in any age from newborns to nonagenarians. The essential histologic features are densely packed spindle cells forming interlacing fascicles, cytoplasm containing myofibrils, nuclei which are hypertrophic and hyperchromatic with blunt ends, and mitoses. Cellular pleomorphism, necrosis, and invasiveness are variable (91). Endobronchial tumors confined to the bronchial wall behave in a relatively indolent manner, as do pulmonary leiomyosarcomas in children. Intrapulmonary tumors in adults behave with a degree of malignancy proportional to their size. They may occupy an entire lobe and invade pleura and chest wall. The mitotic rate has prognostic value. Tumors with 8 or less mitoses per 10 high power fields remain stationary or grow slowly, those with 12 or more mitoses per 10 high power fields metastasize, and those with 8 to 12 mitoses per 10 high power fields fall into an indeterminate group (49). Bronchopulmonary leiomyosarcomas may metastasize widely but, characteristically, not to hilar or mediastinal lymph nodes (107).

Leiomyomas also occur in the lung. Solitary benign leiomyomas may be intrabronchial or intrapulmonary (137). Multiple pulmonary leiomyomas or leiomyomatous hamartomas occur almost exclusively in middle-aged women, most of whom have or had uterine leiomyomas or leiomyosarcomas (122,124). This condition of multiple nodules of benign-appearing smooth muscle is presumed to develop from pulmonary implantation of uterine smooth muscle cells. A very few cases have occurred in males with leiomyosarcomas of vein, diaphragm, or soft tissue. Bronchiolar epithelium may become enveloped by the smooth muscle proliferation. When numerous and large, these nodules create a dramatic radiograph but enlarge lanquidly and rarely cause symptoms.

Diffuse proliferation of smooth muscle in walls of pulmonary and pleural lymphatics occurs in lymphangiomyomatosis (33,104). Lymphatic channels in the mediastinum and retroperitoneum are also involved. Pneumothorax and chylothorax occur. The disease may terminate in honeycomb lung and respiratory insufficiency (68,133). Like histology may be found in the lung in tuberous sclerosis.

Fibrosarcoma

Fibrosarcoma primary in the lung is less common than fibrosarcoma metastatic to the lung, but approximately 100 cases of bronchopulmonary fibrosarcoma have been reported. Grossly, fibrosarcoma may arise from the wall of a bronchus and have an endobronchial or exobronchial component or both, may be intrapulmonary with attachment to pleura, or may be intrapulmonary without attachment to either bronchus or pleura. The essential histologic features are the same as those for fibrosarcoma arising elsewhere in the body, i.e., invasive borders, dense cellularity, spindle-shaped cells, scant and undifferentiated cytoplasm, hyperchromatic and pleomorphic nuclei. Most pulmonary fibrosarcomas have grown slowly before and after surgery. Large intrapulmonary fibrosarcomas cause death by invading pleura, chest wall, and mediastinum and filling the thorax (49). Small intrapulmonary fibrosarcomas are more likely to metastasize when they contain more than 8 mitoses per 10 high power fields (49). Overall, distant metastases occur in one-third of cases (64,67).

Since certain carcinomas may have large areas composed of spindle-shaped cells, one must extensively sample a spindle-cell malignancy and search for areas of squamous cell carcinoma, large cell carcinoma, or carcinosarcoma before considering a diagnosis of fibrosarcoma. Plasma cell granuloma (fibrous histiocytoma) may contain a vigorous fibroblastic proliferation including many mitoses and then be difficult to distinguish from fibrosarcoma.

Bronchial Hamartoma

Bronchial hamartoma is the most common benign lung neoplasm. Two types exist: central and peripheral. The central type arises in large bronchi, grows as an endobronchial polyp covered by intact mucosa, and generally causes a cough. The peripheral type arises in small bronchi, grows as a discrete nodule in the parenchyma, and generally causes no symptoms (24). Grossly, the peripheral type has a white bosselated surface and, when extracted from the lung parenchyma, resembles a piece of popped popcorn. Central and peripheral hamartomas have similar histology and histogenesis (15,16). The essential histologic feature is a localized proliferation of mature mesenchyme, most commonly cartilage but also fibrous tissue, smooth muscle, and fat. Calcification and ossification are often present and may be detected radiologically. When cartilage has been absent, the tumors have been called intra-bronchial lipomas, fibromas, myxomas, leiomyomas, or fibroadenomas, depending on the predominant tissue, but such examples are all variations on the same theme. As it expands outward from the bronchus, the mesenchymal proliferation surrounds adjacent alveoli, and the hamartoma then appears to include clefted air spaces lined by respiratory epithelium which may be cuboidal, columnar, hyperplastic or papillary. Nuclear pleomorphism and aggressive behavior occur extraordinarily. Although the term hamartoma implies that these tumors are developmental malformations, they are rarely detected in children. Bronchial hamartomas may be multiple and constitute one element of the syndrome of gastric epithelioid leiomyosarcoma, extra-adrenal paraganglioma, and multiple pulmonary chondro-hamartomas (27).

VASCULAR TUMORS

Sclerosing Epithelioid Angiosarcoma

Sclerosing epithelioid angiosarcoma of the lung is a rare multicentric tumor of low grade malignancy. It occurs in young or middle-aged women, and has a slow but inexorable clinical progression. Patients die of hemoptysis, intercurrent infection, or respiratory failure as the lungs fill with tumor. Occasionally the tumor metastasizes to liver, bone, and other viscera.

A few or several nodules averaging 1 cm are scattered through the lung on the initial chest radiograph. Later the nodules increase in number and size. Grossly they are scirrhous. Microscopically each nodule has three concentric zones. In the peripheral zone compact, polypoid tufts of small, polygonal tumor cells fill alveoli. In the middle zone alveoli lined by cuboidal, benign pneumocytes are entrapped by interstitial, hyaline sclerosis and infiltrating tumor cells. Toward the central zone sclerosis increases, tumor cells decrease, and necrosis and calcification may be found. The sclerosis is presumably a reaction to the malignant cells. An elastic tissue stain of the sclerotic area will reveal blood vessels lined or plugged by the malignant cells. Cytologically the malignant cells have pale, oval nuclei but enlarged nucleoli. They appear deceptively innocuous and may resemble chondrocytes. The bosselated contour of a nodule, the entrapped airspaces with hyperplastic pneumocytes, and the inconspicuousness of the tumor cells within abundant hyaline stroma can contribute to a common misdiagnosis of bronchial hamartoma.

This tumor was originally called "intravascular sclerosing bronchoalveolar" carcinoma, because it was thought to be an unusual variant of bronchoalveolar carcinoma with a propensity to invade blood vessels early. It is now known to be derived from endothelial cells. It first fills blood vessels and then invades perivascular interstitium and airspace. A similar tumor, usually termed "epithelioid hemangioendothelioma," arises at other sites in the body.

Intimal Sarcoma of Pulmonary Artery

Intimal sarcoma is a distinctive malignant neoplasm which arises in the wall of a major pulmonary artery, the pulmonary trunk, or the pulmonic valve. Intimal sarcomas can also originate in the aorta and in major systemic arteries and veins, but intimal sarcoma of pulmonary artery stands apart from these clinically and pathologically because it so often mimics pulmonary embolism, multiple pulmonary infarctions, and cor pulmonale (3,143). The essential histologic feature is a dense population of malignant spindle cells, which infiltrate the intima and media of a pulmonary artery both circumferentially and longitudinally. Malignant intramural infiltration may extend peripherally into small arteries beneath the pleura and thus appear in an open lung biopsy. Thrombosis of the affected arteries is common. Because the media of the artery is sometimes involved more than the intima and normally contains smooth muscle cells, some examples of this tumor have been diagnosed as leiomyosarcoma, but all probably originate from an undifferentiated mesenchymal cell. A few pulmonary intimal sarcomas have contained cartilage and bone (99) and have been diagnosed as malignant mesenchymoma (52).

Hemangioendotheliomatosis

Hemangioendotheliomatosis is a multifocal or diffuse proliferation of blood vessels with malignant potential. The essential histologic feature is a mass of small, abnormal, blood vessels lined by hyperplastic endothelial cells with hyperchromatic and pleomorphic nuclei. The neoplastic nodules have indistinct and infiltrating borders. If hemangioendotheliomatosis involves several organs concurrently, as is usually the case, one cannot prove whether any one particular lesion is primary or metastatic, or whether the lesions are multicentric in origin (148). When pulmonary involvement has been much greater than extrapulmonary involvement, primary malignant vascular tumor of the lung with extrapulmonary metastasis has been presumed (53). Hemangioendotheliomatosis restricted to the lung can permeate extensively along septa, resulting in pulmonary hemorrhage, hemosiderosis and interstitial fibrosis. Pleural involvement can result in hemothorax (144).

Sclerosing Hemangioma

Sclerosing hemangioma is a benign pulmonary tumor of controversial histogenesis. Clinically, the tumor classically appears as a coin-like lesion on a chest radiograph of a middle-aged woman without symptoms referable to the tumor. Hemoptysis can occur (97). Grossly, sclerosing hemangioma is a firm, discrete, yellow, intraparenchymal nodule without attachment to bronchi or macroscopic blood vessels. The essential histologic features are proliferation of blood vessels with tendency to sclerosis, papillary infolding into terminal air spaces produced by the vascular proliferation, hemorrhage, hemosiderin, and lipid-laden histiocytes (86). Some ultrastructural evidence suggests that pulmonary sclerosing hemangioma includes a proliferation of endothelial cells with secondary inflammatory and fibrotic changes (51,74), but epithelial proliferation also occurs (60). Sclerosing hemangioma will appear fibromatous or xanthomatous if the fibrous or histiocytic elements predominate. The authentically neoplastic cell, which is small, round, clear, massed, and interstitial, has mesothelial characteristics by recent immunopathologic work.

LYMPHOPROLIFERATIVE TUMORS

Lymphoma of Small Cell or Large Cell Type

Non-Hodgkin's lymphoma in the lung may occur either as primary pulmonary lymphoma or as dissemination of nodal lymphoma. Primary pulmonary lymphoma will be clinically unsuspected when it presents as a discrete intraparenchymal mass, but may be clinically suspected when it develops upon a background of a known precursor lesion such as lymphoplasmacytic interstitial pneumonitis, Sjogren's syndrome with pneumonitis, Waldenstrom's macroglobulinemia with pneumonitis, or lymphomatoid granulomatosis (56).

Grossly, primary pulmonary lymphoma may permeate, consolidate or destroy. Histologically, it may be diffuse or nodular and composed of mature, immature or primitive lymphoid cells. Histopathologic distinction of malignant lymphoma from benign or premalignant lymphoproliferative disease may be difficult even with open lung biopsy, particularly when hilar and mediastinal lymph nodes are normal (31,120). Histology of primary pulmonary lymphoma does not permit predicting whether generalized nodal disease will develop, but lymphomatous involvement of hilar and mediastinal lymph nodes presages systemic disease and worsens the prognosis compared with lymphoma confined to the lung. Surgical excision has cured some patients with primary pulmonary lymphoma (117).

Pulmonary involvement occurs ultimately in 20% of cases of generalized, nodal, non-Hodgkin's lymphoma (89). In systemic non-Hodgkins lymphoma, involvement of hilar lymph nodes is more common than involvement of pulmonary parenchyma, whereas the converse is true in systemic Hodgkin's disease. Metastatic lymphoma may form nodules, interstitial infiltrates, alveolar consolidation, or lymphangitic deposition in the pleura or around bronchovascular bundles. Intrathoracic lymphoma responds better to treatment when it is part of the initial presentation of generalized lymphoma then when it first manifests itself during relapse (89).

Hodgkin's Disease

Pulmonary Hodgkin's disease appears in almost one-half of patients with Hodgkin's disease at stage III or IV. Infiltration along bronchovascular bundles is the most common pattern of growth and occurs earlier in the course of the disease than do the less common patterns of parenchymal masses, diffuse interstitial thickening, lobular or lobar consolidation, miliary nodules, or endobronchial tumor with bronchial occlusion and atelectasis (88,116). Pleural nodules and/or pleural effusions occur in one-fifth of these patients. Hodgkin's disease in any of these forms can be localized to one lobe, and in such cases the degree of pulmonary involvement bears no relationship to the rate of spread of Hodgkin's disease in other organs. When the Hodgkin's lesions are found in all lobes, however, prognosis worsens (132). Involvement of pulmonary parenchyma in disseminated Hodgkin's disease occurs more commonly than involvement of hilar lymph nodes (88). Spread of Hodgkin's disease from the pulmonary hila or from mediastinal pleura to the mediastinal lymph nodes is more common than the reverse (132). The lymphocyte predominant type of Hodgkin's disease affects the lung less commonly than do nodular sclerosis, mixed cellularity, or lymphocyte depletion types (88). Primary pulmonary Hodgkin's disease is vanishingly rare (64). Lymphomatoid granulomatosis, angioimmunoblastic lymphadenopathy in the lung, and infectious mononucleosis in the lung all can contain cells which mimic Reed-Sternberg cells, and the diagnosis of primary pulmonary Hodgkin's disease must be made with caution.

Lymphoma of Lymphomatoid Granulomatosis Type

Lymphoma of lymphomatoid granulomatosis type is a malignant, lympho-proliferative, pulmonary disease which over an interval of several months to a few years tends to progressively fill the lung. Almost all of the patients die of the disease, usually because of neoplastic destruction of the lung, sepsis, or hemoptysis. Median survival of these patients from time of histologic diagnosis to death is 14 months (72). The disease is refractory to therapy. The kidney, liver, and central nervous system are each involved in approximately one-fifth of patients. Lymph nodes, spleen, skin and other organs are also occasionally involved.

The essential histologic feature is a mixed infiltrate of large, atypical lymphocytes, immunoblasts, small lymphocytes, and plasma cells, which is lymphangitic, angiocentric, and angiodestructive (84). Other histologic features are cellular infiltration of bronchi, coagulative necrosis, and granulomatous aggregates of histiocytes. Discrete sarcoidal granulomas are rare (119). Grossly, lymphomatoid granulomatosis commonly creates several nodules and uncommonly a single nodule or a permeative infiltrate involving a segment or lobe. Prognosis correlates with the proportion of the infiltrate that is composed of the atypical lymphoid cells (72). Cases with small numbers of atypical cells may be confused with pulmonary Wegener's granulomatosis. However, the distinction is crucial because Wegener's disease responds better to cytotoxic drugs and has a much better prognosis. Cases with large numbers of atypical cells share histologic features with large cell lymphoma or Hodgkin's disease. Lymphomatoid granulomatosis can be considered to be a peculiar, polymorphous lymphoma which usually presents in the lung while sparing lymph nodes. At autopsy, deposits are found, in order of decreasing frequency, in skin, kidney, liver, brain, and lymph nodes (72).

Plasmacytoma

Plasmacytoma is a rare benign tumor of the lung composed of plasma cells. The tumor may be small or so massive it occupies most of a lobe. The plasma cells are generally regular but with some variability in maturation. The clinical hallmark of the tumor is the production of abnormal circulating proteins: surgical excision of the plasmacytoma will result in disappearance of the abnormal serum M-proteins (13,147). Disseminated nodules of multiple myeloma may involve the lung. Morphology alone of a solid mass of plasma cells in the lung usually will not suffice to distinguish between a solitary benign plasmacytoma and a nodule of malignant multiple myeloma.

Plasma Cell Granuloma

Plasma cell granuloma is an inflammatory tumefaction within the pulmonary parenchyma. It is not a neoplasm. A variegated composition of plasma cells, lymphocytes, histiocytes, granulomas, fibrosis, and vascular proliferation accounts for its various names: fibrous histiocytoma, fibroxanthoma, and inflammatory pseudotumor (11,23,146). Plasma cell granuloma may grow either as a large intraparenchymal mass or as a small intrabronchial polyp (58,129). Some lesions contain a large amount of lipid and histologically resemble cholesterol pneumonitis, others contain spindle cells in fascicular array and resemble leiomyoma, and yet others contain sheets of plasma cells and mimic a plasmacytoma. If numerous mitoses are present in a lesion which is predominantly fibroblastic, differentiation from a low-grade fibrosarcoma can prove difficult. Rarely is an etiology determined. Trauma may occasionally play a role. Excision is definitive treatment.

LEUKEMIA

Interstitial infiltration by leukemic cells occurs in approximately one-third of patients dying of leukemia (102,115). Additional cases have obstruction of blood vessels and lymphatics due to leukostasis. Interstitial leukemic infiltration is not closely related to the white blood cell count in the peripheral blood. However, the sequence of mechanical obstruction to blood flow by leukemic cells, interstitial and intra-alveolar edema, and respiratory distress is prone to develop in acute granulocytic leukemia when the circulating white blood cell count rises about 150,000 per mm^3 and more than 80% of the cells are blasts (141). Low deformability of circulating myeloblasts and compaction of cells both play a role (141).

Chemotherapy has not altered the incidence of interstitial leukemic infiltration (115). The incidence is similar in acute lymphocytic and acute myelocytic leukemia. In hairy cell leukemia, however, pulmonary infiltration is the rule rather than the exception (139).

Although 40% of leukemic patients have respiratory impairment, it is rarely due to the leukemic infiltration per se (115). However, respiratory distress ascribed to alveolar-capillary block can be the patient's initial complaint in both acute and chronic leukemia (42,48,11). Radiologically detectable, diffuse, pulmonary infiltrates in leukemic patients will prove to be due to leukemia in 10% of cases (47). Whereas diffuse interstitial infiltration occurs at a late state of disease and is bilateral, pleural effusion may occur selectively at an earlier stage and may be unilateral (128).

REFERENCES

1. Abeloff, M. D., Eggleston, J. C., Mendelsohn, G., Ettinger, D. S., and Baylin, S. B. (1979): *Am. J. Med.*, 66:757–764.
2. Ali, M. Y., and Lee, G. S. (1964): *Cancer*, 17:1220–1224.
3. Al-Saleem, T., and Peale, A. R. (1969): *Am. Rev. Respir. Dis.*, 99:767–772.
4. Al-Saleem, T., Peale, A. R., and Norris, C. M. (1968): *Cancer*, 22:1173–1184.
5. Aranda, C., Sidhu, G., Sasso, L. A., and Adams, F. V. (1978): *Cancer*, 42:1995–1998.
6. Arrigoni, M. G., Woolner, L. B., and Bernatz, P. E. (1972): *J. Thorac. Cardiovasc. Surg.*, 64:413–421.
7. Auerbach, O., Garfinkel, L., and Parks, V. R. (1979): *Cancer*, 43:636–642.
8. Auerbach, O., Saccomanno, G., Kuschner, M., Brown, R. D., and Garfinkel, L. (1978): *Cancer*, 42:483–489.
9. Auerbach, O., Stout, A. P., Hammond, E. C., and Garfinkel, L. (1967): *Cancer*, 20:699–705.
10. Azzopardi, J. G. (1959): *J. Pathol. Bacteriol.*, 78:513–519.
11. Bahadori, M., and Leibow, A. A. (1973): *Cancer*, 31:191–208.
12. Barnard, W. G. (1926): *J. Pathol.*, 29:241–244.
13. Baroni, C. D., Mineo, T. C., Ricci, C., Guarino, S., and Mandelli, F. (1977): *Cancer*, 40:2329–2322.
14. Barson, A. J., Jones, A. W., and Lodge, K. V. (1968): *J. Clin. Pathol.*, 21:480–485.
15. Bateson, E. M. (1965): *Thorax*, 20:477–461.
16. Bateson, E. M. (1973): *Cancer*, 31:1458–1467.
17. Becker, N. H., and Soifer, I. (1971): *Cancer*, 27:712–719.
18. Bedrossian, C. W. M., Weilbaecher, D. G., Bentinck, D. C., and Greenberg, S. D. (1975): *Cancer*, 36:1399–1413.
19. Belsey, R. H. R., and Valentine, J. C. (1951): *J. Pathol. Bacteriol.*, 63:377–387.
20. Bennett, D. E., Sasser, W. F., and Ferguson, T. B. (1969): *Cancer*, 23:431–439.
21. Bensch, K. G., Corrin, B., Pariente, R., and Spencer, H. (1968): *Cancer*, 22:1163–1172.
22. Brereton, H. D., Mathews, M. M., Costa, J., Kent, C. H., and Johnson, R. E. (1978): *Ann. Intern. Med.*, 88:805–806.

23. Buell, R., Wang, N. S., Seemayer, T. A., and Ahmed, M. N. (1976): *Hum. Pathol.*, 7:411–426.
24. Butler, C., II, and Kleinerman, J. (1969): *Arch. Pathol.*, 88:583–592.
25. Cahan, W. G., Castron, E. B., and Hajdu, S. I. (1974): *Cancer*, 33:414–421.
26. Caplan, H. (1959): *Thorax*, 14:89–96.
27. Carney, J. A. (1979): *Cancer*, 43:374–382.
28. Carter, D., Marsh, B. R., Baker, R. R., Erozan, Y. S., and Frost, J. K. (1976): *Cancer*, 37:1389–1396.
29. Chadhuri, M. R. (1971): *J. Thorac. Cardiovasc. Surg.*, 61:319–323.
30. Churg, A. (1978): *Hum. Pathol.*, 9:143–156.
31. Churg, A., and Warnock, M. L. (1976): *Cancer*, 37:1469–1477.
32. Conlan, A. A., Payne, W. S., Woolner, L. B., and Sanderson, D. R. (1978): *J. Thorac. Cardiovasc. Surg.*, 76:369–377.
33. Corring, B., Liebow, A. A., and Friedman, P. J. (1975): *Am. J. Pathol.*, 79:348–382.
34. Cross, K. R. (1957): *Arch. Pathol.*, 63:132–148.
35. Dail, D., and Liebow, A. (1975): *Am. J. Pathol.*, 78:6a–7a.
36. Diaconita, G. (1975): *Thorax*, 30:682–686.
37. Dunn, D., Hertel, B., Norwood, W., and Nicoloff, D. M. (1978): *Ann. Thorac. Surg.*, 26:241–249.
38. Dunn, D., and Dehner, L. P. (1977): *Cancer*, 40:3054–3064.
39. Feyrter, F. (1954): *Virchows Archiv.*, 325:723–732.
40. Fox, B., and Risdon, R. A. (1968): *J. Clin. Pathol.*, 21:486–491.
41. Fung, C. H., Lo, J. W., Yonan, T. N., Milloy, F. J., and Hakami, M. M. (1977): *Cancer*, 39:153–163.
42. Geller, S. A. (1971): *Arch. Pathol.*, 91:573–576.
43. Godwin, J. D., II, and Brown, C. C. (1977): *Cancer*, 40:1671–1673.
44. Gonzalez-Vitale, J. C., and Garcia-Bunel, R. (1976): *Cancer*, 38:2105–2110.
45. Goodner, J. T., Berg, J. W., and Watson, W. L. (1961): *Cancer*, 14:539–546.
46. Gould, V. E., and Cheifec, G. (1978): *Hum. Pathol.*, 9:377–384.
47. Green, R. A., and Nichols, N. J. (1959): *Am. Rev. Respir. Dis.*, 80:833–844.
48. Green, R. A., Nichols, N. J., and King, E. J. (1959): *Am. Rev. Respir. Dis.*, 80:895–901.
49. Guccion, J. G., and Rosen, S. H. (1972): *Cancer*, 836–847.
50. Gullian, R. A., and Zelman, S. (1966): *Am. J. Clin. Pathol.*, 46:427–432.
51. Haas, J. E., Yunis, E. J., and Totten, R. S. (1972): *Cancer*, 30:512–518.
52. Hagstrom, L. (1961): *Acta Pathol. Microbiol. Scan.*, 51:87–94.
53. Hall, E. M. (1935): *Am. J. Pathol.*, 11:343–352.
54. Harbin, W. P., Mark, G. J., and Greene, R. E. (1978): *Radiology*, 129:595–596.
55. Hattori, S., Matsuda, M., Tateishi, R., Nishihara, H., and Horal, T. (1972): *Cancer*, 30:1014–1024.
56. Heitzman, E. R., Markarian, B., and DeLise, C. T. (1975): *Semin. Roentgenol.*, 10:73–81.
57. Hellstrom, H. R., and Fisher, E. R. (1963): *Cancer*, 16:1080–1088.
58. Herczeg, E., Weissberg, D., Almog, C., and Pajewski, M. (1978): *Chest*, 73:669–670.
59. Herman, D. L., Bullock, W. K., and Waken, J. K. (1966): *Cancer*, 19:1337–1346.
60. Hill, G. S., and Eggleston, J. C. (1972): *Cancer*, 30:1092–1106.
61. Hinds, J. R., and Hitchcock, G. C. (1969): *Thorax*, 24:10–17.
62. Hirsch, F., Hansen, H. H., Dombernowsky, P., and Hainau, B. (1977): *Cancer*, 39:2563–2567.
63. Hoch, W. S., Patchefsky, A. S., Takeda, M., and Gordon, G. (1974): *Cancer*, 33:1328–1336.
64. Hochberg, L. A., and Crastnopol, P. (1956): *Arch. Surg.*, 73:74–78.
65. Homma, H., Kira, S., Takahashi, Y., and Imai, H. (1975): *Am. Rev. Respir. Dis.*, 111:857–862.
66. Ioachim, H. L., Dorsett, B. H., and Paulch, E. (1976): *Cancer*, 38:2296–2309.
67. Iverson, L. (1954): *J. Thorac. Surg.*, 27:130–148.
68. Joliat, G., Stadler, H., and Kapanci, Y. (1973): *Cancer*, 31:455–461.
69. Kandawalla, N. M., Kasnic, G., Jr., and Azar, H. Λ. (1977): *Lab. Invest.*, 36:342.
70. Kane, R. D., Hawkins, H. K., Miller, J. A., Noci, P. S. (1975): *Cancer*, 36:1473–1482.
71. Karcioglu, Z. A., and Someran, A. O. (1974): *Am. J. Clin. Pathol.*, 61:287–295.
72. Katzenstein, A. A., Carrington, C. B., and Liebow, A. A. (1979): *Cancer*, 43:360–373.
73. Katzenstein, A., Purvis, R., Jr., Gmelich, J., and Askin, F. (1978): *Cancer*, 41:712–723.
74. Kay, S., Still, W. J. S., and Borochovitz, D. (1977): *Hum. Pathol.*, 8:468–474.
75. Kennedy, A. (1969): *J. Clin. Pathol.*, 22:354–360.

76. Kimula, Y. (1978): *Am. J. Surg. Pathol.*, 2:253–264.
77. King, D. S., and Castleman, B. (1943): *J. Thorac. Surg.*, 12:305–315.
78. Kreyberg, L. (1981): Histological Typing of Lung Tumours. Second ed., World Health Organization, Geneva.
79. Kroe, D. J., and Pitcock, J. A. (1967): *Arch. Pathol.*, 84:539–542.
80. Laubscher, F. A. (1969): *Am. J. Clin. Pathol.*, 52:599–603.
81. Lawthorne, T. W., Jr., Baker, R. R., and Carter, D. (1973): *Hopkins Med. J.*, 133:82–87.
82. LeRoux, B. T., Williams, M. A., and Kallichurum, S. (1969): *Thorax*, 24:673–677.
83. Liebow, A. A. (1960): *Adv. Int. Med.*, 10:329–358.
84. Liebow, A. A., Carrington, C. R. B., and Friedman, P. J. (1972): *Hum. Pathol.*, 3:457–558.
85. Liebow, A. A., and Castleman, B. (1971): *J. Biol. Med.*, 43:213–222.
86. Liebow, A. A., and Hubbell, D. S. (1956): *Cancer*, 9:53–75.
87. Ludington, L. G., Verska, J. J., Howard, T., Kypridakis, G., and Brewer, L. A. (1972): *Chest*, 61:622–628.
88. MacDonald, J. B. (1977): *Thorax*, 32:664–667.
89. Manoharan, A., Pitney, W. R., Schoenell, M. E., and Bader, L. V. (1979): *Thorax*, 34:29–32.
90. Marsh, W. L., Jr., and Allen, M. S., Jr. (1979): *Cancer*, 43:1463–1473.
91. Mason, M. K., and Azeem, P. S. (1965): *Thorax*, 20:13–17.
92. Mason, PNM. K., and Jordan, J. W. (1969): *Thorax*, 24:461–471.
93. McCann, M. P., Fu, Y. S., and Day, S. (1976): *Cancer*, 38:789–797.
94. Meyer, E. C., and Liebow, A. A. (1965): *Cancer*, 18:322–351.
95. Miller, M. A., Mark, G. J., and Kanarek, D. (1978): *Am. J. Med.*, 65:373–378.
96. Morgan, A. D., and MacKenzie, D. H. (1964): *J. Pathol. Bacteriol.*, 87:25–27.
97. Mori, S. (1968): *Dis. Chest*, 54:71–74.
98. Mullins, J. D., and Barnes, R. P. (1979): *Cancer*, 44:315–322.
99. Murthy, M. S., Meckstroth, C. V., Merkle, B. H., Huston, J. T., and Cattaneo, M. (1976): *Arch. Pathol. Lab. Med.*, 100:649–651.
100. Munnell, E. R., Dilling, E., Grantham, R. N., Harkey, M. R., and Mohr, J. A. (1978): *Ann. Thorac. Surg.*, 25:289–297.
101. Nash, A. D., and Stout, A. P. (1958): *Cancer*, 11:369–376.
102. Nathan, D. J., and Sanders, M. (1955): *N. Engl. J. Med.*, 252:797–801.
103. Nixon, D. W., Murphy, G. F., Sewell, C. W., Kutner, M., and Lynn, M. J. (1979): *Cancer*.
104. Nobel, T. A., and Perk, K. (1979): *Am. J. Pathol.*, 95:783–786.
105. Okike, N., Bernatz, P. E., and Woolner, L. B. (1976): *Ann. Thorac. Surg.*, 22:270–277.
106. Oyasu, R., Battifora, H. A., Buckingham, W. B., and Hidvegi, D. (1977): *Cancer*, 39:1119–1128.
107. Ramathan, T. (1974): *Thorax*, 29:482–489.
108. Ramsey, J. H., and Reimann, D. L. (1953): *Am. J. Pathol.*, 29:339–351.
109. Ranchod, M. (1977): *Cancer*, 39:1135–1145.
110. Reinilä, A., and Dammert, K. (1974): *Acta Pathol. Microbiol. Scand. A.*, 82:783–790.
111. Resnick, M. E., Berkowitz, R. D., and Rodman, T. (1961): *Am. J. Med.*, 31:149–153.
112. Reznik-Schüller, H. (1977): *Am. J. Pathol.*, 89:59–63.
113. Rhone, D. P., and Horowitz, R. N. (1976): *Cancer*, 38:1773–1780.
114. Rosenblatt, M. B., Lisa, J. R., and Collier, F. (1967): *Dis. Chest*, 51:587–595.
115. Ross, J. S., and Ellman, L. (1974): *Am. J. Clin. Pathol.*, 61:235–241.
116. Rottino, A., and Hoffman, G. (1955): *Am. J. Surg.*, 89:550–555.
117. Rubin, M. (1968): *J. Thorac. Cardiovasc. Surg.*, 56:293–303.
118. Rubinstein, I., Baum, G. L., Kalter, Y., Pauzner, Y., Lieberman, Y., and Bubis, J. J. (1979): *Am. Rev. Respir. Dis.*, 119:253–261.
119. Saldana, M. J., Patchefsky, A. S., Israel, H. I., and Atkinson, G. W. (1977): *Hum. Pathol.*, 8:391–409.
120. Saltzstein, S. L. (1963): *Cancer*, 7:928–955.
121. Salyer, D. C., Sayler, W. R., and Eggleston, J. C. (1975): *Cancer*, 36:1522–1537.
122. Sargent, E. N., Barnes, R. A., and Schwinn, C. P. (1970): *Radiology*, 110:694–700.
123. Siegenthaler, V. D., Merki, W., Funk, H. W., Hedinger, C., and Pletscher, A. (1965): *Schweiz. med. Wochenschr.*, 95:869–876.
124. Silverman, J. F., and Kay, S. (1976): *Cancer*, 38:1199–1204.
125. Smith, J. F., and Dexter, D. (1963): *Thorax*, 18:340–349.

126. Soga, J., and Tazawa, K. (1971): *Cancer*, 28:990–998.
127. Souza, R. C., Peasley, E. D., and Takaro, T. (1965): *Ann. Thorac. Surg.*, 1:259–268.
128. Spencer, H., and Raeburn, C. (1956): *J. Pathol. Bacteriol.*, 71:145–154.
129. Spoto, G., Jr., Rossi, N. P., and Allsbrook, W. C. (1977): *J. Thorac. Cardiovasc. Surg.*, 73:804–806.
130. Stackhouse, E. M., Harrison, E. G., Jr., and Ellis, F. H. (1969): *J. Thorac. Cardiovasc. Surg.*, 57:385–399.
131. Stanford, W., Spivey, C. G., Jr., Larsen, G. L., Alexander, J. A., and Besich, W. J. (1976): *J. Thorac. Cardiovasc. Surg.*, 72:441–449.
132. Stolberg, H. O., Patt, N. L., MacEwen, K. F., Warwick, O. H., and Brown, T. C. (1962): *Radiology*, 92:96–115.
133. Stovin, P. G. I., Lum, L. C., Flower, C. D. R., Darke, C. S., and Beeley, M. (1975): *Thorax*, 30:497–509.
134. Sweeney, E. C., and Cooney, T. (1978): *J. Clin. Pathol.*, 31:1218–1225.
135. Symmers, W. St. C. (1951): *Am. J. Pathol.*, 27:493–521.
136. Tateishi, R., Horai, T., and Hattori, S. (1978): *Virchows Arch. A Pathol. Anat. Histol.*, 377:203–210.
137. Taylor, T. L., and Miller, D. R. (1969): *J. Thorac. Cardiovasc. Surg.*, 57:284–288.
138. Torikata, C., and Ishiwata, K. (1977): *Cancer*, 40:1194–1201.
139. Vardiman, J. W., Variakigis, D., and Golomb, H. M. (1979): *Cancer*, 43:1339–1349.
140. Vasquez, J. J., Fernandez-Cuervo, and Fidalgo, B. (1976): *Cancer*, 37:2321–2328.
141. Vernant, J. P., Brun, B., Mannoni, P., and Dreyfus, B. (1979): *Cancer*, 44:264–268.
142. Vincent, R. G., Pickren, J. W., Lane, W. W., Bross, I., Takita, H., Houten, L., Gutierrez, A. C., and Rzepka, T. (1977): *Cancer*, 39:1647–1655.
143. Wackers, F. J. T., Van der Schoot, J. B., and Hampe, J. F. (1969): *Cancer*, 23:339–351.
144. Wagenvoort, C. A., Beetstra, A., and Spijker, J. (1978): *Histopathology*, 2:401–406.
145. Wang, N. S., Seemayer, T. A., Ahmed, M. D., and Knaack, J. (1976): *Hum. Pathol.*, 7:3–16.
146. Wentworth, P., Lynch, M. J., Fallis, J. C., Turner, J. P. A., Lowden, J. A., and Conen, P. E. (1968): *Cancer*, 22:345–355.
147. Wile, A., Olinger, G., Peter, J. B., and Dornfeld, L. (1976): *Cancer*, 37:2338–2342.
148. Wollstein, M. (1931): *Arch. Pathol.*, 12:562–571.
149. Woolner, L. B., David, E., Fontana, R. S., Andersen, H. A., and Bernatz, P. E. (1970): *J. Thorac. Cardiovasc. Surg.*, 60:275–290.
150. Yesner, R., Gerstl, B., and Auerbach, O. (1965): *Ann. Thorac. Surg.*, 1:33–49.

Thoracic Oncology, edited by N. C. Choi and
H. C. Grillo. Raven Press, New York © 1983.

Clinical Radiation Biology

Herman D. Suit

*Department of Radiation Medicine, Massachusetts General Hospital,
Harvard Medical School, Boston, Massachusetts 02114*

The observed response to irradiation of an organ or structure is the integrated response of the various tissue and cellular constituents. Cellular responses to radiation may be classed as (a) delay in progression through the cell replication cycle; (b) gross change in chromosome morphology; (c) change in cell size; (d) increased frequency of daughter cell death; and (e) loss of viability, i.e., the loss of the capacity for sustained proliferation. This latter response is the one of greatest interest and concern to the clinician involved in the treatment of the cancer patient. The observable changes in a tissue or structure following irradiation are dependent on the time course of pyknosis or lysis of the various consituent cells and the changes in the proliferation kinetics of those constituent cells. Severe and acute changes are seen in lymphoid, marrow, small intestinal, skin, and mucous membranes, since these tissues are comprised of actively dividing cell populations. Hence, after an appropriate radiation dose, the radiation damage is expressed early and the total cell population becomes grossly depleted. In contrast, tissues such as connective, muscle, peripheral nerves, or central nervous system, exhibit changes at times remote from the event of the irradiation because the cells comprising these tissues are either nonproliferative or are dividing at extremely slow rates. In accordance with these findings on response to radiation of normal tissue, the response of tumor tissue can be predicted with a reasonable accuracy by knowing the proliferative activity of the tumor cells and the nature and abundance of the stroma. For example, a poorly differentiated, very cellular, and actively proliferating tumor cell population (as evidenced by a high mitotic index) would be expected to, and is observed to, regress rapidly following conventional radiation (e.g., oat cell carcinoma or poorly differentiated carcinoma of the nasopharynx). In contrast, a well-differentiated tumor with an extensive and mature stroma but with a low cell number and rare mitotic figures would be expected to regress slowly or not at all (e.g., a well-differentiated chondrosarcoma of the chest wall or well-differentiated squamous carcinoma of the esophagus or bronchus). Marked differences in "response" are expected even though the intrinsic radiation sensitivities of the tumor cells were identical in the various tumors mentioned.

Dr. Suit is Andres Soriano Director of Cancer Management at Massachusetts General Hospital, Harvard Medical School.

RADIATION CELL KILL

In order to appreciate radiobiologic considerations, it is worthwhile to review the definition of cell kill. As stated earlier, loss of cell viability means that as a consequence of the radiation the cell has lost the capacity for sustained proliferation. We note that the definition states sustained proliferation. Indeed, cinephotographic analyses of proliferative activity of mammalian cells grown *in vitro* and subjected to single doses of radiation have shown that a cell may undergo one, two, three, five, or six post-radiation divisions before the progeny of that radiation-killed cell undergoes pyknosis and lysis. Figure 1 is the pedigree of an L59 fibroblast cell that received 216 cGy (8). There was extensive proliferation post-radiation, but all of the progeny eventually died. For the cell to be classed as viable there would have to have been at least one sector along the pedigree that would continue to show cell proliferation and eventually would make a colony. This colony could be transferred repeatedly and a cell line would be established from that original irradiated parent cell. *In vitro* studies by Sinclair (5) established that following irradiation there is an increase in the mean cell cycle time, that the cells in viable colonies are smaller, that there is increased probability of death among progeny of the irradiated cell, and that there may be an increase in the inherent radiation sensitivity. The number of post-radiation divisions an irradiated cell may undergo

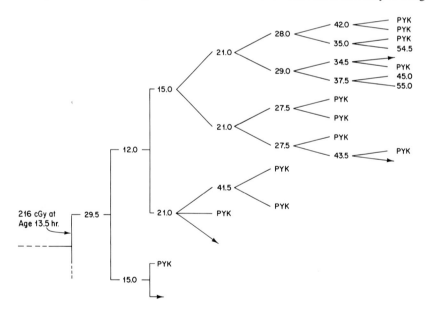

FIG. 1. An L59 cell given 216 cGy at 13.5 hr of age (time after mitosis or its "birth") divided after a total intermitotic time of 29.5 hr. The subsequent division history of its progeny is shown in the pedigree. Note that one of the daughter cells produced two sterile daughters. The other section generated four subsequent divisions before the colony clearly became "abortive," i.e., the cell was killed by the single radiation dose but there were irregular divisions over the next several days.

is cell-type related. For example, the lymphoid or gonadal cell that has been killed by radiation may undergo pyknosis and lysis during interphase, i.e., before the first post-irradiation division is attempted. That is, cells of this origin usually would not be observed to pass through a large number of post-radiation divisions before the progeny died in a metabolic sense. In contrast, cells of mesenchymal or epithelial origin usually will undergo pyknosis and lysis in an attempted mitosis, and many of the radiation-killed cells and their progeny pass through a number of post-radiation divisions before metabolic death, as shown in Fig. 1. Another feature of cell populations undergoing radiation is a suppression of the mitotic index. Cells will often be dealyed in their progression through the cell cylce at G2. Accordingly, after irradiation, as the G2 block is overcome there may be a rebound, with the mitotic index level exceeding control values.

The relationship between dose and loss of cell viability follows a relatively simple exponential function. Figure 2 shows the dose–response curve obtained by Puck and Marcus in 1956 when they measured loss of cell viability versus dose for the HeLa cell line (3). It is of interest to the physician that the first determinations of radiation–cell survival relationships for mammalian cells were performed using cells derived from human tissue and that that tissue was malignant. In this particular instance, the cells were derived from a human squamous cell carcinoma. The curve shown in Fig. 2 is characterized by an initial shoulder region in which dose is relatively ineffective, and then a simple straight line, for a plot of survival fraction versus dose on a log-linear grid. The slope of the straight line portion of the curve is usually taken as a measure of the inherent radiation sensitivity of the cell. This slope is described as D_0 and is the dose which will achieve a reduction in survival by a factor of 0.37. That is, each unit of dose achieves the same fractional decrease in survival. The D_0 for cobalt or supervoltage radiation is approximately 160 cGy. The initial shoulder region indicates that the cell accumulates a certain amount of

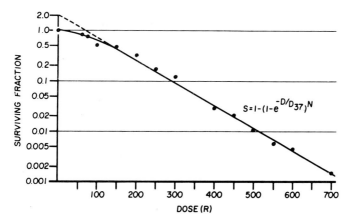

FIG. 2. Cell survival curves for HeLa cells subjected to a single dose of X-radiation. (From Puck and Marcus, ref. 3, with permission.)

radiation damage before damage becomes lethal. To a first approximation, the width of the shoulder region is a reflection of the capacity of the cell to repair radiation damage. Since the publication by Puck and Marcus in 1956, there have been extensive studies on a wide variety of mammalian cells of normal and malignant tissue origin derived from human and various mammalian species; the relationship between survival fraction and dose is very close to that shown in Fig. 2. There has been some variation in the values for the D_0 and the width of the shoulder, but this variation has been relatively small provided one separates out studies on cells derived from lymphoid or gonadal origin. For those cells, the D_0 is smaller, i.e., in the range of 50–100 cGy, and the shoulder width is much smaller or may be absent. For cells of mesenchymal or epithelial origin there is almost always a shoulder, which may be considerably broader than the one shown in Fig. 2, and the D_0 may be in the range of 150–200 cGy (for aerobic cells). Further, there have been studies on a variety of murine tissues *in vivo* by techniques that have not involved disruption of the integrity of the tissues (skin, gastric, jejunal, colonic crypt cell, cartilage). The values of D_0 and the shoulder width for those cell systems have been similar to the values obtained *in vitro*. Important conclusions from these studies have been that radiation is relatively efficient in causing reproductive death of mammalian cells, that the relationship between cell survival and dose is exponential, and that relatively low doses will kill nearly all of the cells (>99%) in the population being irradiated. If the goal is to kill all of the cells (100%) in a large population of cells (for example, a tumor that may contain 1×10^6 to 1×10^8 viable cells), then a large total dose is required. A problem in clinical radiation therapy is administering radiation in such a way that all the cells in the tumor are inactivated with a high probablity, but that the cell kill within the adjacent normal tissue is sufficiently low so that there are sufficient viable cells remaining to repopulate and to reconstitute the normal tissue.

PHYSIOLOGICAL DETERMINANTS OF RADIATION SENSITIVITY

Oxygen Tension

Molecular oxygen has been comprehensively studied as a radiation sensitizer and is now known to be one of the most powerful sensitizers studied to date. For example, the D_0 for hypoxic mammalian cells (< 1 mm Hg) is in the range of 450–550 cGy; that is, the ratio of D_0 values for hypoxic to aerobic cells would be ≈ 3. Of special significance is the fact that oxygen is maximally sensitizing at physiological concentrations. The sensitivity to radiation increases extremely rapidly as P_{O_2} is increased from 1 to 10 mm Hg, but the increase after that is relatively modest. There is little change in sensitivity after P_{O_2} reaches 40 mm Hg. This is judged to be of clinical importance because of the finding of Thomlinson and Gray (7) that areas of necrosis are seen in human bronchogenic carcinomas at distances from capillaries that correspond to the oxygen diffusion length. The oxygen diffusion length was predicted on the basis of oxygen utilization rates, oxygen diffusion coefficients, estimates of blood flow rates through capillaries, and the P_{O_2} of blood at the arterial end of the capillaries. Subsequent studies have confirmed that necrosis is present in almost all tissues in which, for a variety of reasons, the distance between capillaries has become so great that some cells may be at distances from capillaries exceeding the oxygen diffusion length. Of special concern is the fact that adjacent to the necrotic regions there would be viable but hypoxic, and hence radiation-resistant, cells. To the extent that such cells may be present in tumors throughout a course of fractionated irradiation, they would be expected to contribute to clinical radiation resistance and failures of radiation to eradicate the primary tumor. The clinical importance of the hypoxic cell has not been fully established. Intensive clinical and laboratory investigative efforts have been directed toward estimating the significance of hypoxic and viable tumor cells, and a variety of clinical maneuvers have been attempted to overcome or to reduce the importance of such cells in determining success of radiation therapy. These include respiration of pure oxygen at high pressure (3 or 4 atm, absolute), intra-arterial infusions of hydrogen peroxide, the use of chemical agents that selectively sensitize hypoxic cells (e.g., misonidazole), high LET radiation (biological effectiveness is relatively independent of P_{O_2}; e.g., fast neutrons, negative pions, neon and silicone ions), and low LET radiation administered under conditions of tourniquet-induced hypoxia (eliminating the differential in P_{O_2}, which favors tumor).

Proliferative Activity

Radiobiologists Howard and Pelc in 1952 (2) described the cell replication cycle as having four stages: M or mitosis, S or the phase during which chromosomes are replicated, G1 phase (between M and S), and G2 (between S and M). The role of the age of the cell in the cell replication cycle and its effect on radiation sensitivity have now been exhaustively studied. Terasima and Tolmach (6) first showed the marked dependence of radiation sensitivity on position in the cell replication cycle; this has been extensively confirmed by Sinclair (4) and others. Figure 3 is a summary graph of Sinclair (4) showing cell survival curves for Chinese hamster cells irradiated in early S, late S, M, G1, and G2 phases. His findings are that for cells in M the sensitivity is high, i.e., a very low D_0 and a virtually absent shoulder on the survival curve. In contrast, cells in late S have a broad shoulder and a slightly higher D_0. Accordingly, the dependence of sensitivity on cell age is a critical parameter; this is referred to as the age–response function. The cell kill of a specified radiation dose to a cell population with a defined age–response function would, of course, be determined by the distribution of cell ages (or positions in the cell replication cycle). This distribution is referred to as the age–density distribution.

Repair Kinetics

Mammalian cells have varying capacities to repair radiation damage. The magnitude of this repair is most readily demonstrated by comparing the radiation doses required to achieve a given effect when radiation is administered in a series of

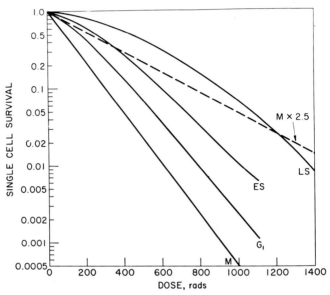

FIG. 3. Cell survival curves for Chinese hamster cells irradiated at M, G1, early S, or late S phase of the cell replication cycle. (From Sinclair, ref. 4, with permission.)

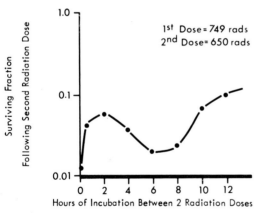

FIG. 4. Repair of radiation damage in cells which have sustained sublethal injury is demonstrated by the marked increase in survival of cells as the time between the first and second radiation doses is increased to 2 hr. There is some decrease in the survival fraction for intertreatment interval at 6 hr; this is due to the progression of cell replication cycle at hour 6. (From Elkind et al., ref. 1, with permission.)

doses, compared with a single dose. Almost invariably, the total radiation dose required to effect a given level of cell kill or a given degree of tissue response increases sharply with the number of fractions. For example, if radiation is given in 30 fractions instead of single dose, the required total radiation dose is increased by a factor of 3–3.5. The conventional approach to clinical radiation therapy has been to administer doses of the order of 200 cGy for 30 to 35 fractions, for total doses of 6,000 to 7,000 cGy. If radiation were to be administered in a single dose, the maximum amount tolerated by the patient would be ≈1600–1800 cGy (this value is not known since there is so little experience with single-dose treatments, except for small skin cancers). This fractionation effect is a complex interaction of repair kinetics and altered distribution of cells within the cell replication cycle at each treatment session. Laboratory demonstration of the rate and magnitude of repair of radiation damage is shown in Fig. 4 (1). For this experiment, radiation was given in two equal doses, with inter-treatment intervals of up to 24 hr. If the radiation was administered as a single dose, i.e., zero time interval between fractions, survival fraction was 0.01, whereas if 2–4 hr were allowed to pass between dose 1 and dose 2, survival fraction was greater by a factor of about 5.

Factors Determining Response of Tissues to Radiation

The physical factors that are important determinants of tissue response are total dose, dose per fraction, dose rate, and time interval between fractions. Effectiveness per unit dose decreases (total dose must be raised) as number of fractions and or time interval between fractions increases, and the effectiveness decreases as dose rate is reduced, especially below a few cGy per minute. The important consideration for the clinician is not the total dose employed but the differential response of tumor and normal tissue. The highly fractionated therapy is more effective clinically than the single dose treatment, i.e., a higher likelihood of destruction of tumor for a specified degree of damage to normal tissue.

Biological factors that determine the response of tissues to radiation include (a) the fraction and the absolute number of cells surviving radiation. This will be determined by the distribution of D_0 and n values throughout the cell population of interest, which will be influenced, of course, by the distributions of Po_2 values, the age–response function, and the age–density distribution; (b) the time distribution of pyknosis and lysis, and of removal of the cellular debris; (c) the ability of the surviving cells to proliferate and reconstitute tissue; (d) the presence of an effective host rejection reaction against the tissue. Where there is an effective rejection reaction by the host against the tumor, this would be expected to cooperate with the radiation dose in achieving a greater cell kill or perhaps accomplish a tumor inactivation.

CLINICAL APPLICATIONS OF RADIATION BIOLOGY

Several important considerations from radiation biology have had direct and important implications in clinical radiation therapy. The first of these has been to make clear that there is an orderly relationship between radiation dose and probablity of inactivation of all the cells in a tumor cell population. That is, as the radiation dose is increased, the probablity of inactivation of a tumor is increased in a sensible manner. As a corollary, any particular radiation dose level (total dose applied in a specified number of fractions over a given total time) will yield a particular frequency of tumor inactivation. That is, there is no validity to the concept of a "tumoricidal" dose; a particular treatment schedule merely yields a given probability of tumor eradication.

Second, efforts to improve the dose distribution so that higher radiation doses can be employed should be pursued. In point of fact, there is abundant evidence supporting the validity of this concept: as supervoltage radiation was introduced (replacement of orthovoltage), much higher radiation doses were employed. This achieved major increases in tumor control frequencies with similar or lesser damage to normal tissues. The resultant increase in cure was related strictly to the higher radiation doses employed, i.e., there was no radiobiological advantage in the higher energy photons. Third, radiation doses should be distributed throughout the tumor-bearing tissue in accordance with the probable distribution of tumor cell number. Early in radiation therapy, single square or rectangular fields were applied and these were used throughout the course of treatment. Because of the increased awareness of cell-survival curve shape, etc., treatment techniques have been widely adopted that employ the "shrinking field technique." That is, for the initial component of treatment, the radiation is given to a large volume of tissue, i.e., the volume of tissue that contains the clinically or radiographically evident tumor plus all tissues suspected, to a clinically important probability, of involvement by subclinical or microscopic disease. For the final component of treatment, portals are redesigned to include only the obvious mass. The result is a higher dose to the principal tumor mass than was feasible with the older approach. Fourth, radiation dose levels are planned in relationship to the tumor size (9). Small lesions (T1) are treated to lower dose than locally advanced (T3–T4). Fifth, a strong rationale for combining radiation and surgery has developed. Well-tolerated radiation doses are judged to be effective in the destruction of tumor extending beyond the clinically evident mass, and surgery is regularly successful in resection of the evident mass. This means that less than radical surgery or radiation can be employed with good expectation of accomplishing at least as good a result as either modality applied radically and alone. There is active clinical evaluation of these combined approaches.

REFERENCES

1. Elkind, M. M., Alescio, T., Swain, R. W., Moses, W. B., and Sutton, H. (1964): Recovery of hypoxic mammalian cells from sublethal X-ray damage. *Nature*, 202:1190–1193.
2. Howard, A., and Pelc, S. R. (1952): Synthesis of deoxyribonucleic acid in normal and irradiated cells and its relation to chromosome breakage. *Heredity*, (Suppl. 6):261.
3. Puck, T. T., and Marcus, P. I. (1956): Action of X-rays on mammalian cells. *J. Exp. Med.*, 103:653.
4. Sinclair, W. K. (1968): Cyclic X-ray response to mammalian cells in vitro. *Radiat. Res.*, 33:620–643.
5. Sinclair, W. K. (1964): X-ray induced heritable damage (small colony formation) in cultured mammalian cells. *Radiat. Res.*, 21:584.
6. Terasima, T., and Tolmach, L. J. (1963): Variations in several responses of HeLa cells to x-irradiation during the division cycle. *Biophys. J.*, 3:11.
7. Thomlinson, R. H., and Gray, L. H. (1955) The histological structure of some human lung cancers and possible implications for radiotherapy. *Br. J. Cancer*, 9:539.
8. Thompson, L. H., and Suit, H. D. (1969): Proliferation kinetics of x-irradiation mouse L cells studies with time-lapse photography. *Int. J. Rad. Biol.*, 15:347–363.
9. Withers, H. R., and Peters, L. J. (1980): Basic clinical parameters. In: *Textbook of Radiotherapy*, edited by G. H. Fletcher, pp. 180–218. Lea & Febiger, Philadelphia.

Thoracic Oncology, edited by N. C. Choi and
H. C. Grillo. Raven Press, New York © 1983.

Radiological Studies of Thoracic Neoplasms

Reginald Greene

Department of Radiology, Harvard Medical School, Boston, Massachusetts 02114

Diagnostic radiology contributes to the detection, diagnosis, staging, treatment planning, and follow-up of malignant lung neoplasms. Some new radiologic techniques, such as computerized tomography, have had a major impact on pre- and post-treatment evaluation. This chapter summarizes basic aspects of the use of modern radiologic technology in the management of primary malignant thoracic neoplasms.

Detection of lung cancer involves two distinct groups of patients: asymptomatic individuals with tumors discovered by screening studies, and patients with tumor-related symptoms. An almost certain presumptive diagnosis of malignancy can frequently be made from radiologic images alone, but proof of diagnosis is usually required before a treatment program can be undertaken. The necessary cytologic or histologic proof of diagnosis can be provided by a number of different techniques, including radiologic percutaneous needle biopsy under fluoroscopic or computerized tomographic control. Radiologic studies are essential to establish the extent of tumor spread and to help indicate the most appropriate next step in patient management. Periodic radiologic examinations are also standard components of treatment planning and post-treatment follow-up. The contributions of radiologic studies to each step of the evaluation of patients with primary malignant thoracic neoplasms will be discussed in this chapter.

DETECTION OF LUNG CANCER

Radiologic characteristics of lung cancers at the time of initial detection depend on the presence or absence of symptoms, the histologic type of the tumor, and the location and extent of the tumor. Radiographic abnormalities on presentation can be caused by the primary tumor itself, secondary effects on non-tumor-invaded structures, regional tumor spread, and distant metastases. Clinicians must become familiar with the most common clinical and/or radiological presentation of lung cancer as well as occasionally bizarre initial manifestations.

Screening

The vast majority of lung cancers are detected because of tumor-related symptoms. However, experienced clinicians have long been aware, from reviewing old chest radiographs of newly discovered neoplasms, that quiescent lung cancers are often present for many years before symptoms develop (1). The small but significant number of "silent" lung cancers (probably less than 10% of the total) that can be discovered by incidental or "routine" radiographic studies is important because it is believed that the chance for cure diminishes if treatment is delayed until symptoms appear (2). However, screening programs for silent lung cancers have produced such disappointing results thus far that the American Cancer Society believes the yield does not justify the cost and radiation exposure (3–5).

Several important issues need to be examined before one can establish the utility of lung cancer screening programs. Is chest radiography sensitive enough to detect lung cancers before they cause symptoms? Is the time interval between initial radiographic detectability and the onset of symptoms long enough to make radiographic screening practicable? How often should screening be performed? How should subjects be selected for screening? How effective is radiographic screening compared to other procedures, e.g., sputum cytology? Finally, does treatment of cancers discovered through radiographic screening actually improve survival or does it only discover cancers earlier in their unaltered natural history?

Some insight into the potential utility of screening high risk groups with combined sputum and radiographic examinations is provided by data from the Mayo Lung Project (6). Males, 45 years old or older, who smoked 20 or more cigarettes per day participated in a program of annual or every fourth month (hereafter "fourth-month") chest X-rays and sputum examinations. In a study group, the lung cancer prevalence rate of these 10,000 men was about 9 in 1,000 on the initial chest radiographic study. Sixty-one percent of the cancers were detected by radiography only and 19% were detected only with sputum cytology. Radiography was three times more sensitive than cytology in detecting prevalence cancers. As one would expect, radiography primarily detected peripheral tumors, particularly adenocarcinoma and large cell undifferentiated carcinoma, whereas cytology primarily detected central epidermoid carcinoma. The radiographic indicators of lung cancer were as follows: peripheral nodule (54%), central or perihilar density (39%), and pneumonitis (7%). More than one-half of prevalence cancers qualified for curative-type surgical resection. Based on clinical staging data, the 5-year survival that could be expected from surgical resection of prevalence cancers was 60% for radiographically detected tumors and 93% for the cancers detected by sputum cytology.

The yield of "incidence" lung cancers, i.e., cancers that are found with periodic screening after elimination of the "prevalence" cancers detected with the initial screen was 5 cancers per 1,000 man years with fourth-month surveillance. Small cell carcinomas tended to be much more common among the incidence than prevalence cancers. Ninety percent of the cancers detected in the annual screening group were not discovered by the screening studies but by symptoms that developed between examinations. In contrast with the experience of the annual screening group, only 13% of cancers in the fourth-month screening group were not discovered by the screening studies themselves. Lung cancers were much more often stage 1 if they were detected in the fourth month than in the annual program (60% vs. 25%). The fourth-month radiographic and sputum surveillance program might ultimately prove to be of benefit to high lung cancer risk groups. However, the relatively high proportion of small cell carcinomas in high lung cancer risk populations may negate much of the potential benefit of screening (7).

Tumor Histology

The four major histologic types of lung cancer that account for more than 90% of lung cancers (epidermoid carcinoma, adenocarcinoma, small cell undifferentiated, and large cell undifferentiated carcinoma) have diverse but more or less characteristic radiologic appearances on presentation (Table 1) (8–12). Other types of malignant lung neoplasms are also important, and tend to have specific radiologic characteristics, including, for example, bronchoalveolar cell carcinoma, giant cell carcinoma, and carcinoid tumors (13).

Epidermoid carcinoma, which accounts for nearly one-half of all lung cancers, usually originates in the central surface epithelium of the bronchial tree. The tumor, therefore, tends to present relatively early, with symptoms caused by bronchial obstruction or erosion, e.g., cough, hemoptysis, and pneumonia. The common radiological presentations are pneumonia, atelectasis and hilar enlargement (Fig. 1). Only one-quarter of epidermoid carcinomas arise in the lung periphery, and 10% undergo cavitation (Fig. 2).

Adenocarcinoma, which characteristically presents as a nodule or mass in the lung periphery, tends to remain clinically quiescent until regional spread or metastases occur. Adenocarcinoma nodules may be uniformly solid or contain central inhomogeneities that simulate cavitation (Fig. 3). A slowly growing peripheral tumor nodules is the type of lung cancer that is best suited to detection by radiographic screening. Only 25% of adenocarcinomas originate in the central bronchial tree. Adenocarcinoma does not appear to be statistically related to smoking, but the relative incidence of this type of lung cancer appears to be rising. Expected survival after resection is similar to that for epidermoid carcinoma if the tumor is localized, but is much worse if there is evidence of regional spread.

TABLE 1. *Frequency of radiographic presenting signs (%)[a]*

	All types of lung cancer	Epidermoid	Adeno-carcinoma	Large cell undifferentiated	Small cell undifferentiated
Peripheral opacity	49	31	74	65	32
Atelectasis	21	37	10	13	18
Consolidation	21	20	15	25	24
Hilar enlargement	42	40	18	32	78
Mediastinal enlargement	6	2	3	10	13
Multiple abnormalities	42	36	30	42	62

[a]Data adapted from Byrd et al. (1968): *Mayo Clinic Proc.*, 43:327. Byrd et al. (1968): *Mayo Clinic Proc.*, 43:337. Lehar et al. (1967): *Am. Rev. Resp. Dis.*, 96:245. Byrd et al. (1968): *Mayo Clinic Proc.*, 43:333.

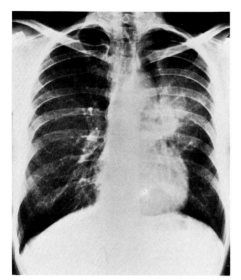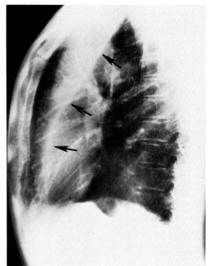

FIG. 1. The left hilar mass *(left)* and left upper lobe atelectasis *(right, arrows)* are typical findings of central endobronchial epidermoid carcinoma.

Small cell undifferentiated or *oat cell carcinoma* is the third most common and most malignant variety of primary lung cancer. Constitutional symptoms and/or signs of distant metastases are usually present when the tumor is first detected. Screening studies for this type of malignancy are ineffective because the tumor grows so rapidly that symptoms usually develop in the interval between the last negative radiographic screening study and the next one, even when screening is carried out at very short intervals. The tumor tends to originate in the central bronchial tree. Marked mediastinal lymph node enlargement and multiple abnormalities including atelectasis, consolidation, and pleural effusion are characteristic radiologic abnormalities at the time of detection (Figs. 4 and 5). *Large cell undifferentiated carcinoma* is very similar to adenocarcinoma in its histologic ultrastructure, survival statistics, and radiological manifestations.

Bronchoalveolar cell carcinoma is considered a variant of adenocarcinoma and shares some of its characteristics. The tumor tends to occur in the lung periphery, especially in the vicinity of scars (14). The radiographic presentation is varied and includes the solitary peripheral pulmonary nodule (indistinguishable from adenocarcinoma), lobar lung consolidation (indistinguishable from pneumonia), and diffuse miliary nodules (indistinguishable from miliary tuberculosis or metastatic thyroid carcinoma) (Figs. 6 and 7).

Occasionally, all three of these radiographic forms are seen sequentially in the same patient. *Giant cell carcinoma* is a relatively rare and highly malignant variant of adenocarcinoma. The histology that defines this tumor consists of unusual, bizarre, cannibalizing giant cancer cells. The characteristic radiologic presentation of this tumor is a triad of a large lung mass, peripheral location, and involvement

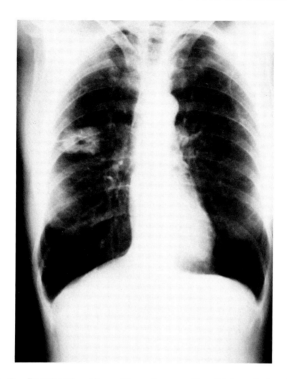

FIG. 2. Peripheral epidermoid carcinoma with a thick-walled cavity.

of the chest wall (15) (Fig. 8). Patient survival after detection is similar to that for small cell undifferentiated carcinoma. *Bronchial carcinoid* is a slow-growing low-grade malignancy of the glandular bronchial epithelium that tends to occur in the central bronchial tree. Clinical presentation is usually related to bronchial obstruction or surface erosion causing hemoptysis, pneumonia, or atelectasis (Fig. 9). Tumor-related symptoms are often present for many years prior to diagnosis of this slowly growing neoplasm. At the time of detection, these patients are on average 10 years younger than patients with other lung cancers. Regional metastases to hilar lymph nodes are not uncommon, but distant metastases and the carcinoid syndrome are rare. Presenting radiologic signs include atelectasis, consolidation, bronchiectasis, and hilar mass (16) (Fig. 10). Fewer than 10% of carcinoids occur in the lung periphery. Atypical carcinoids may secrete ACTH.

Tumor-Related Symptoms that Initiate Radiologic Studies

The vast majority of lung cancers are discovered by studies that are ordered to workup tumor-related symptoms (17). Symptoms may be caused by local effects of the primary tumor, secondary (nonmalignant) effects of the primary tumor, regional spread, distant metastases, or paramalignant syndromes. The most common presenting chest symptoms related to the primary tumor and its secondary (non-

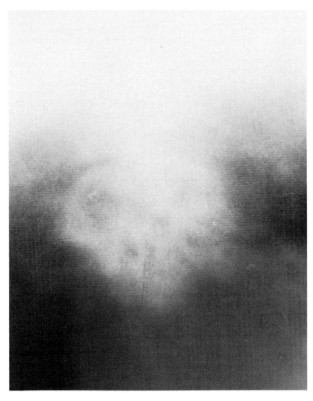

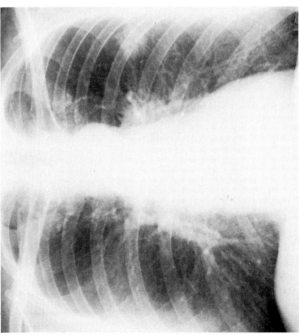

FIG. 3. Peripheral lung opacity characteristic of peripheral adenocarcinoma *(left panel)*. Central lucency of scar emphysema within the tumor simulates cavitation *(right panel)*.

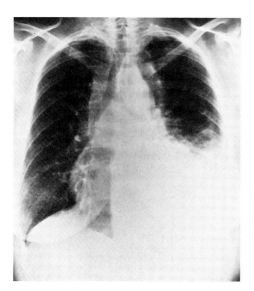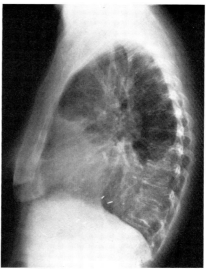

FIG. 4. Multiple abnormalities on the initial examination of patient with small cell undifferentiated carcinoma. Note a left pleural effusion, enlargement of the heart silhouette secondary to pericardial effusion, and massive adenopathy in superior mediastinum and subcarinal regions *(arrows).*

malignant) effects include cough (75%), hemoptysis (50%), chest pain (18%), shortness of breath, wheezing, and stridor. Regional metastases to the mediastinum are responsible for hoarseness, dysphagia, superior vena cava obstruction, and Horner's syndrome. Up to one-fourth of patients with lung cancer present with symptoms and signs that indicate extrathoracic metastatic disease, especially to bone and brain (19). Paramalignant syndromes cause systemic symptoms and signs not related to metastases. These include endocrine-metabolic disorders such as hypertrophic pulmonary osteoarthropathy, hypercalcemia, Cushing's syndrome, inappropriate antidiuretic hormone, gynecomastia, hyperthyroidism, and various neuromyopathies (including the myasthenia gravis-like Eaton–Lambert syndrome) (20). Presenting symptoms and signs are important clues to the most appropriate radiographic studies that should be undertaken.

Radiologically Occult Lung Carcinomas

Intensive sputum cytology screening of high risk patients has detected a number of radiologically occult carcinomas (21). The Mayo Clinic Lung Project, for instance, found 15 cases of occult lung cancer over a 15 month period. Although prompt excision of radiographically occult carcinoma promises prolonged survival, the high incidence of multiple carcinomas in this group (as high as 20%) is cause for pessimism (21–23). Radiographically occult carcinomas usually arise in the proximal bronchial tree and tend to be best localized with bronchoscopy. Truly

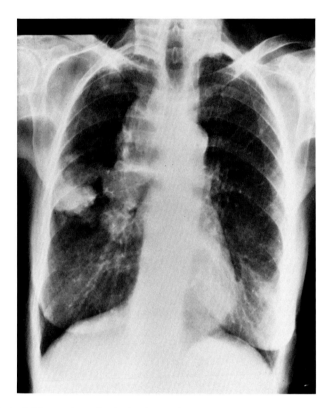

FIG. 5. Marked hilar and mediastinal adenopathy on presentation of peripheral small cell undifferentiated carcinoma. Only 10% of small cell tumors present with a peripheral lung mass.

occult carcinomas are very uncommon and are to be differentiated from tumors that are "occult" only because of inadequate radiologic examination or observer error (Fig. 11).

Peripheral Lung Opacities

One-third of all lung cancers present as peripheral lung opacities, especially in the upper lobes. Adenocarcinoma and large cell undifferentiated carcinoma characteristically present in this way. The edge and density characteristics of benign and malignant peripheral opacities vary greatly. Some cancers have sharply defined margins and others have lobulated or irregularly striated edges. Rounded contours are frequently flattened when tumors abut against pleural fissures. Some peripheral lung cancers, especially bronchoalveolar cell carcinomas, have indistinct margins more suggestive of consolidation than tumor. When cancers have central lucencies suggestive of air bronchograms, the appearance may closely simulate consolidation. Most truly cavitated carcinomas are of the epidermoid type. Peripheral lung cancers may have the appearance of lung cysts when they occur adjacent to preexisting

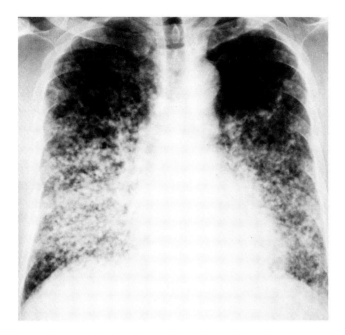

FIG. 6. Diffuse miliary nodules in advanced bronchoalveolar cell carcinoma simulating advanced miliary tuberculosis and metastases to lungs.

cysts and bullae and when the tumor undergoes cavitation and scarring (24). Some cancers closely simulate pleural abnormalities and therefore present great difficulty in differential diagnosis (Fig. 12).

Peripheral nodules that are less than 1 cm in diameter often go undetected on conventional chest radiographs because the tumor density causes too little contrast to be detected with film. Computerized tomography and other new digital techniques significantly increase the ability to detect the density of small cancer nodules.

About one-half of newly detected noncalcified solitary pulmonary nodules are primary pulmonary malignancies. Although all newly discovered noncalcified lung nodules are highly suspicious for lung cancer, a definite diagnosis cannot usually be made on the radiological characteristics alone. Both benign or malignant pulmonary opacities can have smooth or irregular outlines, be solid or cavitated and have stellate extensions or satellite densities. Both benign and malignant nodules may be very large or very small. However, nodules less than 1 cm in diameter and easily visible on chest radiographs are likely to be diffusely calcified and therefore unlikely to be malignant. One-third of epidermoid and large cell undifferentiated carcinoma and two-thirds of adenocarcinomas and small cell undifferentiated carcinomas are less than 4 cm in diameter when first detected (11,12,25).

Only two radiographic characteristics dependably differentiate between benign and malignant pulmonary opacities: long-term size stability and calcification. Lesions that remain absolutely unchanged for 2 years or more are very unlikely to be

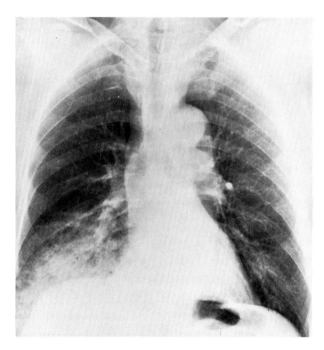

FIG. 7. Bronchoalveolar cell carcinoma of the right lower lobe causing consolidation, indistinguishable from pneumonia.

malignant. However, it should be understood that a small diameter increase indicates a much larger volume change. Small changes in film density can strongly influence apparent nodule size. Dark films decrease the radiographic size of nodules and light films do the opposite. Certain types of calcification indicate benignity (diffuse, popcorn-type or target calcification) (Fig. 13). Calcification in asymmetrical nodules is no assurance of benignity because scar cancers can occur adjacent to calcified granulomas. Low kilovoltage radiographs and computed tomography help to identify diffuse calcification, but in most cases careful inspection of the initial film will suggest calcification. In cases where there is significant doubt about the nature of a pulmonary nodule, percutaneous or open lung biopsy is warranted. All nodules that lack typical characteristics of benign lesions should be regarded as potential lung carcinomas.

Atelectasis and Consolidation

Atelectasis and/or consolidation are the initial manifestations of almost one-half of lung cancers, especially central, endobronchial epidermoid carcinoma. Consolidation distal to central carcinomas may be due to direct tumor spread or noncancerous pneumonia distal to bronchial obstruction. Atelectasis and/or consolidation are common manifestations of both lung cancer and simple pneumonia. All consolidations and atelectasis thought to be noncancer-related pneumonias should be

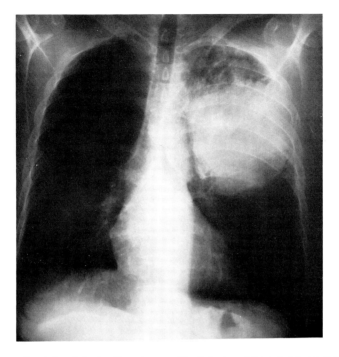

FIG. 8. Largest peripheral giant cell carcinoma of the left upper lobe extending into the pleura.

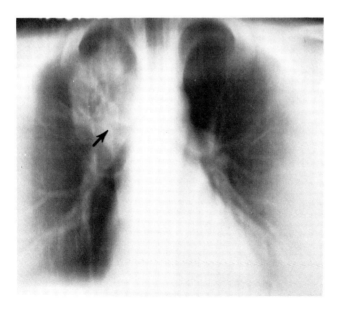

FIG. 9. Right upper lobe consolidation secondary to bronchial obstruction by carcinoid tumor *(arrow).*

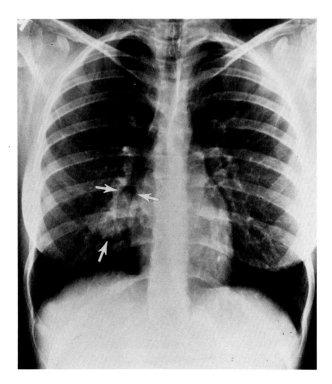

FIG. 10. Right hilar mass secondary to carcinoid tumor occluding the lower lobe bronchus *(arrows)*. Collateral ventilation maintains aeration of the lower lobe distal to the occlusion.

followed to complete clearing. If a suspected pneumonia does not clear appropriately, additional studies to examine the bronchial tree should be undertaken, including high penetration grid films, fluoroscopic spot films, tomography, computerized tomography, bronchography or bronchoscopy. Sequelae of total or partial bronchial obstruction by tumor include mucus plugging, bronchiectasis and lung abscess. Incomplete bronchial obstruction can cause decreased or delayed ventilation, or air-trapping. Total bronchial obstruction may not cause atelectasis when collateral ventilation from other lung segments is adequate to maintain lung volume. Local ventilation disturbances are best evaluated by dynamic studies, such as fluoroscopy, expiration radiography or ventilation/perfusion radionuclide scanning.

Mediastinal and Hilar Enlargement

Almost one-half of lung cancers have evidence of mediastinal or hilar enlargement on presentation (9–12) (Table 1). The proportion is much higher in small cell undifferentiated carcinomas. Hilar enlargement can be simulated by enlarged pulmonary arteries and by lung masses that overlie the hila. Hilar enlargement is manifested by abnormal soft tissue lobulations superimposed on the hilar vessels. Multiple radiographic views, tomography, and computerized tomography with con-

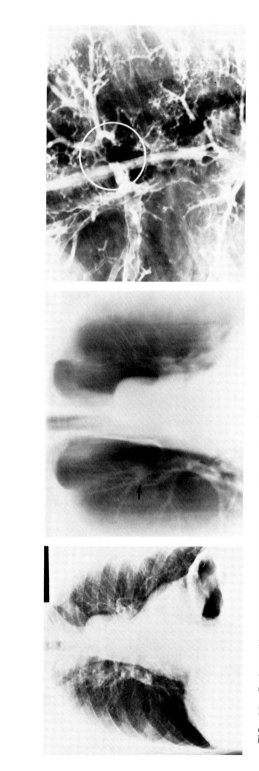

FIG. 11. Patient with a new cough and right upper lobe epidermoid carcinoma was originally thought to have a negative chest radiograph *(left panel)*. However, a right suprahilar mass was confirmed by tomography *(center panel)*. A subsequent lateral bronchogram demonstrated an endobronchial mass at the origin of the posterior segmental bronchus *(right panel)*.

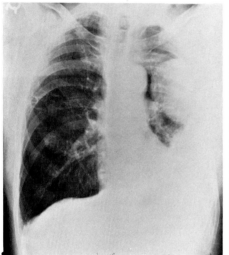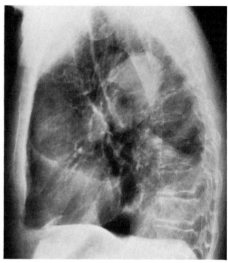

FIG. 12. Undifferentiated carcinoma of the lung with a radiographic presentation simulating empyema.

trast help to document hilar lymph node enlargement. Patients that have mediastinal enlargement on presentation usually have undifferentiated tumors. Mediastinal enlargement frequently goes undetected on frontal and lateral radiographs until it becomes large enough to encroach on the lung fields. In this respect, computerized tomography is much more sensitive in detecting mediastinal enlargement because it can detect masses within the mediastinum before they encroach on the lung fields. In some areas, especially in subcarinal and paraesophageal locations, mediastinal metastases are better detected with simple barium swallow fluoroscopic spot films than with computerized tomography. Paratracheal lymphadenopathy is often visible on plain radiography or conventional tomography. However, computerized tomography is better able to detect small retrocaval, paratracheal and prevascular lymph nodes that do not project into the lung fields. Subaortic lymph node enlargement, especially when it is suspected in patients with newly developed hoarseness, can be corroborated with plain radiography as well as conventional computerized tomography (Fig. 14). Direct tumor extension into the mediastinum is as important as lymph node metastases in determining appropriate management.

Other Radiological Findings

Pleural abnormalities are present in about 10% of initial lung cancer studies. Small pleural effusions are occasionally detectable in patients with primary lung carcinomas but their significance is not certain. Pleural effusion usually, but not always, indicates pleural spread or unresectable tumor (26–28). According to the TNM staging system, pleural effusion, whether malignant effusion or not, places the tumor in an unfavorable survival category. All patients with lung cancer and

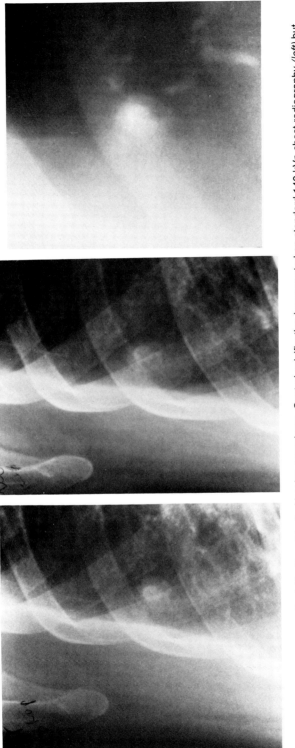

FIG. 13. Dense central calcification of typical benign granuloma. Central calcification is suspected on standard 140 kVp chest radiography *(left)* but better shown with 80 kVp radiographs *(center)* and 80 kVp tomography *(right)*.

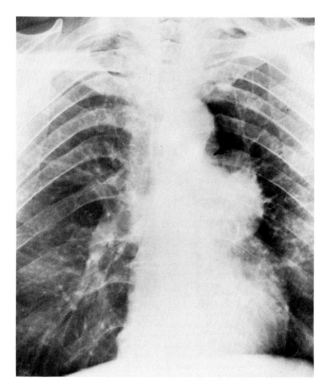

FIG. 14. Enlargement of aorticopulmonary (Botallo) lymph node *(arrow)* and left hilus in patient with newly acquired hoarseness and cough. These findings suggest carcinoma of the left upper lobe with mediastinal metastasis causing vocal cord palsy.

pleural effusions should be carefully studied for evidence of regional spread, subpleural thickening, and lymphatic permeation adjacent to the tumor mass. Decubitus radiography, fluoroscopic spot films, and computerized tomography are all sensitive methods of detecting pleural effusions. Pneumothorax is a rare presenting sign of lung cancer (29,30).

Chest wall invasion by lung cancer usually occurs with undifferentiated peripheral cancers. Patients who present with chest pain should be carefully examined for rib cage involvement with detailed radiographs, tomography, and/or radionuclide imaging. The most distinctive type of chest wall involvement occurs with superior sulcus (or Pancoast) syndrome (Fig. 15). These tumors cause brachial plexus and sympathetic disturbances.

STAGING OF TUMOR EXTENT

The role of radiology in lung cancer management does not end with the detection or diagnosis of lung cancer. In many respects, the most important contributions of radiology follow the detection of the tumor. Radiologic assessment is an integral part of the TNM staging system that has been adopted by the American Joint Committee for Lung Cancer Staging and End-Results Reporting (28). This clas-

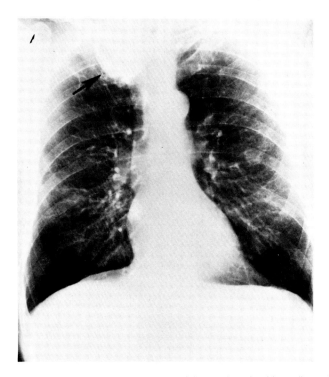

FIG. 15.   Epidermoid (Pancoast) carcinoma *(arrow)* detected on shoulder radiographs obtained for severe, unremitting shoulder pain.

sification helps to predict outcome and select the most appropriate mode of treatment. Survival after treatment depends not only on tumor histology but also on the location, size, and extent of the primary tumor (T), the presence and location of lymph node metastases (N), and the presence of distant metastases (M). Small cell undifferentiated carcinoma is the only cancer cell type in which survival is not dependent on clinical staging. Almost all small cell carcinomas behave as if they are widespread on discovery. Clinical TNM staging is carried out prior to specific treatment and includes all aspects of the patient's history, physical examination, and laboratory as well as radiographic assessment. Surgical staging includes all of the above, plus information based on surgical observations and procedures. Post-surgical staging includes information obtained after complete examination of the resected specimen.

An orderly radiologic staging program must be tailored to the specific circumstances of each patient. No uniform protocol is appropriate for every patient. However there are certain guidelines to follow. The best method of carrying out radiologic staging is to follow a series of directed questions pertaining to primary tumor extent (T), regional metastases (N), and widespread dissemination (N).

The following questions that pertain to the primary tumor itself (T) are directed at determining whether lung cancer is likely to be present. (i) How long has the lesion been present? (ii) Has it increased in size? (iii) Is the lesion an artifact such as a button density, skin mole, nipple or hair braid? (iv) Is the lesion intrathoracic but extrapulmonary, such as a benign rib bone island, pleural plaque, or traumatic extrapleural hematoma related to rib fracture?

These questions are best answered by reviewing all previous radiographs. Reading radiographic reports is no substitute for reviewing the actual studies themselves. A careful review of multiple view radiographs, tomography or fluoroscopy, usually clarifies the situation.

The next series of questions is directed at determining the exact location number and extent of the lung lesion. (i) What is the lobar or bronchopulmonary segmental location of a pulmonary lesion? (ii) Is the lesion solitary? (iii) Is the tumor in the mediastinum or does it arise from the lung and lie in a juxtamediastinal position? (iv) Does the lesion extend from the lung into the mediastinum or vice versa? (v) What are the morphologic characteristics of the lesion? Does the lesion contain benign calcification? Is the lesion surrounded by lung and contained within intact visceral pleura (T1)? (vi) What is the proximal extent of endobronchial lesions (T1 vs. T2 or T3). Does the lesion extend to within 1 cm of the lobar bronchus (T2) (Fig. 16) or within 1 cm of the carina (T3) (Fig. 17). (vii) Does the lung lesion extend into the chest wall or the mediastinum (T3)? Is there pleural effusion?

Extension of tumor into the mediastinum and chest may be inferred by clinical findings attributable to mediastinal nerve invasion or chest wall destruction. Doc-

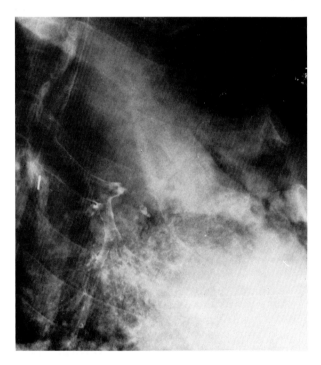

FIG. 16. Bronchography shows occlusion of the left upper lobe bronchus within 1 cm of its origin, which indicates T2 staging of this epidermoid carcinoma.

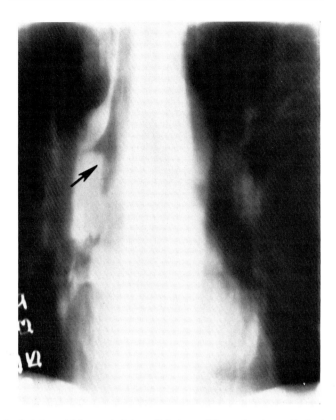

FIG. 17. An endobronchial mass bulging within 1 cm of the carina *(arrow)* indicates T3 staging of this adenocarcinoma.

umentation of recurrent laryngeal nerve or phrenic nerve palsy can be easily accomplished with fluoroscopic observation of the vocal cords and diaphragm. Conventional tomography and high penetration plain grid films can produce detailed studies of mediastinal and chest wall anatomy. Computerized tomography is especially useful in detecting both mediastinal invasion and adenopathy. Pulmonary arteriography or computerized tomography with contrast are the best methods of excluding direct vascular involvement by centrally located tumors. Carcinomas of the medial part of the right upper lobe may be unresectable because of involvement of the intrapericardiac portion of the anterior ramus of the right pulmonary artery (Fig. 18). Vascular indications of inoperability include occlusion of the superior vena cava, concentric narrowing of the left main pulmonary artery, complete or partial occlusion of the right pulmonary artery at or near its bifurcation, occlusion of the right ascending pulmonary artery branch in combination with any abnormality of the superior vena cava, occlusion of the pulmonary veins and vascular involvement in the contralateral lung (31). Ventilation/perfusion scanning has been useful primarily in assessing functional deficit prior to surgery, but the extent of tumor involvement of the thorax can also be estimated by this technique.

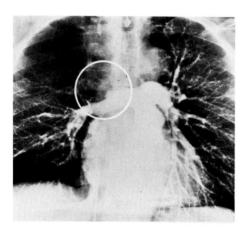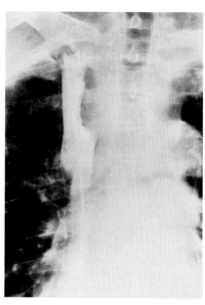

FIG. 18. Angiographic evidence of amputation of upper lobe pulmonary artery *(left)* in combination with deformity of superior vena cava *(right)* indicates inoperability of right upper lobe carcinoma.

The answers to questions relating to primary tumor extent (T) may require different radiological methods depending on the patient's presentation, available equipment, and the precise question being addressed. Often, very simple techniques provide very accurate answers; at other times, more complicated techniques are needed. In each case, there should be a review of all previous studies and an up-to-date study. The latter should include multiple radiographs with grid technique (posteroanterior, lateral, and both oblique views). Fluoroscopic observation of a suspect density can clarify whether it is pulmonary or extrapulmonary by observing characteristically different excursions during breathing. Conventional or computerized tomography are often indispensable in determining the precise location of tumors, in documenting that they are solitary, and in excluding invasion of vital structures. Proximal extent of endobronchial tumor can sometimes be inferred from dynamic studies. For instance, upper lobe atelectasis indicates a bronchial occlusion in or around the upper lobe bronchus. An additional finding of air trapping of the lower lobe implies that the tumor also extends into or partially obstructs the lower lobe bronchus as well (Fig. 19).

The next staging questions pertain to the presence of lymph node metastases. (i) Is there ipsilateral hilar (N1)? (ii) Is there contralateral hilar adenopathy (N2) adenopathy? (iii) Is there mediastinal (N2) adenopathy? (iv) Is the lymph node enlargement cancerous or reactive?

Radiologic evaluation of the hilar and mediastinal regions requires knowledge of the location of lymph node groups and careful attention to detail. Hilar lymph nodes surround the hilar bronchi, especially at bifurcations. The greatest difficulty in recognizing lymph node enlargement is differentiation from enlarged hilar vas-

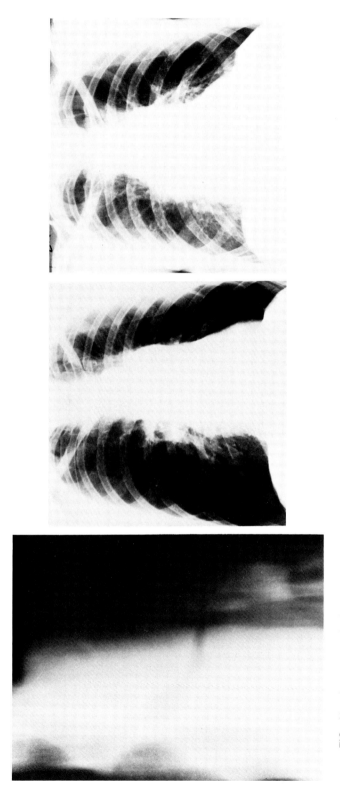

FIG. 19. A tomogram *(left)* of the left bronchus in patient with left upper atelectasis *(center)* shows an abnormal distal mainstem bronchus *(arrow)*. Expiration view shows air-trapping of left lower lobe and confirms partial occlusion of lower lobe bronchus in association with total occlusion of left upper lobe bronchus *(right)*.

culature. Hilar lymph node enlargement is usually indicated by added soft tissue lobulation around the hilar pulmonary artery outline or nonvascular soft tissue masses at bronchial bifurcations. Conventional plain films and tomography are well suited to detecting hilar lymph node enlargement (Fig. 20). Bilateral hilar enlargement implies involvement of the subcarinal group as well. Hilar lymph node enlargement does not necessarily indicate unresectability but it often indicates the need for pneumonectomy rather than lobectomy.

Tumor involvement of the mediastinum, however, is tantamount to inoperability. Subcarinal and paraesophageal adenopathy are most easily detected with barium swallow fluoroscopic spot films. Conventional and especially computerized tomography are sensitive methods of detecting paratracheal, periaortic, paravertebral, and prevascular lymphadenopathy. Detection of lymphadenopathy in the aortopulmonary window in patients with newly acquired hoarseness suggests the presence of mediastinal metastasis. The results of carefully performed radiological studies of the mediastinum correlate fairly well with those of mediastinoscopy (32,33). Detection of enlarged lymph nodes is not equivalent to diagnosing metastases because noncancerous node enlargement, such as from reactive lymphadenitis in nodes draining tumor-related consolidations frequently occurs. Biopsy proof or other strong clinical evidence is required before radiological lymph node enlargement can be equated with mediastinal metastasis.

The next question that deals with the presence of metastases usually involves nonthoracic radiologic studies and other clinical assessment: Is there evidence of distant metastatic disease (M1)?

Clinical studies play a central role in documenting metastases, but various radiological modalities, including radionuclide bone scanning, ultrasound abdominal

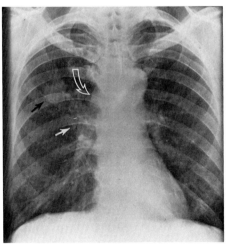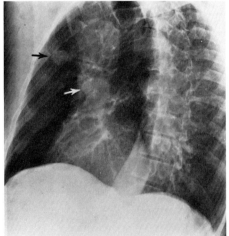

FIG. 20. Enlargement of a right hilar lymph node *(white arrows)* indicates N1 staging and enlargement of the azygos lymph node indicates N2 staging *(open arrow)* in this patient with right upper lobe epidermoid carcinoma *(black arrows)*.

studies, and computerized tomography of the abdomen and brain are also important. Radiologic tests are most likely to be fruitful when there are symptoms or signs to suggest an organ abnormality or when the primary tumor is undifferentiated or locally extensive. Gallium scanning for mediastinal metastases has been found to have a sensitivity of 89% and a specificity of 67% (34). However, gallium scanning is not widely advocated as a routine method of detecting mediastinal metastases (35). In general, there is little benefit to be derived from routine bone, liver, and brain scans in staging of lung cancer except in patients with clinical evidence of metastases (36–39). Computerized tomographic examination of the upper abdomen for liver and adrenal metastases has produced promising results in nonoat cell carcinomas (40,41). However, routine computerized tomography of the brain has proven to be of limited value in documenting metastases of small cell carcinoma. Computerized tomography of the upper abdomen appears to be useful in finding metastases in oat cell carcinoma (42,43).

COMPUTERIZED TOMOGRAPHY AND OTHER TECHNIQUES IN LUNG CANCER STAGING

No advance in radiologic technology since the discovery of the X-ray itself has had a greater impact on the diagnosis and staging of lung cancer than computerized tomography (CT). The technique cannot be matched for its ability to characterize lung lesions, detect occult lesions, detect and characterize mediastinal abnormalities, and assess the lung and mediastinum deep to overlying pleural abnormalities (44).

In the detection and evaluation of peripheral pulmonary lesions, CT has made unique contributions. The powerful contrast resolution and transverse section perspective of the technique give it a superior ability to detect small pulmonary nodules (45,46) (Fig. 21). Lesions posterior to the heart, in the posterior recesses of the lung and subpleural locations are better shown with CT than any other method (47,48). Before the general availability of CT, full chest tomography was the best method of excluding the presence of second or third lesions in patients with presumed primary lung cancers. Conventional full chest tomography has been shown to be 1.5 times as sensitive as plain radiography in detecting additional lesions (49–52). CT has also proven to be about 1.5 times as sensitive as conventional tomography in detecting small pulmonary lesions (47). However, the specificity of additional findings detected by CT appears to be low. Twenty-four to 60% of the added findings with CT in assessing pulmonary metastases have been found to be false positives, e.g., benign granulomas (47). Additional lesions detected by CT tend to be smaller than those detected by conventional tomography. CT can detect 78% of all nodules over 3 mm in diameter (47).

Increased contrast resolution not only helps CT to be more sensitive in detecting small peripheral nodules, it also helps to differentiate calcified benign granulomas from malignant deposits. Calcification of pulmonary nodules that cannot be demonstrated by conventional means can be identified by quantitative determination of CT density (53) (Fig. 22). However, many workers have not found CT assessment

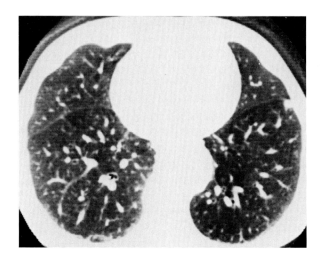

FIG. 21. A subpleural metastatic nodule 4 mm in diameter is well shown by CT *(arrows)* but was not detected with standard studies. Because of powerful contrast resolution, CT is the most sensitive method of detecting small peripheral tumor nodules.

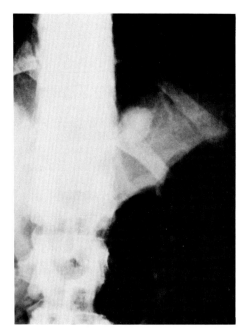

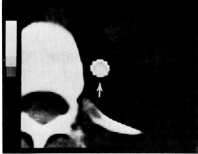

FIG. 22. Granulomatous calcification, suspected on plain radiography *(left)*, is definitely determined by quantitative CT measurements in this benign lesion.

of density to be a great value in differentiating benign from malignant lesions (54). Many radiologists find that CT characterization of lung nodule density is subject to significant machine error and inconsistency. Others find that most nodules shown to be calcified by CT were suspected of calcification on previous conventional studies (55,56). Nodules that are suspected of calcification with standard high kilovoltage radiography can be shown to be calcified by simply obtaining low kilovoltage plain radiography or tomography. If the presence of calcification is still in doubt, thin-section CT may prove useful in confirming the presence of calcification. The safety of assessing nodule density with CT rests on the fact that errors tend to lower the apparent density of benign calcified lesions rather than increase the apparent density of malignancies.

CT has had an even more spectacular impact on the mediastinum than on the lung. A growing number of studies show that CT is superior to both conventional plain film and tomographic methods in evaluating the mediastinum for invasion and metastases (32,33,57–59).

The sensitivity of CT is much higher (90%) than conventional tomography (33%) in the detection of mediastinal lymph node metastases (33). Some studies document a high degree of specificity (94%) and sensitivity (88 to 89%) in identifying mediastinal lymph node metastases (32,33,60). However, other studies have found a considerably lower specificity (62%) to mediastinal findings in lung cancer staging (57). The latter study indicates the need to corroborate CT evidence of lymph node enlargement with independent proof of cancer involvement. However, it can now be concluded that CT is a clearly more sensitive staging modality than conventional radiography (Fig. 23). Resectability can be correctly predicted in 93% of cases, i.e., no mediastinal lymph nodes detected greater than 1 cm in diameter (58). Nonresectability for cure can be predicted in 100% of cases, i.e., demonstration of direct tumor extension into mediastinum or detection of mediastinal lymph nodes greater than 2 cm in diameter (58). In 35% of cases with inconclusive findings, i.e., detection of mediastinal lymph nodes of 1–2 cm in diameter and no definitive evidence of mediastinal or chest wall invasion, the resectability rate was about 50%

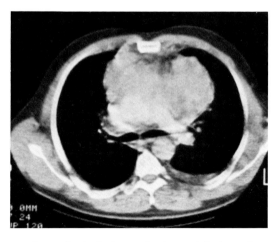

FIG. 23. Massive anterior mediastinal adenopathy *(arrows)* displaces the tracheal carina posteriorly in a patient with small cell undifferentiated carcinoma. Loss of sharply defined tissue planes around the pericardium indicates that pericardial invasion was likely.

(58). CT can detect about 95% of carcinomatous mediastinal lymph nodes as compared to 60% by plain chest radiographs with oblique views (61).

The superiority of CT over conventional methods in evaluation of hilar lymph nodes is not so certain (32,62–64). Plain radiography is more sensitive in detecting right than left hilar lymphadenopathy (Fig. 24). Both plain radiography and CT have been reported to have a sensitivity of about 60% (32). However, some reports suggest that CT is superior to standard radiography of the hila (65). Welsh et al. found that cancerous hilar lymph node chest radiographs were positive in 53%, whereas CT was positive in 83% (65).

False negative CT studies of the mediastinum tend to occur in the subcarinal, periesophageal, and inferior pulmonary ligament regions. Barium esophagrams under fluoroscopy are therefore valuable supplements to CT staging of the periesophageal mediastinum.

TRANSTHORACIC NEEDLE ASPIRATION BIOPSY IN CANCER DIAGNOSIS

Percutaneous needle aspiration biopsy of the lung occupies a preeminent position in the nonsurgical diagnosis of small peripheral pulmonary lesions. The technique is safe and produces a high diagnostic yield in lung cancer. Positive diagnoses are obtained in 90 to 95% of lung cancers with near zero risk of fatality or tumor implantation (66). The false negative rate varies from 5 to 20%. The major value of needle aspiration biopsy is in the diagnosis of new peripheral pulmonary lesions or lesions of unknown growth history. These lesions are difficult to diagnose by techniques other than open thoracotomy. Percutaneous biopsy is especially well suited to evaluating patients who are not in good medical condition for diagnostic thoracotomy, patients who have presumably incurable cancers, and patients in good general health with lesions that are unlikely to require therapeutic resection. Transthoracic needle aspiration biopsy has added a degree of certainty in the evaluation

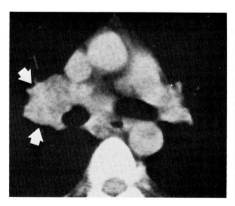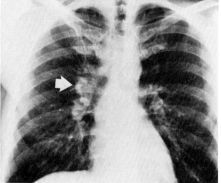

FIG. 24. A tomogram *(left)* and plain radiograph *(right)* both show right hilar enlargement in patient with right upper lobe carcinoma *(arrows)*.

of the pulmonary nodule that was previously absent. It has reduced the number of patients who have to be managed with ill-advised "wait and see" programs, on the one hand and ill-advised precipitous thoracotomy on the other (Fig. 25). New technical advances of the fine needle aspiration biopsy method now can provide intact histological samples as well as cytologic material for diagnosis (Fig. 26). This important advance has helped to improve the accuracy of cancer cell type designation and to identify specific benign conditions in cancer-negative biopsies (67).

Contraindications of percutaneous biopsy include inadequate radiologic localization, abnormal bleeding factors, pulmonary microvascular hypertension, severe pulmonary functional insufficiency, and suspected echinococcus cyst or thoracic extension of liver or kidney and vascular lesions. Local bullous disease is not a categorical contraindication of percutaneous biopsy.

The primary clinical applications of transthoracic needle aspiration biopsy include: (i) evaluation of undiagnosed lung lesions in patients for whom the hazard of diagnostic thoracotomy is higher than normal (Fig. 27); (ii) evaluation of lesions that are not likely to require resection or treatment, such as pneumonia; (iii) evaluation of patients who are very likely to have an inoperable or metastatic carcinoma in the lung; (iv) evaluation of multiple pulmonary nodules with or without a past history of cancer; (v) evaluation of two or more undiagnosed lung lesions in different lungs or lobes; (vi) evaluation of lung lesions that are likely to require pneumonectomy for resection.

The most suitable radiographic targets for needle aspiration biopsy include: small peripheral lesions, lesions with asymmetrical calcifications, large pulmonary masses, cavitated lesions, superior sulcus lesions, and chest wall lesions. Mediastinal lesions, pleural lesions, and diffuse lung abnormalities are less suitable candidates for percutaneous biopsy. Mediastinal masses can be successfully biopsied, particularly under CT control. Mediastinal biopsy can be useful in diagnosing mediastinal cysts and metastases. However, mediastinal lymphomas, thymomas and teratomas are less suitable targets for percutaneous biopsy because surgical excision assures more accurate histologic diagnosis. Except for metastatic implants, pleural lesions are not particularly suitable to percutaneous biopsy because radiologic localization and histologic characteristics are often too complex for the technique. It is most difficult to establish a diagnosis of malignant mesothelioma with transthoracic percutaneous needle aspiration biopsy. Diffuse lung diseases are best diagnosed by transbronchial or open lung biopsy, but transthoracic needle biopsy is occasionally useful in diagnosis.

Fatal complications from percutaneous needle aspiration biopsy are extremely rare. It has been estimated that the mortality rate is considerably less than 0.02% (66). Pneumothorax, by far the most common complication of needle aspiration biopsy, is easily managed. The post-needle biopsy incidence of pneumothorax is about 20% when a fine needle is used. One quarter of patients who develop pneumothoraces ultimately require thoracotomy tube drainage. Hemoptysis and local hemorrhage after needle biopsy (2% incidence) are usually transient and mild. There

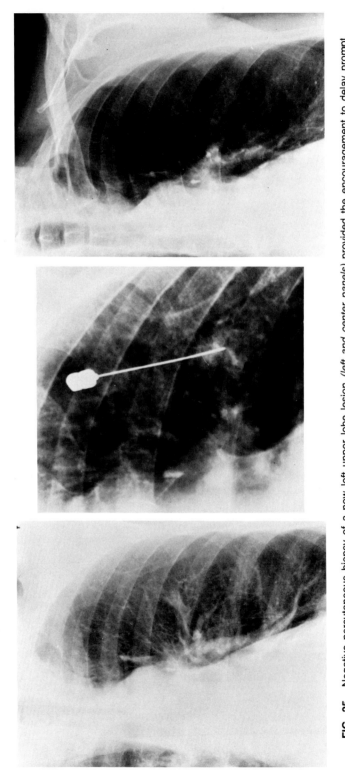

FIG. 25. Negative percutaneous biopsy of a new left upper lobe lesion *(left and center panels)* provided the encouragement to delay prompt thoracotomy in a frail elderly man. Followup radiography 6 months later showed complete clearing of a presumed pneumonitis *(right panel)*.

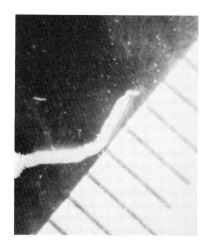

FIG. 26.   A ½-cm-long tissue core suitable for histology obtained by percutaneous aspiration with a modified 23 gauge needle.

are rare reports of air embolism and tumor cell implantation after percutaneous biopsy.

In almost 1000 biopsies at the Massachusetts General Hospital with 22 or 23 gauge fine needle, the false positive rate is less than 1%, false negative rate is 10 to 15%, and the specific benign diagnosis rate in negative biopsies is 10 to 20% (66). The diagnostic yield of transthoracic needle biopsy greatly depends on careful attention to detail and accurate radiologic localization of pulmonary targets.

RADIOLOGY FOLLOW-UP OF THE TREATED
LUNG CANCER PATIENT

The major clinical problems encountered after treatment of lung cancer are persistent or recurrent tumor; regional lymph node metastases; disseminated tumor; complications of treatment; and intercurrent disease. Radiologic studies play an important role in the diagnosis of each of these problems.

Persistent or Recurrent Tumor

Recurrent disease at the bronchial stump after lung resection is often heralded by hemoptysis and can generally be seen bronchoscopically or demonstrated with well-penetrated grid radiographs. Hemoptysis after treatment for lung carcinoma requires complete clinical evaluation of upper food and air passages and the lung because multiple primary carcinomas are common. Recurrence of the primary tumor often presages tumor dissemination.

Careful review of pretreatment studies is needed if tumor response to treatment is to be accurately assessed and if recurrence and complications are to be recognized. Undifferentiated small cell tumors frequently show a rapid lymphoma-like response to irradiation or chemotherapy. Atelectasis distal to a cancer occluded bronchi can clear rapidly after irradiation. Local recurrence of undifferentiated tumors is com-

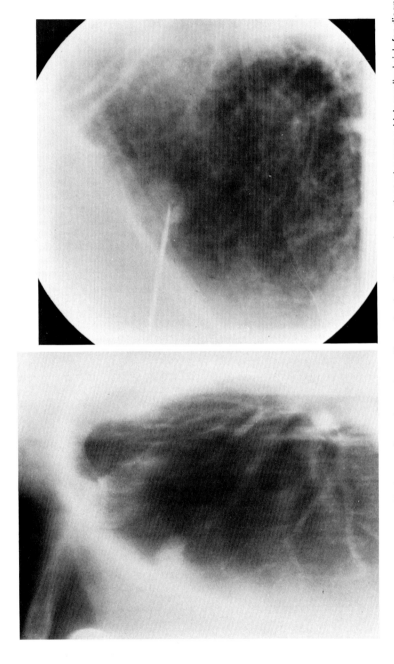

FIG. 27. Percutaneous biopsy provided a certain prethoracotomy diagnosis of malignancy in a patient who was a high medical risk for diagnostic thoracotomy.

mon. Separation of metal clips at the surgical site occasionally aids in the detection of tumor or lymph node recurrence.

Regional Lymph Node Metastases

The development of regional lymph node metastases is often heralded by symptoms. Bulky periesophageal lymph node metastases may be signalled by the development of dysphagia (Fig. 28). Choking during eating or drinking requires evaluation for tracheoesophageal fistula. Cancerous enlargement of mediastinal lymph nodes often occurs after successful local treatment of the tumor. Tumor involvement of subcarinal nodes or recurrent mainstem bronchial cancer may extend locally into the mediastinum and result in tracheoesophageal fistula or other disastrous events.

Disseminated Disease

Malaise, weight loss, fever and cough after treatment for lung cancer may be the result of tumor extension, radiation/chemotherapy effects, postsurgical infection, disseminated tumor, or intercurrent disease. Associated symptoms often help to make this differentiation. Bone pain suggests the development of disseminated tumor

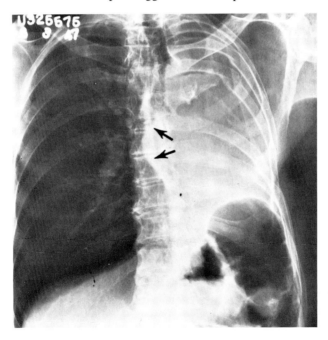

FIG. 28. Bulging of mediastinal pleura *(arrow)* after left pneumonectomy for lung cancer indicates recurrent tumor. The bulge was caused by periesophageal metastases in this patient who complained of dysphagia.

or chest wall tumor extension. Radionuclide studies and CT are of great help in detecting metastasis, especially bony and cerebral metastases. Multiple pulmonary metastases are uncommon, late developments in disseminated lung cancer.

Complications of Treatment

Empyema or bronchopleural fistula are unusual late complications of bronchial stump leaks. Persistent air-fluid levels in a post-lung resection hemithorax may herald empyema. Late empyemas developing a year or more after surgery are difficult to recognize radiologically unless air enters the pleural space from a bronchopleural communication. Since the mediastinum becomes relatively fixed postoperatively, no contralateral mediastinal shift occurs to signal the development of empyema.

Large-field irradiation of the lung inducing pneumonitis can be recognized by its geographic distribution and its temporal relationship to radiotherapy (Fig. 29). The earliest radiologic sign of radiation effect is peribronchial cuffing followed by consolidation. The first radiographic manifestation often occurs near the termination of treatment. Later in its course, radiation effects are manifest by more cicatricial and bronchiectatic changes.

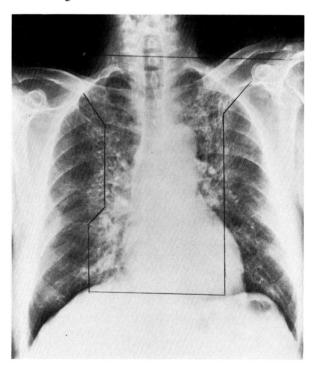

FIG. 29. Geographic lung opacities that conform to treatment portals *(black lines)* are characteristic of radiation pneumonitis.

Intercurrent Disease

Noncancerous disease such as pulmonary embolism, myocardial infarction, stroke, and pneumonia are sometimes mistaken for the effect of treatment of lung cancer. Proper use of radiologic studies such as pulmonary arteriography and biopsy procedures can accurately establish the true identity of radiologic lesions that appear after tumor treatment.

Mediastinal Malignancies

The mediastinum is an important anatomic site, not only of secondary deposits of lung cancer but also of primary malignancies and secondary malignancies of extrathoracic origin (66). Secondary tumor involvement of the mediastinum is actually more common than involvement with primary tumors (Fig. 30). The most common extrapulmonary neoplasms to cause mediastinal metastases include melanoma and malignant tumors of the breast, stomach, colon, kidney, uterus, and thyroid. Sometimes the mediastinal metastases are discovered before the primary tumor is identified. The majority of primary mediastinal malignancies are lymphomas, thymomas, teratomas, and tumors of tracheal, esophageal, and neurogenic origin. The first three occur in the anterior mediastinal compartment, the second two in the middle compartment, and the last in the posterior compartment. Secondary malignancies can involve all mediastinal compartments.

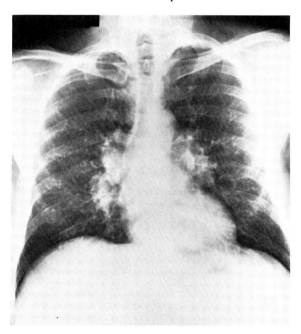

FIG. 30. Bilateral hilar lymphadenopathy on presentation of a newly discovered renal cell carcinoma is secondary to hilar metastases.

Primary mediastinal malignancies occur in characteristic locations. For diagnostic considerations, it is convenient to divide the mediastinum by the pericardium and great vessels into anterior, middle, and posterior compartments.

Malignancies of the *anterior mediastinum* (primarily metastases, teratomas, thymomas, and lymphomas) are frequently perceived only on lateral radiographic studies until they develop enough bulk to project into the lungs on the frontal view (Fig. 31). Strategically located masses may displace, compress, or invade the trachea, esophagus, great vessels, and phrenic or recurrent laryngeal nerves. Thy-

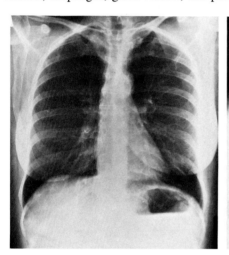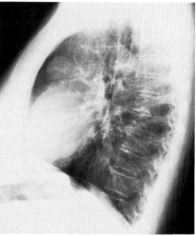

FIG. 31. There is no convincing evidence of tumor on frontal radiography but an anterior mediastinal thymoma is clearly visible on the lateral view. The subtle double contour of the aortic arch is the only manifestation of the tumor on the frontal view.

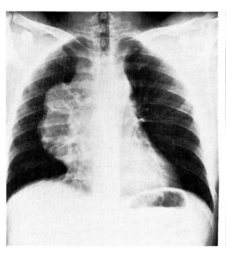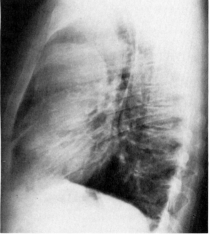

FIG. 32. Large lobulated anterior mediastinal mass is caused by malignant teratoma.

moma is one of the most common tumors of the anterior compartment. About 50% of patients with thymomas have myasthenia gravis and about 15% of patients with myasthenia gravis have thymomas. Grading the anatomic extent of tumor is important because 10-year survival is approximately 90% when thymomas are not associated with either myasthenia gravis or evidence of gross tumor extension into adjacent structures, about 50% if either myasthenia gravis or invasion is present, and very low if both factors are present (69,70). Teratomas occur with about the same frequency in the anterior mediastinum as thymomas and have a very similar appearance (Fig. 32).

The common malignant tumors of the anterior mediastinal compartment (lymphoma, teratoma, thymoma) must be differentiated from the common benign lesions that occur in that location, i.e., goiters, thymic hyperplasia, thymic or bronchogenic cysts, dermoids, and benign vascular tumors. Goiters generally elevate with swallowing, frequently contain calcium, and displace the trachea up to the larynx. Rapid goiter enlargement from internal hemorrhage is often misinterpreted as a rapidly growing malignancy. In the pediatric age group, thymic enlargement is often caused by thymic hyperplasia. Benign cysts can often be differentiated from solid malignant lesions by CT when the density of the contents is very low (Fig. 33). This is particularly true of pericardial (spring water) cysts but not so true of bronchogenic cysts that often contain high density material. Occasionally, large amounts of mediastinal fat accumulate in the mediastinum and simulate malignant masses. The fat generally extends symmetrically through all of the mediastinal compartments and is easily identified by CT. Malignancies of the anterior compartment may also involve the middle mediastinum, especially lymphomas and carcinomas. Malignancies of juxtamediastinal lung cancers in the anterior segments of the upper lobe can closely simulate mediastinal malignancies. Differentiation between juxtamediastinal lung lesions and mediastinal masses can be made with CT or fluoroscopic observation during breathing.

Malignancies of the *middle mediastinum* are caused by primary mediastinal tumors, lymphomas, and metastases from lung cancers and extrathoracic malignancies. Primary middle mediastinal malignancies are more often detected by symptoms rather than radiographic bulk. Tracheal malignancies are often missed on radiographs unless there is a considerably bulky extraluminal component or lobar atelectasis (71–73) (Fig. 34). Esophageal carcinoma is only occasionally bulky enough to be detected with plain radiographic studies, except in the bulky carcinosarcoma type of malignancy. Malignancies of the middle mediastinum are more often secondary than primary. Lung cancers and extrapulmonary malignancies commonly metastasize to the middle mediastinum.

Malignancies of the *posterior mediastinum* are primarily caused by metastases and primary tumors of the esophagus and nerves. These tumors present radiographically as mass lesions adjacent to the aorta and spine. Neurogenic tumors often have associated deformities of the neural foramina. These tumors can be well shown with CT (Fig. 35). Tumors of the posterior mediastinum (neurogenic, esophageal, and lymph nodes) must be differentiated from benign lesions such as neuroenteric,

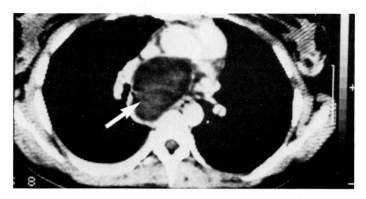

FIG. 33. Subcarinal bronchogenic cyst shown by CT to have characteristic mixed high density and a low density contour *(arrow)*.

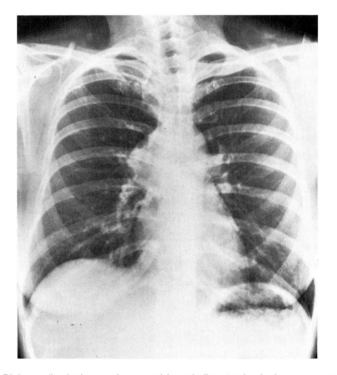

FIG. 34. Right mediastinal mass is caused by a bulky extraluminal component of adenoid cystic carcinoma of the trachea. The intraluminal component is not visible and there is no associated atelectasis.

bronchogenic, and duplication cysts. These can sometimes be identified by CT or percutaneous biopsy. Other benign lesions of the posterior compartment include neurogenic tumors and paraspinal infections. Esophageal carcinomas are identified with barium studies.

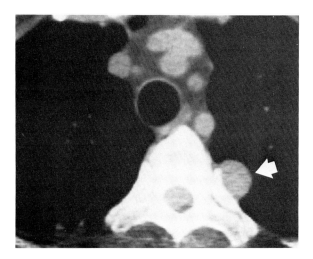

FIG. 35. Left paravertebral mass displacing the spinal cord to the right *(white arrow)* is characteristic of dumbbell-shaped schwannoma.

The differential diagnosis of mediastinal masses is particularly challenging because both benign and malignant solid masses need to be differentiated from each other and from vascular lesions. Almost 10% of patients with primary mediastinal tumors are at first considered to have vascular abnormalities (74). Because the management of vascular and solid lesions of the mediastinum differ so greatly, each must be identified early in the patient workup. CT with contrast is the ideal method of differentiating vascular from nonvascular lesions. CT is an essential part of evaluating the density characteristics and extent of all mediastinal neoplasms. It is a particularly useful method of identifying fat accumulations and cysts, detecting and determining the extent of malignant thymomas, and the extent of esophageal carcinoma (75,76) (Fig. 36).

The anterior compartment may be encroached upon by various dilated normal vascular structures such as pericardium, right ventricle, ascending aorta and internal mammary arteries. The middle mediastinum can also become enlarged by vascular abnormalities such as pericardial effusion, brachiocephalic or aortic aneurysm and pulmonary varix. Masses caused by dilatation of the superior vena cava and azygos vein can be identified by radiographic or fluoroscopic findings. CT with contrast and angiography are certain methods of identifying these structures. Simple blood pool radionuclide studies are an alternative simple method of diagnosis. Aneurysm of the descending aorta, the primary vascular cause of enlargement in the posterior compartment, is often difficult to distinguish from solid tumors without the use of CT or angiography. Solid tumors can be differentiated from vascular lesions by their ability to concentrate isotopes (77). Goiters can sometimes be identified by their ability to concentrate isotopes such as technetium or iodine. CT can dependably identify the fatty density of a herniated omental sac (Fig. 37). Roentgen evaluation of mediastinal masses should begin with a review of all retrievable previous chest

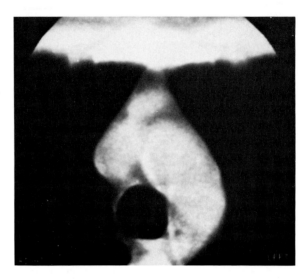

FIG. 36. Rounded soft tissue density of thymoma in anterior mediastinum of patient with myasthenia gravis is well shown by CT but occult by standard radiography.

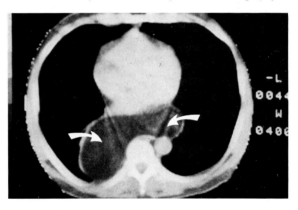

FIG. 37. Diagnosis of large posterior mediastinal mass is clarified by CT which shows typical fat density of omental herniation *(arrows).*

examinations. Fluoroscopy is invaluable in the assessment of dynamic events such as diaphragmatic and vocal cord movement. Barium swallow will also aid in the evaluation of middle mediastinal masses. Tomography and low kilovoltage radiographs can help to identify calcifications within the lesions.

Malignant Mesothelioma

Malignant mesothelioma is the most important primary malignancy of the pleura. Extensive adenocarcinoma involving the pleura, benign asbestos-related pleural effusion, and enlarging benign pleural plaques can closely simulate the radiographic appearance of this tumor. Malignant mesothelioma is closely linked to asbestos

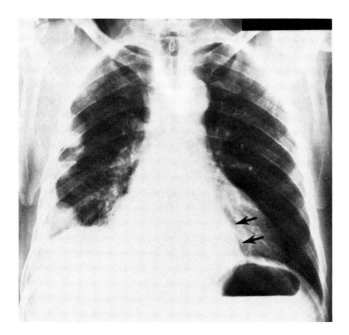

FIG. 38. Nodular right pleural masses are characteristic of malignant mesothelioma. The left chest density projecting behind the heart indicates tumor extension across the mediastinum from the right chest (arrow).

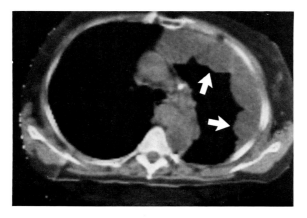

FIG. 39. Lobulated pleural masses characteristic of malignant mesothelioma encase and constrict the left hemithorax (arrows).

exposure, but a significant minority of patients with the tumor have no known exposure to asbestos. The tumor usually develops following a long latency after asbestos exposure (approximately 25–40 years).

The primary clinical finding is pain. The major radiographic findings are pleural effusion, pleural thickening, constriction of the thorax, encasement of the lung, and lobulated pleural masses (Fig. 38). Because percutaneous biopsy is not usually a dependable method of establishing the diagnosis, open lung biopsy is usually necessary. The primary purpose of staging studies is to exclude extension of tumor into the mediastinum, peritoneum, lung or contralateral chest (Fig. 39). Metastases to bone are known to occur. The best method of assessing tumor extent is with CT.

REFERENCES

1. Garland, L. H., Coulson, W., and Wollin, E. (1963): The rate of growth and apparent duration of untreated primary bronchial carcinoma. *Cancer*, 16:694.
2. Smith, R. A. (1966): Development and treatment of fresh lung carcinoma after successful lobectomy. *Thorax*, 21:1.
3. (1980): Guidelines for the cancer-related checkup: recommendations and rationale. *CA-A Cancer J. Clinicians*, 30:194–240.
4. Boucot, K. R., and Weiss, W. (1973): Is curable lung cancer detected by semiannual screening? *J.A.M.A*, 224:1361–1365.
5. Brett, G. Z. (1969): Earlier diagnosis and survival in lung cancer. *Br. Med. J.*, 4:260–262.
6. Fontana, R. S. (1977): Early diagnosis of lung cancer. *Am. Rev. Resp. Dis.*, 116:399–402.
7. Heelan, R. T., Melamed, M. R., Zaman, M. B., Martini, N., and Flehinger, B. J. (1980): Radiologic diagnosis of oat cell cancer in a high-risk screened population. *Radiology*, 136:593–601.
8. Kreyberg, L. (1967): *Histological Typing of Lung Tumours*. World Health Organization, Geneva.
9. Byrd, R. B., Miller, W. E., Carr, D. T., et al. (1968): The roentgenographic appearance of squamous cell carcinoma of the bronchus. *Mayo Clin. Proc.*, 43:327.
10. Byrd, R. B., Miller, W. E., Carr, D. T., et al. (1968): The roentgenographic appearance of small cell carcinoma of the bronchus. *Mayo Clin. Proc.*, 43:337.
11. Lehar, I. J., Carr, D. T., Miller, W. E., et al. (1967): Roentgenographic appearance of bronchogenic adenocarcinoma. *Am. Rev. Resp. Dis.*, 96:245.
12. Byrd, R. B., Miller, W. E., Carr, D. T., et al. (1968): The roentgenographic appearance of large cell carcinoma of the bronchus. *Mayo Clin. Proc.*, 43:333.
13. Greene, R., McLoud, T. C., and Stark, P. (1977): Other malignant tumors of the lung. *Semin. Roentgenol.*, XII:225–237.
14. Campobasso, O. (1968): The characteristics of peripheral lung tumours that suggest their bronchioloalveolar origin. *Br. J. Cancer*, 22:655.
15. Razzuk, M. A., Lynn, J. A., Kingsley, W. B., et al. (1970): Giant cell carcinoma of the lung. *J. Thorac. Cardiovasc. Surg.*, 59:574–580.
16. Bower, G. (1965): Bronchial adenoma. A review of twenty-eight cases. *Am. Rev. Resp. Dis.*, 92:558–563.
17. Gupta, A. K., Pryce, D. M., and Blenkinsopp, W. K. (1965): Pre-operative length of history and tumour size in central and peripheral bronchial carcinomata. *Thorax*, 20:398.
18. Cohen, S., and Hossain, M. S. A. (1966): Primary carcinoma of the lung: A review of 417 histologically proven cases. *Chest*, 49:67.
19. Selawry, O. S., and Hansen, H. H. (1973): Lung cancer. In: *Cancer Medicine*, edited by Holland, J. R. and Frei, E. Lea & Febiger, Philadelphia.
20. Rassan, J. W., and Anderson, G. (1975): Incidence of paramalignant disorders in bronchogenic carcinoma. *Thorax*, 30:86.
21. Sanderson, D. R., Fontana, R. S. Woolner, L. B., et al. (1974): Bronchoscopic localization of radiographically occult lung cancer. *Chest*, 65:608.
22. Stark, P. (1982): Multiple independent bronchogenic carcinomas. *Radiology*, 145:599–601.
23. Woolner, L. B., David, E., and Fontana, R. S. (1970): In situ and early invasive bronchogenic carcinoma: Report of 28 cases with post operative survival data. *J. Thorac. Cardiovasc. Surg.*, 60:275.
24. Aronberg, D. J., Sagel, S. S., LeFrak, S., Kuhn, C., and Susman, N. (1980): Lung carcinoma associated with bullous lung disease in young men. *A.J.R.*, 134:249–252.
25. Weiss, W., Boucot, K. R., and Cooper, D. A. (1966): The survival of men with measurable proved lung cancer in relation to growth rate. *Am. J. Roentgenol. Radium Ther. Nucl. Med.*, 98:404.

26. Salyer, W. R., Elleston, J. C., and Erozan, Y. S. (1975): Efficacy of pleural needle biopsy and pleural fluid cytopathology in the diagnosis of malignant neoplasm involving the pleura. *Chest*, 67:536–539.
27. Decker, D. A., Dines, D. E., Pyne, W. S., et al. (1975): The significance of a cytologically negative pleural effusion in bronchogenic carcinoma. *Chest*, 69:934–941.
28. The American Joint Committee for Cancer Staging and End Results Reporting (1974): Clinical staging system for carcinoma of the lung. *CA*, 24:87.
29. Laurens, R. G., Pine, J. R., and Honig, E. G. (1983): Spontaneous pneumothorax in primary cavitating lung carcinoma. *Radiology*, 146:295–297.
30. Mahajan, V., Kupferer, C. F., and Van Ordstrand, H. S. (1975): Pneumothorax: A rare manifestation of primary lung cancer. *Chest*, 68:730–732.
31. Abrams, H. L., ed. (1971): *Angiography*. Little, Brown and Company, Boston.
32. Faling, L. J., Pugatch, R. D., Jung-Legg, Y., Daly, B. D. T., Hong, W. K., Robbins, A. H., and Snider, G. (1981): Computed tomographic scanning of the mediastinum in the staging of bronchogenic carcinoma. *Am. Rev. Respir. Dis.*, 124:690–695.
33. Lewis, J. W., Madrazo, B. L., Eyler, W. R., Gross, S. C., Magilligan, D. J., and Rosen, R. A. (1982): The value of computed tomography and conventional laminography in the staging of lung carcinoma. Presented at the Society of Thoracic Surgeons.
34. Mintz, U., DeMeester, T. R., Golomb, H. M., et al. (1979): Sequential staging in bronchogenic carcinoma. *Chest*, 76:653–657.
35. Froehlich, G., Inoue, Y., and Magnus, H. E. (1973): The use of GA67 citrate application in the diagnosis of tumors of the chest. *Fortschr. Geb. Roentgenstr. Nuklearmed.*, 119:578–587.
36. Wittes, R. E., and Yeh, S. D. (1977): Indications for liver and brain scans. Screening tests for patients with oat cell carcinoma of lung. *J.A.M.A.*, 238:506–507.
37. Muggia, F., and Schereu, L. R. (1974): Lung cancer: Diagnosis in metastatic sites. *Semin. Oncol.*, 1:217–228.
38. Johnson, P. M., and Sweeney, W. A. (1967): The false positive hepatic scan. *J. Nucl. Med.*, 8:451–460.
39. Castagna, J., Benfield, J. R., Yamada, H., et al. (1972): The reliability of liver scans and function tests in detecting metastases. *Surg. Gynecol. Obstet.*, 134:463–466.
40. Chapman, G. S., Kumar, D., Redmond, J., and Gandara, D. R. (1982): Upper abdominal CT scanning in staging non-oat-cell lung carcinoma. *N. Engl. J. Med.*, 307:189.
41. Sandler, M. A., Pearlberg, J. L., Madrazo, B. L., Gitschlag, K. F., and Gross, S. C. (1982): Computed tomographic evaluation of the adrenal gland in the preoperative assessment of bronchogenic carcinoma. *Radiology*, 145:733–736.
42. Johnson, D. H., Windham, W. W., Allen, J. H., and Greco, F. A. (1983): Limited value of CT brain scans in the staging of small cell lung cancer. *A.J.R.*, 140:37–40.
43. Dunnick, N. R. (1979): Abdominal CT in the evaluation of small cell carcinoma of the lung. *A.J.R.*, 133:1085–1088.
44. Society for Computed Body Tomography (1979): Special report: New indications for computed body tomography. *A.J.R.*, 133:115.
45. Muhm, J. R., Brown, L. R., Crowe, J. K., Sheedy, P. F., Hattery, R. R., and Stephens, D. (1978): Comparison of whole lung tomography and computed tomography for detecting pulmonary nodules. *A.J.R.*, 131:981–984.
46. Muhm, J. R., Brown, L. R., and Crowe, J. K. (1977): Detection of pulmonary nodules by computed tomography. *A.J.R.*, 128:267–270.
47. Schaner, E. G., Chang, A. E., Doppman, J. L., Conkle, D. M., Flye, M. W., and Rosenberg, S. A. (1978): Comparison of computed and conventional whole lung tomography in detecting pulmonary nodules: A prospective radiologic-pathologic study. *A.J.R.*, 131:51–54.
48. McLoud, T. C., Wittenberg, J., and Ferrucci, J. T. (1979): Computed tomography of the thorax and standard radiographic evaluation of the chest. A comparative study. *J. Comput. Assist. Tomogr.*, 3:170–180.
49. Sindelar, W. F., Bagley, D. H., Felix, E. L., Doppman, J. L., and Ketcham, A. S. (1978): Lung tomography in cancer patients. *J.A.M.A*, 240:2060–2063.
50. Didolkar, M. S., Cedemark, B. J., Goel, I. P., Takita, H., and Moore, R. H. (1977): Accuracy of roentgenograms of the chest in metastases to the lungs. *Surg. Gyn. Obstet.*, 144:903–905.

51. Polga, J. P., and Watnick, M. (1976): Whole lung tomography in metastatic disease. *Clin. Radiol.*, 27:53–57.
52. Neifeld, J. P., Michaelis, L. L., and Doppman, J. L. (1977): Suspected pulmonary metastases: Correlation of chest x-ray, whole lung tomograms and operative findings. *Cancer*, 39:383–387.
53. Siegelman, S. S., Zerhouni, E. A., Leo, F. P., Khouri, N. F., and Stitik, F. P. (1980): CT of the solitary pulmonary nodule. *A.J.R.*, 135:1–13.
54. Holle, R. H., Carnes, J., Mack, L. A., and Figley, M. M. (1982): CT scanning of the solitary pulmonary nodule in Seattle. *Invest. Radiol.*, 17:S2.
55. Levi, C., Gray, J. E., McCullough, E. C., and Hattery, R. R. (1982): The unreliability of CT numbers as absolute values. *A.J.R.*, 139:443–447.
56. Godwin, J. D., Speckman, M. J., Fram, E. K., Johnson, G. A., Putman, C. E., Korobkin, M., and Breiman, R. S. (1982): Distinguishing benign from malignant pulmonary nodules by computed tomography. *Radiology*, 144:349–351.
57. Osborne, D. R., Korobkin, M., Ravin, C. E., et al. (1982): Comparison of plain radiography, conventional tomography, and computed tomography in detecting intrathoracic lymph nodes metastases from lung carcinoma. *Radiology*, 142:157–161.
58. Baron, R. L., Levitt, R. G., Sagel, S. S., White, M. J., Roper, C. L., and Marbarger, J. P. (1982): Computed tomography in the preoperative evaluation of bronchogenic carcinoma. *Radiology*, 145:727–732.
59. Shevland, J. E., Chiu, L. C., Shapiro, R. L., Young, J. A., and Rossi, N. P. (1978): The role of conventional tomography and computed tomography in assessing the resectability of primary lung cancer: A preliminary report. *CT*, 2:1–19.
60. Rea, H. H., Shevland, J. E., and House, A. J. S. (1981): Accuracy of computed tomographic scanning in assessment of the mediastinum in bronchial carcinoma. *J. Thorac. Cardiovasc. Surg.*, 81:825–829.
61. Friedman, P. J., Feigin, D. S., Liston, S. E., Alazraki, N. P., Haghighi, P., and Peters, R. M. (1982): Sensitivity of radiography, computed tomography and gallium scanning to mediastinal metastasis of lung carcinoma. Presented at the Radiological Society of North America Annual Meeting.
62. Heitzman, E. R. (1981): Computed tomography of the thorax: Current perspectives. *A.J.R.*, 136:2–12.
63. Mintzer, R. A., Malave, S. R., Neiman, H. L., Lawrence, L. M., Vanecko, R. M., and Sanders, J. H. (1979): Computed versus conventional tomography in evaluation of primary and secondary pulmonary neoplasms. *Radiology*, 132:653–659.
64. Hirleman, M. T., Yiu-Chiu, V. S., Chiu, L. C., and Schapiro, R. L. (1980): The resectability of primary lung carcinoma: A diagnostic staging review. *CT*, 4:146–163.
65. Webb, W. R., Gamsu, G., and Speckman, J. (1981): CT of the pulmonary hilum in patients with bronchogenic carcinoma. Presented at the Radiological Society of North America Annual Meeting.
66. Greene, R. (1981): Transthoracic needle aspiration biopsy. In: *Interventional Radiology*, edited by Athanasoulis, C., Pfister, R., Greene, R., and Roberson, G. W. B. Saunders, Philadelphia.
67. Greene, R., Isler, R. J., Szyfelbein, W., and Jantsch, H. (1983): Histologic and cytologic samples from transthoracic fine needle aspiration. *A.J.R.*, (submitted).
68. Joseph, W. L., Murray, J. E., and Mulder, D. G. (1966): Mediastinal tumors—problems in diagnosis and treatment. *Chest*, 50:150.
69. Jamplis, R. W., and Cressman, R. L. (1959): Current concepts of thymomas. *Am. J. Surg.*, 98:202.
70. Wikins, E. W., Edmunds, L. H., and Castleman, B. (1966): Cases of thymoma at the Massachusetts General Hospital. *J. Thorac. Cardiovasc. Surg.*, 52:322.
71. Houston, H. E., Pyne, W. S., Harrison, E. J., et al. (1969): Primary cancer of the trachea. *Arch. Surg.*, 99:132.
72. Grillo, H. C. (1972): Benign and malignant diseases of the chest. In: *General Thoracic Surgery*, edited by Shields, T. W., pp. 555–575. Lea & Febiger, Philadelphia.
73. Janower, M. L., Grillo, H. C., MacMillan, S., et al. (1970): The radiological appearance of carcinoma of the trachea. *Radiology*, 96:39.
74. Brown, L. R., Muhm, J. R., Sheedy, P. F., Unni, K. K., Bernatz, P. E., and Hermann, R. C. (1983): The value of computed tomography in myasthenia gravis. *A.J.R.*, 140:31–35.

75. Picus, D., Balfe, D. M., Koehler, R. E., Roper, C. L., and Owen, J. W. (1983): Computed tomography in the staging of esophageal carcinoma. *Radiology*, 146:433–438.
76. Oldham, H. N., and Sabiston, D. C. (1968): Primary tumors and cysts of the mediastinum. *Arch. Surg.*, 96:71.
77. Ito, Y., Okuyama, S., Awano, T., et al. (1971): Diagnostic evaluation of 67Ga scanning of lung cancer and other disease. *Radiology*, 101:255.

Thoracic Oncology, edited by N. C. Choi and
H. C. Grillo. Raven Press, New York © 1983.

Assessment of Pulmonary Function in Lung Cancer

David J. Kanarek

*Pulmonary Unit, Department of Medicine, Massachusetts General Hospital,
Boston, Massachusetts 02114*

Cancer of the lung often occurs in a setting of diffuse obstructive airways disease. Cigarette smoking is the usual culprit, being strongly related both to the development of chronic bronchitis and emphysema and to lung cancer. Occasionally, the cancer may also be complicated by accompanying conditions such as asthma, bronchiectasis, or interstitial fibrosis, and special considerations may need to be applied to the assessment of lung function under these circumstances. In the great majority of cases, however, one is dealing with lung cancer superimposed on chronic bronchitis and emphysema, whose physiological consequence is severe reduction in airflow rate.

When faced with such a patient several questions may arise: Is this a surgically resectable tumor? If so, how much loss of lung function will occur as a result of either a lobectomy or pneumonectomy? What is the consequent risk of respiratory failure, and (less often asked) how will exercise tolerance be affected subsequent to recovery? What is the risk of atelectasis or infection occurring postoperatively? What will be the effect of radiotherapy on lung function, and what are the risks of respiratory failure supervening during or following the radiotherapy? To each of these questions there are answers based on clinical and physiological evaluation; however, these answers must be tempered by the clinical judgment of the physician and the needs and wishes of the patient. One can provide accurate guidelines and raise physiological red flags, but only rarely can the final decision be based on the functional assessment alone.

This chapter will cover the factors that must be taken into account before resection is attempted in patients with lung cancer. First, the complications are outlined whose occurrence and impact preoperative assessment attempts to predict and minimize. Next will follow a discussion of the clinical observations that can be used to aid the process of assessment, followed by a discussion of the laboratory tests and their use in evaluating pulmonary pathophysiology. An extensive discussion of the use of regional functional assessment will be included, because it is our belief that this has provided major assistance in predicting the risks associated with the various surgical procedures. Specific, if arbitrary, guidelines that have been found useful will be listed in this section. Finally, a brief discussion of radiotherapy will be provided.

COMPLICATIONS

There are four general complications that must be considered in advance of all thoracic surgery: (a) atelectasis, (b) infection, (c) early respiratory failure, and (d) postoperative exertional dyspnea and late respiratory failure. There are other complications that can affect the postoperative course, such as hemorrhage and pneumothorax, but they will not be considered here because physiological evaluation cannot predict the occurrence or extent and therefore the effects of such incidents.

Both atelectasis and infection occur more commonly in patients who are obese or elderly or who have preexisting lung disease (9), whether the disease is diagnosed by clinical features or by lung function tests. This is particularly true for thoracic or upper abdominal surgery. The predisposing factors include poor cough, decreased clearance of secretions, deficient mucociliary function, early airway closure (elevated closing volume) with distal gas absorption, reduced lung compliance, and pain. Detection of symptoms and signs or abnormal pulmonary function should lead to the institution of intensive preoperative preparation, including antibiotics, bronchodilators, and physical therapy where indicated, measures that have been shown to markedly reduce the incidence of atelectasis and infection (8).

The incidence of atelectasis and infection is increased even in the presence of mild pulmonary symptoms or dysfunction, and it is not tightly linked to the degree of abnormality, so that all patients with pulmonary abnormality should be considered at risk for these complications (9). This is in contrast to the development of respiratory failure, where accurate assessment of functional status preoperatively is of critical importance; in the immediate postoperative period there is a further decline in ventilatory capacity of about 50%.

CLINICAL OBSERVATIONS

Several clinical observations must be sought in each case, because they reflect directly on the risks and complications related to the surgery. These include the presence and nature of cough and sputum production, any wheezing or background of asthma, evidence of cor pulmonale or clinical signs of pulmonary hypertension, and the degree of exercise capability. Excessive sputum production predisposes to postoperative atelectasis and infection and requires preoperative interventions such as cessation of smoking, sputum culture and antibiotic therapy where applicable, and chest physical therapy. The preoperative meeting of the patient and the physical therapist serves two functions: reduction of secretion volume and instruction in the postoperative maneuvers that may be required to prevent or treat atelectasis. Wheezing is often an indication of the presence of reversible airway obstruction, and bronchodilators may improve ventilatory capacity. Direct measurements of exercise capability will be discussed later; however, during the initial clinical evaluation, specific questions relating to exercise tolerance, such as the number of stairs that can easily be negotiated, are very important to gain some insight into overall cardiopulmonary reserve and integration. Often there has been a recent decline in exercise tolerance when the tumor has caused lobar obstruction or atelectasis. In these cases, inquiry into exercise tolerance perhaps 3 months prior to the current admission frequently provides a much better appreciation of overall cardiopulmonary performance. It is important to do an informal exercise tolerance study by accompanying the patient while climbing stairs or walking rapidly in a corridor. Observation of the degree of dyspnea and changes in cardiac and respiratory rates gives valuable, if imprecise, information about the ability of the cardiopulmonary system to tolerate a load. Good exercise capability usually implies that the patient will be able to tolerate at least a lobectomy; however, for patients who have severe obstructive lung disease it is unwise to use this as the sole criterion, because the distributions of pulmonary perfusion and ventilation are unknown, and the function that will be lost following resection can be determined only by scanning techniques, as will be discussed later. In addition, patients who have kept themselves physically fit, either by the nature of their occupations or by regular exercise, may appear to perform very well, when, in fact, they are working to the limits of their tolerance. They may continue to exercise even while direct measurements show a marked fall in the partial pressure of oxygen (PO_2) and a rise in the partial pressure of carbon dioxide (PCO_2) in the arterial blood. Conversely, obese, sedentary individuals who take very little exercise may perform poorly under these circumstances and yet be capable of tolerating resection easily. Climbing stairs at normal speed requires an oxygen uptake of about 1.5 to 2 liters per minute, which is a considerable degree of exercise, particularly for the elderly, and a severe test of cardiopulmonary capability and general neuromuscular conditioning.

COMMON PULMONARY FUNCTION TESTS

Pulmonary function is complex, and no single test gives information on the entire pulmonary system. Moreover, pulmonary function must be considered in association with cardiac function, making the evaluation potentially very complicated. Nevertheless, the system can be divided into workable subsections for the purpose of function testing (Table 1). Because the major impact of chronic bronchitis and emphysema is on the airways, limiting the volume and rate of air exchange, and

TABLE 1. *Tests used in evaluating patients with lung cancer and impaired function*

Ventilatory function:	FEV_1, VC, MBC
Gas exchange:	PO_2, PCO_2, $A\text{-}aDO_2$, diffusing capacity
Circulatory studies:	EKG, vascular pressures, cardiac output, scanning techniques
Integrated function:	exercise evaluation
Regional pulmonary function:	quantitative ventilation-perfusion isotope scans

on the parenchyma, affecting the transfer of oxygen and carbon dioxide, selective studies of airflow and gas exchange usually provide the information required for an evaluation of current and potential pulmonary function. Severe disease also involves the pulmonary vasculature, with secondary effects on cardiac function. However, this is almost always reflected in severe ventilatory or gas-exchange abnormalities, and although there are opinions to the contrary (1), it has been our experience that specific studies of the lesser circulation are seldom required. It should be emphasized that all function studies should be carried out and used to make final decisions only when the patient is in optimal condition. This may require a period of waiting while antibiotics, bronchodilators, or other indicated therapies are administered.

Table 1 lists and categorizes the important tests that can be used in evaluating patients with lung cancer and impaired function. Of these tests, the forced expired volume in 1 sec (FEV_1) gives the most valuable information, because it describes not only the mass volume of air that can be moved but also the speed with which it can be moved. When expressed as an absolute volume and as a percentage of the predicted value, it gives information about potential ventilatory exchange, together with an estimate of the actual loss of function that has resulted from the obstructive pulmonary disease. Generalizing, when the FEV_1 has fallen to about 0.8 liter, there is an increased risk of developing carbon dioxide (CO_2) retention and increasing loss of exertional tolerance. This is because a minimum alveolar ventilation is required for the removal of CO_2 produced at rest and exercise and for the maintenance of alveolar oxygen tension under the same conditions. For light to moderate exercise there is a linear relationship between O_2 uptake, CO_2 production, and minute ventilation. A reduced alveolar ventilation limits the maximum oxygen uptake and therefore the maximum exercise capability. If the alveolar ventilation is severely reduced, the PCO_2 may rise with exercise, the individual being unable to cope with the increased metabolic load of CO_2. Clearly there is marked variability in function between individuals for any given level of FEV_1, because many subjects are still quite active at low levels, whereas others already have CO_2 retention. Nevertheless, an FEV_1 of 0.8 liter has proved a reasonable, if arbitrary, value to use as a lower permissible limit of postoperative function in a complex situation in which only guidelines, rather than absolute certainty, can be developed.

The maximum breathing capacity (MBC) has often been used as an alternative to the FEV_1; however, it is a more difficult test for the patient to carry out, it is broadly limited by the same factors that limit the FEV_1, and, in any case, it can usually be estimated by multiplying the FEV_1 by 35. Moreover, the most important advance in preoperative assessment, the accurate estimation of the potential functional loss using radioisotopic split function scanning, cannot be directly calculated from the preoperative MBC. The vital capacity has the inherent problem that it does not provide an estimate of the degree of obstruction, because it does not relate to flow rate. The vital capacity may be relatively normal in the face of severe obstruction.

The Po_2 in the systemic circulation and the gradient between alveolar and arterial oxygen pressure ($A\text{-}aDo_2$) represent the efficiency of oxygen transport from lung to blood. When the Po_2 is reduced, this is generally due to a combination of low-ventilation-perfusion regions and shunt. General hypoventilation, manifested by a raised Pco_2, will also reduce the Po_2. However, an elevated Pco_2 should be regarded as an absolute contraindication to resection, and the presence and evaluation of hypoxemia are of little consequence if the Pco_2 is elevated. In general, a Po_2 less than 50 mm Hg should be a strong relative contraindication. However, when there is atelectasis of one or more lobes because of tumor obstructing a bronchus, venous blood shunting through the collapsed lobe may be largely responsible for the hypoxemia, and removal of the collapsed lung often leads to an increase in Po_2. In the absence of atelectasis or gross consolidation, a Po_2 less than 50 mm Hg is usually associated with such severe obstructive airway disease, cor pulmonale, or gross restriction of exercise tolerance that it is clear that surgery is not feasible. Usually, the Po_2 is unchanged or higher after surgery than prior to the operation. There is no specific study relating directly to the Po_2 and the feasibility of surgery in obstructive airway disease.

The single-breath diffusing capacity for carbon monoxide ($DLco$) is a good indication of the amount of alveolocapillary surface available for gas transfer, both relative to normal lungs and in absolute terms. Because the diffusing capacity is particularly sensitive to the loss of vasculature, it provides valuable evidence of the amount of lung involved by emphysema, in which the pathology consists of alveolar wall and capillary destruction. The diffusing capacity is relatively normal in chronic bronchitis and often elevated in asthma. Both these diseases involve the airways, leaving the alveolocapillary region, the site of gas transfer, intact.

The pulmonary circulation is difficult to study without resorting to invasive procedures to measure the cardiac and vascular pressures and cardiac output directly. Clues to pulmonary hypertension due to vascular obliteration, emboli, or active constriction may be obtained from clinical examination and EKG evaluation. In the future, scanning by blood pool isotopes using indices such as the right ventricular ejection fraction may be of some help. Unless the pulmonary hypertension is due to pulmonary emboli, there usually is sufficient concomitant evidence from ventilatory studies, the diffusing capacity, blood gases, and exercise tolerance evaluation to suggest that there is severe vascular disease present. Studies that have suggested that direct measurement of pulmonary artery pressure is valuable in the decision regarding resection either have failed to show that a single value consistently predicts the likelihood of suffering severe postoperative mortality or morbidity or have been carried out in patients with pulmonary hypertension without marked airway obstruction (1,6). The latter is not the usual situation facing the surgeon, and we have rarely used such measurements or found that they add significantly new insight to difficult problems. Mean pulmonary artery pressures of 30 mm Hg at rest, rising during exercise or with ligation of a pulmonary artery, and elevated pulmonary vascular resistance that does not fall with exercise (1,6) have been indications of a poor prognosis.

SPLIT FUNCTION STUDIES

Split function studies are critical to the process of estimating the lung function loss that will result from any proposed lung resection. The importance of this technique lies in the fact that all other measurements of lung function provide either a mean flow rate, such as the FEV_1, or a total volume, such as the vital capacity, but do not distinguish the contributions of various regions of the lungs to these values. For example, for a given FEV_1, it is possible that from 5% to 95% of that value could come from the lung that contains the tumor, and a pneumonectomy could have the consequence of loss of 5% to 95% of the FEV_1. It is the postoperative lung function that determines whether a patient will go into respiratory failure or will have severe postoperative exercise difficulty. Hence it is the aim of these studies to split the total values measured for both lungs by standard preoperative testing such as FEV_1 and vital capacity into regional values. From these data the percentage of overall function contributed by the area to be resected can be calculated, and the ventilatory capacity that will remain after the resection can be estimated.

The technique is identical to that of the standard ventilation-perfusion lung scan used for the detection of pulmonary emboli in which the distribution of perfusion is depicted by a gamma or positron camera following the infusion of radioactive isotopes such as labeled albumin or ^{13}N, with the distribution of ventilation being demonstrated by inhalation of a full vital capacity of air enriched with radioactive gas. An additional step requiring simple, readily available computer techniques is added in which the perfusion or ventilation image is divided into a number of segments (Fig. 1). The total number of radioactive counts composing the image is measured, and the counts in each segment are expressed as a percentage of the total number of counts. This information, using a simple formula, can then be used to identify the contribution of any specific area to the overall function.

Figure 1 provides an example of this technique. The X-ray shows an atelectatic left upper lobe, demonstrated by bronchoscopy and biopsy to be caused by a proximal obstructing squamous cell carcinoma of the left upper lobe bronchus. No metastatic lesions were identified. The FEV_1 was 1.10 liters. The ventilation scan shows that only about 4% of the total function is in the region of the left upper lobe. However, 35% of function is within the left lung. The formula used to calculate the postoperative function is as follows: predicted postoperative FEV_1 = preoperative $FEV_1 \times$ % function that will remain (3,5). Thus, from Fig. 1, the calculation for a lobectomy: postoperative FEV_1 = $1.1 \times 96/100$ liters = 1.056 liters. However, if pneumonectomy is required, the postoperative FEV_1 will be $1.1 \times 65/100$ liters = 0.72 liter.

Thus, using the general cutoff level that a postoperative FEV_1 greater than 0.8 liter is a reasonable postoperative value, one might conclude that a lobectomy would be well tolerated by this patient and would affect exercise tolerance very little, whereas a pneumonectomy would pose a considerable risk of postoperative respiratory failure and might lead to a very significant increase in exertional dyspnea.

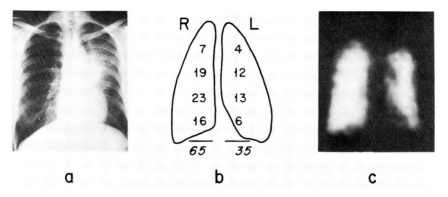

FIG. 1. **(a)** Chest X-ray showing left hilar tumor and left upper lobe atelectasis; **(b)** percentage regional distribution of inhaled isotope; **(c)** image of inhaled isotope from which the regional distribution was derived.

Once again, there is no definitive study showing the precise FEV_1 that will divide the subjects into those who will tolerate surgery well and those who will suffer severe complications. The FEV_1 of 0.8 liter has been chosen arbitrarily, based on the known function of patients with chronic obstructive pulmonary disease. Below this level there is an increasing likelihood of CO_2 retention, and exercise tolerance becomes increasingly limited because of the severe ventilatory restriction.

The accuracy of such calculations has been well established by a number of studies (3,5) and confirmed by our own experience, using either the simple formula given earlier or variations of it. Postoperative values measured 3 to 6 months after surgery tend to be slightly higher than the predicted value, perhaps because the removal of mass from the thoracic cavity permits expansion of the remaining lung and traction on the airways. This dilatation leads to increases in vital capacity and flow rate, in a manner analogous to the situation following surgical removal of a large bulla.

The validity of this approach has not been demonstrated by any comparative trials, nor is it likely that such trials will be carried out. However, several large studies (4, 10) in which patients with obstructive lung disease underwent pulmonary resection without regional studies having been carried out showed a mortality that ranged from 20% to 35%, and these studies generally concluded that pulmonary function data helped little, if at all, in preoperative assessment. Moreover, a number of deaths were due to respiratory failure. It is likely that one reason for this was the assumption that patients with similar preoperative standard pulmonary function data had similar preoperative distributions of regional function. Figure 2 illustrates the fallacy of this assumption. In this case the patient was shown to have a fairly central squamous cell carcinoma of the right lower lobe. The preoperative FEV_1 was 1.4 liters. However, as shown by the quantitative regional scan, 61% of function was in the right lung. Hence a right pneumonectomy would have resulted in a postoperative FEV_1 of only 0.56 liter, a situation that could well be disastrous. Being prewarned, one can elect alternative approaches to treatment, such as radio-

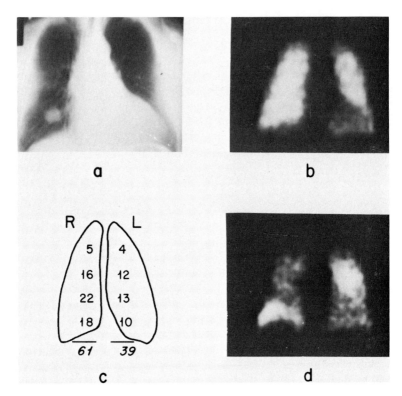

FIG. 2. **(a)** Tomogram showing right lower lobe mass; **(b)** scan showing distribution of inhaled isotope (ventilation); **(c)** percentage regional distribution of ventilation; **(d)** washout image after 2 min of tidal breathing of room air showing poor ventilation of right lower zone and left upper zone and midzone.

therapy, or the surgeon can be warned that a lobectomy is feasible but that a pneumonectomy carries too high a risk. In the case of Fig. 2, a lobectomy would have resulted in a postoperative FEV_1 of 0.92 liter.

The major reason that an even distribution of function in the two lungs cannot be assumed is the inhomogeneous nature of obstructive lung disease. Large, poorly ventilated bullae may be situated predominantly in the lung contralateral to the tumor, so that the major preoperative contribution to ventilatory capacity may be from the lung with the tumor. In such a situation, a pneumonectomy may be potentially disastrous because of "unexpected" postoperative respiratory failure or severe exertional limitation, even though the initial FEV_1 may appear adequate. Radiological techniques may also fail to identify the bullae, and, in any case, they give no information on the functional effect of bullae.

Figure 2 also illustrates a technique for examining the quality of the regional ventilation in the lung without a tumor and identifying areas of particularly poor ventilation. The patient breathes from a spirometer containing radioactive gas until equilibration is reached between lungs and spirometer. The patient then exhales normal tidal volumes to room air, while images of the lung are produced every 30 sec. Areas of poor ventilation are seen in these so-called washout pictures by retention of gas in these areas for prolonged periods of time. Techniques of quantifying the washout phase are available, such as the regional time to wash out 50% of the counts; however, simple inspection usually suffices to recognize these regions. In Fig. 2 it can be seen from picture (d) not only that the majority of function is in the right lung but also that clearance of the gas is slower in the left lung than the right lung, making the disparity in function even greater. This type of information is not available from standard function studies, which are inadequate for final decisions in patients with impaired function. Information is insufficient to apply precise values. However, in borderline cases, knowledge of the quality of ventilation in the remaining lung does provide further useful prognostic data.

Occasionally, following a lobectomy, there is a recurrence of apparently resectable tumor in the remaining lung. Because there may be a redistribution of function following the initial surgery due to expansion of the remaining lung to fill the space previously occupied by the resected lobe, it is important to restudy the case fully and not assume an unchanged regional distribution of function.

Lung scans sometimes help in deciding whether or not a tumor is resectable. It has been shown that when the perfusion to one lung is less than one-third of the combined perfusion to both lungs, it is unlikely that the tumor will be resectable (7). However, this is not invariable and cannot be used unequivocally. This severe loss of perfusion frequently is due to direct proximal vascular involvement making resection difficult. Occasionally the scans are also of help in planning radiotherapy fields and minimizing damage to functioning lung tissue, because the tumor may be immediately adjacent to the region with a large percentage of total function.

Not all patients require split function studies. It is rare to lose more than 500 cc of the FEV_1 following a lobectomy. However, a pneumonectomy may result in loss of 70% or more of total function. Hence, reasonable guidelines for split function studies are the following: (a) an $FEV_1 < 1.5$ liters when only a lobectomy is contemplated; (b) an $FEV_1 < 2$ liters when a pneumonectomy may be required; (c) $FEV_1/FVC < 50\%$.

If the calculated postoperative FEV_1 is less than 0.8 liter, exceptional circumstances will be required before proceeding with surgery, because the increased risk of mortality and morbidity quite probably will exceed the chances of a cure being obtained. As noted previously, an elevated PCO_2 is an absolute contraindication, whereas a PO_2 less than 50 mm Hg in the absence of a shunt is a strong contraindication.

It should be emphasized that these studies do not take into account any complications that might occur. Moreover, the smaller the reserve capacity following resection, the more likely it is that a superimposed complication will precipitate respiratory failure or cor pulmonale. This is particularly important in elderly and relatively debilitated patients, in whom respiratory muscles and cardiac status may be unable to support increased ventilatory or cardiac demands. Within our own institution, any degree of postoperative assisted ventilation for longer than 24 hr postoperatively, using these guidelines, is rare, unless a significant postoperative complication has occurred.

RADIOTHERAPY

The effects of radiotherapy on pulmonary function are variable; however, in general, there is little loss of function as a result of therapy (2). In fact, in some cases there may be substantial improvement in ventilatory function, either because occluded airways are opened or because fibrosis and contraction of the irradiated region cause traction on the remaining lung, dilating airways, similar to the effect of a surgical bullectomy. Arterial blood gases also remain unchanged. In addition, the region being irradiated often has little perfusion or ventilation in any case. Finally, it should be noted that radiotherapy avoids the immediate early loss of ventilatory function that results when the surgical incision causes pain and disruption of the mechanical integrity of the chest wall. This usually amounts to about 50% of the vital capacity in the first 2 or 3 days, slowly improving over the next 6 weeks. It is seldom, if ever, that impaired physiological function contraindicates radiotherapy for lung cancer, particularly if split function studies are used as an aid in planning the radiation fields to avoid damaging areas of the lung with significant ventilation and perfusion.

CONCLUSION

A good clinical evaluation, a simple ventilatory study emphasizing the FEV_1, and determination of arterial blood gases, followed by the judicious use of split function radioisotope studies, should serve to reduce to a very small number those patients who suffer respiratory failure or severe postoperative disability as a result of surgical resection or radiotherapy. It must be emphasized, however, that good results in patients with severe obstructive lung disease are entirely dependent on experienced and highly competent personnel in the surgical, radiotherapy and post-operative intensive care services. Patients with little reserve tolerate complications poorly; the most intensive preoperative evaluation serves only to help select those patients who, although physiologically disabled, can tolerate the therapy most likely to effect a cure. Their actual course depends heavily on the manner in which they are handled subsequent to their physiological evaluation. Conscientious surgeons and physicians must work together to take all the relevant factors into account.

REFERENCES

1. Fee, H. J., Holmes, E. C., Gewirtz, H. S., Ramming, K. P., and Alexander, J. M. (1978): *J. Thorac. Cardiovasc. Surg.*, 75:519–524.
2. Kanarek, D. J., Choi, N. C., Ahluwalia, B., Latty, A., and Kazemi, H. (1977): *Am. Rev. Respir. Dis.*, 115:128.
3. Kristerson, S., Lindell, S., and Svanberg, L. (1972): *Chest*, 62:694–698.
4. Larsen, N. C., and Clifton, E. E. (1965): *Dis. Chest*, 47:585–594.
5. Olsen, G. N., Block, A. J., Swenson, E. W., Castle, J. R., and Wynne, J. W. (1975): *Am. Rev. Respir. Dis.*, 111:379–387.

6. Rams, J. J., Harrison, L. W., Fry, W. A., Moulder, P. V., and Adams, W. E. (1962): *Dis. Chest*, 41:85–90.
7. Secker Walker, R. H., and Provan, J. L. (1969): *Br. Med. J.*, 3:327–330.
8. Stein, N., and Cassara, E. L. (1970): *J. A. M. A.*, 211:787–790.
9. Tisi, G. N. (1979): *Am. Rev. Respir. Dis.*, 119:293–310.
10. Van Nostrand, D., Kjelsberg, M. O., and Humphrey, E. W. (1968): *Surg. Gynecol. Obstet.*, 127:306–312.

Thoracic Oncology, edited by N. C. Choi and
H. C. Grillo. Raven Press, New York © 1983.

Surgery for Lung Cancer: The Massachusetts General Hospital Experience

Earle W. Wilkins, Jr. and Salvatore Saita

Department of Surgery, Harvard Medical School; and General Thoracic Surgical Unit and General Surgical Services, Massachusetts General Hospital, Boston, Massachusetts 02114

The role of surgery in the management of patients with primary carcinoma of the lung has conventionally been one of (a) diagnosis and (b) therapy. Surgical methods of diagnosis have included bronchoscopy, lymph node biopsy techniques, and exploratory thoracotomy. Therapeutic efforts have involved resectional techniques, from pneumonectomy to segmental or localized excisions. The technique of implantation of radiation-producing agents has not been used in this hospital. In the decade of the 1970s an added role for surgery has been its contribution to clinical staging. According to the Clinical Staging System for Carcinoma of the Lung (American Joint Committee for Cancer Staging and End-Results Reporting), clinical classification is based on the anatomic extent of disease, which may be detected by such surgical techniques as bronchoscopy, esophagoscopy, mediastinoscopy, mediastinotomy, thoracentesis, needle aspiration biopsy, and thoracoscopy.

This chapter will be concerned primarily with the development of surgery for carcinoma of the lung at the Massachusetts General Hospital (MGH), a teaching institution of more than 1,000 beds. It will include a thorough assessment of the results of resection in the four decades 1930–1970 and a description of more recent directions and developments in the past decade. We have recently seen the 50th anniversary of the first resection for carcinoma of the lung at MGH, a right lower lobectomy performed in 1930 by Dr. Edward D. Churchill, chief of surgical services. The first pneumonectomy, the first reported right pneumonectomy in America, was carried out in 1933 by Dr. Churchill. Other chapters in this volume will deal with extended methods of resection, including those for superior sulcus carcinomas (Chapter 8) and those involving the chest wall or diaphragm (Chapter 16). There has been considerable experience with both of these specific problems of lung carcinoma at MGH.

Facts to be recalled in the total comprehension of this chapter include the timing of introduction of mediastinoscopy as a diagnostic and staging tool and the development of a formal general thoracic teaching service. Prior to 1970 there had been fewer than a dozen mediastinoscopies. This technique has gradually received acceptance, more or less according to the indications of Pearson and associates (15). Although noncardiac thoracic surgery had been a very active facet of general surgery under Drs. Edward D. Churchill and Richard H. Sweet, a formal thoracic surgical unit was not established until 1973. These two developments have resulted in a more standardized application of surgical efforts, which will be presented in the final section.

SURGICAL EXPERIENCE 1930–1970

In the four decades spanning 1930 to 1970 a vast experience was accumulated at MGH with carcinoma of the lung. The World Health Organization classification (11) of primary lung carcinomas has served as the basis for pathologic subtyping: squamous cell, adeno-, large cell undifferentiated, small cell undifferentiated (including oat cell), and bronchoalveolar carcinomas. Excluded have been all cases of secondary carcinoma of the lung and specific primary tumors of the lower airway, including carcinoid adenoma, adenoid cystic carcinoma, and mucoepidermoid carcinoma. Now, a half century after the initial resection for carcinoma and 10 years following the final resection in that four-decade experience, it is pertinent to review the surgical statistics. The primary purpose of such a review is not to cite mere statistics but to search for progress in the application of such surgical experience in terms of increased survival during that era (17).

The total resection experience in the years 1930 to 1970 totals 820: 392 pneumonectomies, 419 lobectomies and 9 segmentectomies. The term *radical pneumonectomy* has been sufficiently confusing that it is not used in this analysis. Intrapericardial division of pulmonary artery and/or veins was accomplished only when the extent of the tumor so required. Peribronchial lymphadenectomy was, in general, carried out in both pneumonectomies and lobectomies; actual mediastinal lymph node dissection was done sufficiently infrequently to discount any impact.

The frequency with which pneumonectomy has been carried out has fallen with each decade of experience (Table 1). The principle of conservancy of parenchymal resection was practiced earlier at MGH than elsewhere nationally and was the topic of considerable adverse criticism in a 1950 article by Churchill and his colleagues (4). The percentage of 32 in the final of the four decades may indeed be anticipated to drop even further, perhaps to a range of 20% to 25%, but the size and extent of carcinoma should preclude further reduction so long as pneumonectomy is considered a reasonable operative technique. A major reason for conservancy of resection, in addition to retention of improved physiologic respiratory function, has been the increased risk of mortality in patients undergoing pneumonectomy. Allowing for

TABLE 1. *Incidence of pneumonectomy*

Decade	Pneumonectomy	All resections	Percent
1931–1940	23	31	73
1941–1950	116	182	63
1951–1960	145	271	54
1961–1970	108	336	32

From ref. 17, with permission of the publisher.

the high mortality from pneumonectomy in the developmental decade of the 1930s, there has been a surprisingly gradual and minimal decline in mortality between 1940 and 1970 (Table 2). One might have expected greater improvement in these figures considering the refinements in anesthesia and transfusion techniques and the introduction of antibiotics during the period. The unexpected rise in mortality from lobectomy in the 1960s (Table 3) may, in part, reflect utilization of that procedure in poorer-risk patients who in earlier decades would have undergone pneumonectomy or no resection at all. That particular trend merits scrutiny when the fifth decade of experience is available. An editorial comment is entered here: The risk of mortality should be maintained below 10% for pneumonectomy and 5% for lobectomy.

Mortality

More commonly in the literature on the statistics of resection for bronchogenic carcinoma, emphasis is placed on survival. Only infrequently are studies directed toward mortality. Hence, attention is devoted to operative mortality in the final decade of this review, the 1960s. Operative mortality is defined as death in the hospital, no matter how long after surgery in continuous hospitalization, or death anywhere within 30 days of resection. The causes of death in the 32 cases (12 pneumonectomy and 20 lobectomy patients) were determined from autopsy in 22 cases (69% autopsy rate) or by appraisal of the clinical record by an independent observer (a thoracic surgeon other than the operating surgeon). In each case, although the clinical course may have been complex, one principal cause of death was assigned (Table 4).

The deaths resulting from technical mishaps are considered preventable. Three resulted from postresection intrathoracic bleeding. In an effort to lessen this hazard,

TABLE 2. *Hospital mortality after pneumonectomy*

Decade	No. of cases	Hospital deaths	Mortality (%)
1931–1940	23	13	56.5
1941–1950	116	17	14.7
1951–1960	145	20	13.8
1961–1970	108	12	11.1

From ref. 17, with permission of the publisher.

TABLE 3. *Hospital mortality after lobectomy*

Decade	No. of cases	Hospital deaths	Mortality (%)
1931–1940	8	3	37.5
1941–1950	66	7	10.4
1951–1960	126	6	4.7
1961–1970	219	20	9.1

From ref. 17, with permission of the publisher.

TABLE 4. *Postresection mortality from carcinoma of the lung*

Pneumonia	7
Thromboembolism	6
Coronary artery disease	6
Technical[a]	5
Respiratory insufficiency	3
Cardiac failure	3
Cerebrovascular disease	2

[a]Hemorrhage 3, stump leak 1, prolapse right atrium 1.

recent trends have been toward oversewing of the stump of the main pulmonary artery in pneumonectomy patients rather than ligature techniques. (The stapler was not used in this institution.) It is noteworthy that there was only one fatal bronchial stump leak in the decade of 327 resections. All bronchial stumps were closed by interrupted nonabsorbable sutures, reinforced with a rotated flap of parietal pleura. The final death due to a technical problem, prolapse of the right atrium through a pericardial defect following right pneumonectomy, resulted in lacerations of both venae cavae. When a chest tube is used for postpneumonectomy drainage, it should not be placed on suction, particularly if the pericardium has been opened.

The principal cause of death for all other patients was cardiorespiratory, a fact that places appropriate emphasis on the preoperative evaluation of the cardiac and pulmonary systems. Postoperative pneumonia (5 cases occurring in pneumonectomy patients) was a particular hazard. The prophylactic use of antibiotics, vigorous preoperative and postoperative chest physiotherapy, and avoidance of aspiration are important considerations. Venous thromboembolic disease is more common than usually anticipated in this country. Clarke (6) emphasized the hazard of pulmonary emboli in the Coventry conference in 1973. Early ambulation is advisable. Anticoagulant therapy, although receiving increased attention, was not used routinely in this decade. There were three deaths resulting from postresection respiratory insufficiency. These, assessed as errors in judgment in advising surgery, call attention to the need for careful preoperative respiratory physiologic evaluation. Ventilation-perfusion scanning is proving particularly helpful in the succeeding decade. Finally, the 11 instances of cardiovascular deaths presumably reflect the fact that carcinoma of the lung is a disease of older people who tend, in significant numbers, to have simultaneous major cardiac disease. This requires close collaboration with the internist, cardiologist, and/or pulmonary physician.

Survival

The average age of the 820 patients at time of resection is presented in Table 5. Only in the category of males undergoing lobectomy has there been a statistically significant shift: approximately one-half decade of increase in age. There was a slight shift in distribution by sex: from 89% males prior to 1958 (5) to 82% in the

TABLE 5. Average patient age at resection[a]

Decade	Pneumonectomy		Lobectomy	
	Male	Female	Male	Female
1941–1950	58 (104)	62 (12)	58 (59)	62 (7)
1951–1960	59 (135)	59 (10)	61 (112)	61 (14)
1961–1970	60 (95)	54 (13)	64 (172)	59 (47)

From ref. 17, with permission of the publisher.
[a]Figures in parentheses are numbers of patients.

TABLE 6. Cumulative survival at 5 years

Decade	Pneumonectomy (%)	Lobectomy (%)	All resections (%)
1941–1950	26.7	37.9	30.7
1951–1960	25.5	27.8	26.6
1961–1970	24.0	32.8	29.5

From ref. 17, with permission of the publisher.

decade through 1970. The incidence of rate of resectability in patients undergoing thoracotomy increased from 64% prior to 1958 to 76% in the decade through 1970, this without any direct effort at clinical staging.

Cumulative survival for succeeding decades of experience in pulmonary resection is presented in Table 6. The initial decade of 23 resections, with a 56.5% hospital mortality, was not subjected to this analysis because of small numbers and a high risk in this "learning curve" aspect of resection. The overall 5-year survival for the three decades 1941–1970 was 28.9%. There was no improvement in survival following lung resection, for either lobectomy or pneumonectomy, in these decades. The statistics may then be viewed as a consistent and solid basis for comparison with any later cohort being managed in different fashion.

In addition, cumulative survival has been calculated for the extent of pulmonary resection versus carcinoma cell type and lymph node metastases. No attempt was made to distinguish the level of node involvement, whether bronchial, hilar, or mediastinal. These statistics are presented in Tables 7 and 8. The best results are obtainable in squamous cell carcinoma with negative lymph nodes, whether the resection be lobectomy or pneumonectomy (a total of 104 survivors at 5 years in 269 resections, or 38.7%). Lobectomy for other cell types, except small cell carcinoma, is equally effective provided the regional lymph nodes are negative (52 survivors at 5 years in 128 resections, or 40.6%). However, if lymph nodes are involved with carcinoma, in any cell type, or if pneumonectomy is necessary in the nonsquamous carcinoma groups, 5-year survival drops, rather precipitously. There were indeed 52 survivors in 237 resections for squamous carcinoma in which positive nodes were encountered, or 21.9%. (An indeterminate number received postresection mediastinal radiation, although this was not routine.) Finally, there

TABLE 7. Cumulative survival versus cell type after lobectomy

	Uninvolved nodes		Involved nodes	
	No.	%	No.	%
Squamous	60/158	38	13/76	17
Adenocarcinoma	19/61	31	4/31	13
Undifferentiated	22/46	48	4/20	20
Alveolar cell	11/21	52	0/1	0
Small cell	0/2	0	0/4	0

From ref. 17, with permission of the publisher.

TABLE 8. Cumulative survival versus cell type after
pneumonectomy

	Uninvolved nodes		Involved nodes	
	No.	%	No.	%
Squamous	44/111	40	39/161	24
Adenocarcinoma	3/18	17	2/38	5
Undifferentiated	2/11	18	2/31	6
Alveolar cell	0/2	0	0/2	0
Small cell	2/3	67	0/15	0

From ref. 17, with permission of the publisher.

were only 4 survivors in 86 pneumonectomy operations in the nonsquamous car-cinomas with positive lymph nodes, only 4.7%. Lymph node metastasis continues to be the most ominous predictor of potential survival after pulmonary resection for carcinoma.

STAGING

In 1973 the American Joint Committee for Cancer Staging and End-Results Reporting produced an acceptable clinical staging system for carcinoma of the lung (1). The principle of the TNM system has been used, in which the letter T represents the primary tumor, with separate numerals describing increasing size and/or exten-sion of tumor; the letter N represents lymph node involvement, with numbers indicating absence of metastasis or degree of involvement; the letter M represents distant metastasis, with numbers representing the absence or presence thereof only.

In order to provide an accurate and thorough understanding of clinical staging, a verbatim description of the T, N, and M categories is presented here (Table 9). Each case is assigned the highest category of T, N, and M that describes the full extent of the disease. The stage grouping then becomes as follows:

Stage   I: T1 N0 M0, T1 N1 M0, or T2 N0 M0
Stage   II: T2 N1 M0 (ipsilateral nodes only)
Stage III: T3 with any N or M
           N2 with any T or M
           M1 with any T or N

TABLE 9. *Definitions of T, N, and M categories for carcinoma of the lung[a]*

T: Primary tumors

   T0   No evidence of primary tumor.

   TX   Tumor proven by the presence of malignant cells in bronchopulmonary secretions but not visualized roentgenographically or bronchoscopically.

   T1   A tumor that is 3.0 cm or less in greatest diameter, surrounded by lung or visceral pleura and without evidence of invasion proximal to a lobar bronchus at bronchoscopy.

   T2   A tumor more than 3.0 cm in greatest diameter, or a tumor of any size that, with its associated atelectasis or obstructive pneumonitis, extends to the hilar region. At bronchoscopy the proximal extent of demonstrable tumor must be at least 2.0 cm distal to the carina. Any associated atelectasis or obstructive pneumonitis must involve less than an entire lung, and there must be no pleural effusion.

   T3   A tumor of any size with direct extension into an adjacent structure such as the chest wall, the diaphragm, or the mediastinum and its contents, or demonstrable bronchoscopically to be less than 2.0 cm distal to the carina; any tumor associated with atelectasis or obstructive pneumonitis of an entire lung or pleural effusion.

N: Regional lymph nodes

   N0   No demonstrable metastasis to regional lymph nodes.

   N1   Metastasis to lymph nodes in the ipsilateral hilar region (including direct extension).

   N2   Metastasis to lymph nodes in the mediastinum.

M: Distant metastasis

   M0   No distant metastasis.

   M1   Distant metastasis such as in scalene, cervical, or contralateral hilar lymph nodes, brain, bones, lung, liver, etc.

From ref. 1, with permission.
[a]Each case must be assigned the highest category of T, N, and M that describes the full extent of disease in that case.

An operative-pathologic staging can be developed after resection. This provides an often useful skill tool in assessing purely clinical evaluation or staging that, by custom, is permitted to include information before definitive treatment is instituted. Thus, as stated earlier, endoscopic techniques of bronchoscopy, esophagoscopy, mediastinoscopy and thoracoscopy, anterior mediastinotomy, thoracentesis and/or needle aspiration biopsy, and bronchial brushing may be used in clinical staging.

DIAGNOSIS

Preoperative diagnosis is accomplished whenever possible using one or more of the customary techniques: sputum cytology, bronchoscopy, bronchial brushing, and needle aspiration biopsy. The yield of positive diagnosis by cytologic methods depends on techniques and timing of material collection. The likelihood of nonbronchoscopic cytologic diagnosis is enhanced by sputum collection at the time of chest physiotherapy (introduced at MGH in 1959) and by submission of freshly collected specimens to the cytology laboratory.

When bronchoscopy is carried out, the specimen most likely to provide cytologic diagnosis is the initial postbronchoscopy coughed sputum. The yield of bronchoscopic histologic diagnoses is enhanced, in turn, by the use of both rigid and fiberoptic flexible techniques. The Storz lens magnification has been particularly helpful in locating small or unsuspected endobronchial carcinoma. Groups at Johns Hopkins Hospital (2) and the Mayo Clinic (7) have been active in applying these techniques to the prospective evaluation of individuals at unusually high risk for bronchogenic carcinoma.

The techniques of bronchial brushing and needle aspiration biopsy, both for cytologic determination, have been used primarily under fluoroscopic guidance and have therefore become radiologic methods of diagnosis. Success with needle aspiration as a definitive method for presurgical diagnosis has been particularly gratifying. Greene et al. (8) at MGH have reported an almost 95% positive statistic in patients ultimately proved to have primary carcinoma of the lung, using the Nordenstrom needle aspiration technique.

The variety of methods by which lymph node metastases can be assessed preoperatively merit particular emphasis. Conventional mediastinoscopy is most commonly practiced according to the original technique of Carlens (3). By this method, access is possible in peritracheal planes along both sides of the trachea, into the subcarinal area, and on to the proximal segments of both main bronchi, thus to sample pretracheal, paratracheal, subcarinal, and proximal bronchial lymph nodes. Pearson (14) has pointed out three distinct lymph node groups that are not accessible to mediastinoscopic biopsy: anterior mediastinal, posterior subcarinal, and subaortic. The direction of the trachea takes one into the middle mediastinum during mediastinoscopy; the left innominate vein precludes getting far enough anteriorly to gain access to the anterior mediastinum. Posterior subcarinal nodes are accessible only at thoracotomy; however, their presence may be suspected by extrinsic compression visible at esophagoscopy or at barium esophagogram. Subaortic node access requires left anterior mediastinotomy or transpleural minithoracotomy. Transpleural access to parenchymal lung carcinoma is possible at mediastinoscopy by deliberate transgression of the mediastinal pleura; this may be useful for histologic proof of diagnosis in carcinomas located against the suprahilar mediastinal pleura. McNeill and Chamberlain (13) introduced the concept of access to the anterior and middle mediastinum by an anterior parasternal approach. This can be carried out on either side, most often resecting the second costal cartilage, although the approach may be conducted intercostally using the mediastinoscope. The so-called Chamberlain technique is an extrapleural approach to the mediastinal lymph-node-bearing area. On the right side the dissection is carried out medial to the superior vena cava. More commonly, a direct transpleural approach is now used in the so-called modified Chamberlain or anterior minithoracotomy. This provides particularly good access to the subaortic area on the left and allows a route to the right paratracheal nodes from lateral to the superior vena cava. Direct lung biopsy is easily performed for anteriorly placed tumors, i.e., in anterior segments of the upper lobes. The mediastinoscope can be used to reach more remotely placed tumors.

In a consideration of routes of lymph node metastasis as originally presented by Rouvière (16), one need sample only subcarinal and both paratracheal lymph nodes in staging carcinomas of the left lower lobe; in this situation, thorough staging requires either mediastinoscopy or bilateral mediastinotomy. For carcinoma of the left upper lobe, the principal area to be investigated is the subaortic group of nodes, which can be reached only by left anterior mediastinotomy, not mediastinoscopy. In carcinomas of the right lung, it is less important to check for left paratracheal node involvement, although mediastinoscopy provides this opportunity, which ipsilateral mediastinotomy alone does not.

Among thoracic surgeons there is wide variance in practice relative to surgical staging techniques and indications therefor. There is agreement that large, centrally placed tumors, ones that likely would require pneumonectomy and ones that have adenopathy visible by mediastinal tomographic X-rays, should be investigated by these staging techniques. If the histologic nature of the primary tumor is known, as by sputum cytology, bronchoscopy, or needle aspiration biopsy, all but the squamous carcinomas require surgical staging. This is because lymph node metastases in the nonsquamous groups connote an ominous prognosis, no matter what the size or location of the primary carcinoma. The finding of a metatasis to any lymph node in any location in small cell carcinoma is an indication of inoperability. I (EWW) believe that a squamous cell carcinoma that can be resected by lobectomy does not require mediastinoscopy if tomograms do not suggest adenopathy. The unexpected finding of positive nodes in this circumstance may logically be managed by postresection mediastinal radiation.

The risks of mediastinoscopy must be counted. It is not a procedure without hazard, particularly in the hands of the uninitiated. The principal risk is bleeding. All nodes should be aspirated prior to biopsy. The azygos vein is the structure most liable to inadvertent biopsy. Azygos or other venous hemorrhage usually is controllable by pressure. Systemic arterial bleeding, on the other hand, usually requires median sternotomy for control. The possibility of pneumothorax should be checked by a postmediastinoscopy chest film. Infection is uncommon, but there has been one instance of clostridial mediastinitis in the MGH experience. In patients with achalasia or other esophageal dilatation, care must be taken in subcarinal node biopsy; esophagomediastinal fistula has resulted from inadvertent esophageal trauma thereby.

Finally, a comment is necessary relative to the place for supraclavicular or scalene node biopsy. The only indication is palpable adenopathy in that area. Cervicomediastinal exploration as described by Harken et al. (9) has largely been replaced by mediastinoscopy and mediastinotomy.

SURGICAL EXPERIENCE 1971–1979

An incomplete analysis of the surgical management of carcinoma of the lung in the decade of the 1970s is presented as one method of counting the changes in the present-day approach in comparison with the earlier four decades of experience. The principal difference has been the acceptance of surgical staging as a significant indicator of operability. Other major changes include (a) the development of a noncardiac, general thoracic service with residency training program, (b) improved preoperative physiologic determination of patient competence to tolerate pulmonary resection, including exercise tolerance evaluation and ventilation-perfusion scanning, and (c) the provision of postoperative intensive care in the respiratory unit as long as required and then intermediate-level attention in a specialized thoracic surgical unit.

No detailed protocol is used for surgical staging. In fact, there have been substantial theoretical differences in indications for mediastinoscopy among the five thoracic surgeons involved. The principal difference has involved the need for the procedure in peripheral lesions, one that could be presumed to be manageable by lobectomy. Here, perhaps the significant differences in approach concerned the capability of mediastinal tomographic roentgenographic study to assess mediastinal adenopathy. Agreed indications for mediastinoscopy, often with left anterior mediastinotomy for left upper lobe lesions, now include (a) radiologic definition of mediastinal adenopathy, (b) central tumors, (c) any tumor likely to require pneumonectomy, (d) tumors greater than 5 cm in maximal diameter in any location, (e) superior sulcus tumors, and (f) small cell undifferentiated or oat cell carcinomas. Standard so-called categoric contraindications to resection, except for specific palliation, have eliminated the necessity for mediastinoscopy except to obtain pathologic histologic sections; these contraindications include bloody or cytologically positive pleural effusion, recurrent nerve involvement, main bronchial extension by carcinoma within 1 cm of the carina, angiocardiographic involvement of the pulmonary artery within 1.5 cm of its origin from the main pulmonary truncus (12), postoperative respiratory expectation of an FEV_1 less than 800 cc (10), carcinomatous involvement of ribs to the articulation with vertebral bodies, and any distant metastasis.

From the beginning of 1971 to mid-1979 there were 417 cases of primary lung carcinoma seen by the general thoracic or the teaching general surgical services. Of these, 268 (64.3%) were subjected to surgical staging; 149 (35.7%) were not. The exact method of surgical staging is presented in Table 10. The types of carcinoma encountered in the 88 patients found by these operative studies to be in the N2 category are presented in Table 11. Thus, there were 180 staged patients who had negative nodes at operative staging (Table 12).

The total of 88 patients categorized as N2 by surgical staging and the 162 staged patients subjected to thoracotomy provided 250 patients for comparison of radiologic and postsurgical staging processes. Thus, of the 250 such patients, 106 ultimately were found to have N2 lesions (42.4%). Eighteen patients were found to have mediastinal tumor-involved nodes despite negative mediastinoscopy and/or mediastinotomy (11.1% false negative). Eight of these false negative patients were among those who had left upper lobe carcinomas subjected to mediastinoscopy

TABLE 10. *Surgical staging*

Procedure	No. of patients	
Mediastinoscopy	201	
Negative	153	(76.1%)
Positive	48	(23.9%)
Mediastinotomy (modified		
Chamberlain technique)	34	
Negative	5	(14.7%)
Positive	29	(85.3%)
Mediastinoscopy and mediastinotomy	33	
Negative	22	(66.7%)
Positive	11[a]	(33.3%)

[a]In 10 of these, the carcinoma lay in the LUL.

TABLE 11. *Types of carcinoma in N_2 patients*

Ca type	No. of patients
Oat cell	28
Adenocarcinoma	21
Squamous	20
Undifferentiated	17
Bronchoalveolar	2
	(88)

TABLE 12. *Fate of negative mediastinoscopy/mediastinotomy patients*

Procedure	No. of patients
Thoracotomy	162
Exploration/biopsy	16 (9.9%)
Lobectomy	104 (64.2%)
Pneumonectomy	42 (25.9%)
No thoracotomy[a]	18
	(342)

[a]Reasons: inadequate pulmonary function (8), oat cell carcinoma otherwise detected (4), distant metastases (4), and T_3 tumors (2).

only. There were 68 patients called negative by roentgenographic study who ultimately were positive at postsurgical staging, a false negative X-ray rate of 27.2%.

In the group of 149 nonstaged patients, all lesions were resectable, 127 by lobectomy and 22 by pneumonectomy. It is not possible to tell in all cases, but it is presumed that lobectomy had been intended preoperatively in the 22 who had pneumonectomy. The types of carcinoma encountered in these 149 cases are presented in Table 13.

In this subset, there were 17 patients found to have N2 nodal involvement at postsurgical staging, an incidence of 11.4%. Of these, 4 patients had been judged to have positive nodes by radiologic assay, leaving 13 that can then be called false negatives by radiologic methods of survey (9%).

Further statistical evaluation of the MGH experience in the decade of the 1970s will be available at the completion of the half century of resectional experience ending in 1980.

DISCUSSION

A number of conclusions can be drawn from the MGH experience in the surgical management of carcinoma of the lung.

First, perhaps most conclusive, is the fact that there has been no improvement in the cumulative survival of patients undergoing pulmonary resection for bronchogenic carcinoma in the three decades 1941 to 1970. If there is to be an improved survival for the most recent decade, it may well be the result of preoperative clinical staging. Such a phenomenon would not necessarily represent an overall advance in survival of patients with carcinoma of the lung, because the overall resectability rate would necessarily decline.

Second is the well-known fact that, in general, patients with squamous cell carcinoma have a better chance for long-term survival than patients with other carcinoma cell types. This is particularly true if the hilar/mediastinal lymph nodes are positive for carcinoma. The suggestion is that postsurgical radiation therapy is a major factor. There has been no evidence that preoperative radiation enhances survival.

The third finding is that there is continuing need for monitoring mortality from pulmonary resections. The particular focus of this monitoring comes in preoperative physiologic evaluation in terms of respiratory function and cardiovascular stability. Postoperative attention must be continually directed to prevention of pneumonia and pulmonary emboli.

Clinical staging using mediastinoscopy and/or mediastinotomy is a clear advance in determining patient curability. The exact indications of when these staging pro-

TABLE 13. *Histologic carcinoma, nonstaged patients*

Ca type	No. of patients
Adenocarcinoma	64
Squamous	57
Bronchoalveolar	14
Undifferentiated (large cell)	13
Oat cell	1
	(149)

cedures are indicated are not that clear. Patients with peripheral carcinomas and negative mediastinal silhouettes by tomography probably do not require staging. This is especially true if the tumor is known by sputum cytology or needle biopsy to be squamous cell carcinoma.

Finally, surgery, although effective in a certain definable group of patients with carcinoma of the lung, cannot help the vast majority afflicted with this malignancy. The two avenues for further improvement in patient survival remain prevention and the development of another parameter of treatment, such as chemotherapy or immunotherapy.

REFERENCES

1. Anderson, W. A. D., and Carr, D. T. (1973): *Clinical Staging System for Carcinoma of the Lung.* American Joint Committee for Cancer Staging and End-Results Reporting, Chicago.
2. Baker, R. R., Tockman, M. S., Marsh, B. R., Stitik, F. P., Ball, W. C., Jr., Eggleston, J. C., Erozan, Y. S., Levin, M. L., and Frost, J. K. (1979): Screening for bronchogenic carcinoma, the surgical experience. *J. Thorac. Cardiovasc. Surg.*, 78:876.
3. Carlens, E. (1959): Mediastinoscopy: A method for inspection and tissue biopsy in the superior mediastinum. *Dis. Chest*, 36:343.
4. Churchill, E. D., Sweet, R. H., Soutter, L., and Scannell, J. G. (1950): The surgical management of carcinoma of the lung. *J. Thorac. Surg.*, 20:349.
5. Churchill, E. D., Sweet, R. H., Scannell, J. G., and Wilkins, E. W., Jr. (1958): Further studies in the surgical management of carcinoma of the lung. *J. Thorac. Surg.*, 36:301.
6. Clarke, D. B. (1974): Pulmonary embolism after lung surgery. In: *Surgery of the Lung, The Coventry Conference*, edited by R. E. Smith and W. G. Williams, p. 252. Butterworths, London.
7. Fontanna, R. S., Sanderson, D. R., Woolner, L. B., Miller, W. E., Bernatz, P. E., Paine, W. S., and Taylor, W. F. (1975): The Mayo Lung Project for early detection and localization of bronchogenic carcinoma. A status report. *Chest*, 67:511.
8. Greene, R. E. (1982): Transthoracic needle aspiration biopsy. In: *Interventional Radiology*, edited by C. A. Athanasoulis, R. E. Green, R. C. Pfisteo, and G. H. Roberson. W. B. Saunders, Philadelphia.
9. Harken, D. E., Black, H., Claus, R., and Farrand, R. E. (1954): Simple cervicomediastinal exploration for tissue diagnosis of intrathoracic disease: With comments on recognition of inoperable carcinoma of the lung. *N. Engl. J. Med.*, 251:1041.
10. Kanarek, D. J.: *(This volume.)*
11. Kreyberg, L. (1967): *Histologic Typing of Lung Tumors.* World Health Organization, Geneva.
12. Maruyama, Y., Wilkins, E. W., Jr., and Wyman, S. M. (1962): Evaluation of angiocardiography in pulmonary carcinoma with particular emphasis on prognosis. *Radiology*, 79:617.
13. McNeill, T. M., and Chamberlain, J. M. (1966): Diagnostic anterior mediastinotomy. *Ann. Thorac. Surg.*, 2:532.
14. Pearson, F. G. (1968): An evaluation of mediastinoscopy in the management of presumably operable bronchial carcinoma. *J. Thorac. Cardiovasc. Surg.*, 55:617.
15. Pearson, F. G., Nelems, J. M., Henderson, R. D., and Delarue, N. C. (1972): The role of mediastinoscopy in the selection of treatment for bronchial carcinoma with involvement of superior mediastinal lymph nodes. *J. Thorac. Cardiovasc. Surg.*, 64:382.
16. Rouvière, H. (1938): *Anatomy of the Human Lymphatic System* (*Anatomie des Lymphatiques de l'Homme*), translated by M. J. Tobias. Edwards, Ann Arbor.
17. Wilkins, E. W., Jr., Scannell, J. G., and Craver, J. G. (1978): Four decades of experience with resections for bronchogenic carcinoma at the Massachusetts General Hospital. *J. Thorac. Cardiovasc. Surg.*, 76:364.

Thoracic Oncology, edited by N. C. Choi and
H. C. Grillo. Raven Press, New York © 1983.

Role of Postoperative Radiation Therapy in Lung Cancer with Either Metastases to Regional Lymph Nodes (N_1 or Unforeseen N_2) or Direct Invasion beyond Visceral Pleura (T_3)

Noah C. Choi

*Department of Radiation Therapy, Harvard Medical School, and Department of Radiation
Medicine, Massachusetts General Hospital, Boston, Massachusetts 02114*

INTRODUCTION

The interpretation of some data from previous studies (2,23,30) has been incomplete concerning the role of postoperative radiation therapy in the management of patients with resectable carcinoma of the lung. Clarification of these data is urgently needed in light of the prognostic factors defined in more recent studies (4,9,18,19,22,25,28,31). The incidence of involvement of the regional lymph nodes by metastatic carcinoma of the lung has been in the range of 30% to 60% in surgical series, even after thorough staging work-ups including mediastinoscopy (25,31). Autopsy studies have also provided some interesting data showing that the incidence of residual or recurrent non-small cell carcinoma in the mediastinal lymph nodes was 52% (38/72) for patients who had survived for more than 1 month after curative surgery (29), whereas it was only 25% for patients with squamous cell carcinoma when a similar study was done within 1 month after such surgery (21). The fate of patients with positive regional lymph nodes or incomplete surgical resection of the margin has been very poor, with a 5-year survival rate of 0% to 20%. This rate is far lower than the cure rate of 30% to 40% when there is no involvement of the regional lymph nodes or when the resection margins are free of tumor (4,22,25,28,31).

It has been very well demonstrated that radiation therapy is capable of sterilizing carcinoma of the lung at the primary site and the regional lymph nodes when the radiation dose is high, i.e., 5000 to 6000 cGy (TDF 82–99) (5,6,7). Therefore, carefully planned radiation therapy with a moderately high dose (5400–5600 cGy, TDF 89–92) of radiation should be able to convert a surgical resection from incomplete to complete by sterilizing residual microscopic carcinoma at the tumor bed and the regional lymph nodes.

TABLE 1.

TNM Classification	Definitions[a]

Primary Tumor (T)

TX Tumor proven by the presence of malignant cells in bronchopulmonary secretions but not visualized roentgenographically or bronchoscopically, or any tumor that cannot be assessed

T0 No evidence of primary tumor

TIS Carcinoma *in situ*

T1 Tumor 3.0 cm or less in greatest diameter, surrounded by lung or visceral pleura, and without evidence of invasion proximal to a lobar bronchus at bronchoscopy

T2 Tumor more than 3.0 cm in greatest diameter, or a tumor of any size that either invades the visceral pleura or has associated atelectasis or obstructive pneumonitis extending to the hilar region. At bronchoscopy, the proximal extent of demonstrable tumor must be within a lobar bronchus or at least 2.0 cm distal to the carina. Any assoicated atelectasis or obstructive pneumonitis must involve less than an entire lung and there must be no pleural effusion

T3 Tumor of any size with direct extension into an adjacent structure such as the parietal pleura or the chest wall, the diaphragm, or the mediastinum and its contents; or a tumor demonstrable bronchoscopically to involve a main bronchus less than 2.0 cm distal to the carina; or any tumor associated with atelectasis or obstructive pneumonitis of an entire lung or pleural effusion

Nodal Involvement (N)

N0 No demonstrable metastasis to regional lymph nodes

N1 Metastasis to lymph nodes in the peribronchial or the ipsilateral hilar region, or both, including direct extension

N2 Metastasis to lymph nodes in the mediastinum

Distant Metastasis (M)

MX Not assessed

M0 No (known) distant metastasis

M1 Distant metastasis present

Specify sites according to the following notations:

Pulmonary–PUL	Hepatic–HEP	Lymph Nodes–LYM	Skin–SKI	Eye–EYE
Osseous–OSS	Brain–BRA	Bone Marrow–MAR	Pleura–PLE	Other–OTH

Histopathology

Squamous cell carcinoma, adenocarcinoma, undifferentiated large cell, undifferentiated small cell (oat cell cancer)

REAPPRAISAL OF PREVIOUS STUDIES

Critical review of previous studies is very important for further study of the role of postoperative radiation therapy in managing patients with positive regional lymph nodes or incomplete resection margins. These studies must be analyzed thoroughly with respect to the extent of the tumor (TNM stage), histologic types of the tumor, radiation doses, target volume, and radiation-therapy techniques on which the success or failure of treatment depends (1,9). They can be categorized into three groups according to the stages of the tumor or surgical procedures (Tables 1 and 2).

TABLE 1. *(continued)*

TNM Classification		Definitions[a]
Grade		
Well-differentiated, moderately well-differentiated, poorly to very differentiated, or numbers 1, 2, 3, 4		
Stage grouping		
Occult stage	TX N0 M0	Occult carcinoma with bronchopulmonary secretions containing malignant cells but without other evidence of the primary tumor or evidence of metastasis to the regional lymph nodes or distant metastasis
Stage I	TIS N0 M0	Carcinoma *in situ*
	T1 N0 M0 T1 N1 M0 T2 N0 M0[b]	Tumor that can be classified T1 without any metastasis or with metastasis to the lymph nodes in the peribronchial and/or ipsilateral hilar region only, or a tumor that can be classified T2 without any metastasis to nodes or distant metastasis
Stage II	T2 N1 M0	Tumor classified as T2 with metastasis to the lymph nodes in the peribronchial and/or ipsilateral hilar region only
Stage III	T3 with any N or M N2 with any T or M M1 with any T or N	Any tumor more extensive than T2, or any tumor with metastasis to the lymph nodes in the mediastinum, or any tumor with distant metastasis

[a]TNM classification system recommended by the American Joint Committee for Cancer Staging and End-Results Reporting (1).
[b]TX N1 M0 and T0 N1 M0 are also theoretically possible, but such a clinical diagnosis would be difficult if not impossible to make. If such a diagnosis is made, it should be included under stage I.

Postoperative Radiation Therapy for Patients with Early Stages ($T_{1-2}N_0M_0$) of Carcinoma of the Lung

The studies by Van Houtte et al. (30) and Bangma (2) dealt primarily with early stages ($T_{1-2}N_0M_0$) of squamous cell carcinoma of the lung. Postoperative radiation therapy did not effect improvement of survival. Instead, there was a high rate of pulmonary complications related to the radiotherapeutic techniques used. The preliminary report by Israel et al. (15) also showed that patients with early stages (N_0 lesions) of squamous cell carcinoma of the lung did not benefit from radiation therapy with or without chemotherapy and BCG.

TABLE 2. Results of post-operative radiation therapy in selected previous studies

Authors	Stage of Tumors	S	S+RT	Histologic Types	S	S+RT	Radiation Therapy Techniques, Radiation Doses (cGy) and Target Volumes		Survival (%) 1	3	5 yrs.
Paterson & Russell (1955–1958) (23)				Sq Cell Ca	63	64	3-field approach (AP, RPO, LPO) with 10 x 5 cm² field size 4500/3 wk by 4 MeV photon Hilum and adjacent mediastinum	S	–	36.4	–
				Anaplastic	24	26		S+RT	–	38	–
				Ad Ca	5	9					
				Others	1	2					
				No Report	6	2					
Bangma (1958) (2)	$T_{1-2}N_{-}M_{-}$	28	27	Sq Cell Ca	29	27	Rotation or 2--4-field approach 4370-4640/5-5.6 wk Hilum and ipsilateral adjacent mediastinum (small volume)	S	62	–	–
	$T_{1-2}N_1M_0$	7		Small Cell	3	4		S+RT	53	–	–
	$T_{1-2}N_2M_0$	2	5	Large Cell	5	4					
				Ad Ca	0	1					
Green et al (1954–1966) (14)	$T_{1-2}N_0M_0$	64	59	(N_{1-2} groups) Sq Cell Ca	16	28	4400 (3000-6000)/4.4 wk Hilum, mediastinum and supraclavicular areas	S	–	–	22
	$T_{1-2}N_1M_0$ (64)			Ad Ca	6	16		$S+RT(T_{1-2}N_0M_0)$	–	–	27
	$T_{1-2}N_2M_0$ (32)		66	Anaplastic	8	22		S	–	–	3
								$S+RT(T_{1-2}N_{1-2}M_0)$	–	–	35
Kirsh et al (1959–1969) (18)	$T_{1-2}N_2M_0$	20	69	All types			5000-5500/5-5.5 wk Hilum and mediastinum	S	–	–	0
								S+RT	–	–	23
Van Houtte et al (1966–1975) (30)	TNM	39	33	Sq Cell Ca	61	56	3 field approach (AP, RPO, LPO) with 15 x 9 cm² field size 6000/6 wk by Co-60 unit Hilum and mediastinum	S	–	–	43
	$T_2N_0M_0$	39	15	Large Cell	9	6		S+RT	–	–	24
	$T_3N_0M_0$	3	3	Small Cell	7	7					
				Ad Ca	13	14					
				Sarcoma	2	0					
Choi et al (1971–1977) (9)	$T_{1-2}N_1M_0$	38	43	Sq Cell Ca	29	46	AP, PA (3600) plus AP, RPO and LPO (2000) for postlobectomy pts. AP, PA (4400) plus AP, PA oblique opposing portals (1000-1200) for postpneumonectomy pts. 4000-5600/4-5.6 wk+ Hilum, entire mediastinum and both supraclavicular areas	S ⎤ Sq Cell Ca	–	–	33
	$T_{1-2}N_2M_0$	6	25	Ad Ca	21	40		S+RT ⎦	–	–	34++
	$T_3N_0M_0$	6	13	Large Cell and Undiff. Ca	5	7		S ⎤ Ad Ca	–	–	8
	$T_3N_1M_0$	5	9					S+RT ⎦	–	–	43
	$T_3N_2M_0$	0	3								
Israel et al (1973–1976) (15)	N_0	76	66	Sq Cell Ca only			4500-5500/4.5-5.5 wk to tumor bed and mediastinum. Chemotherapy and BCG were also given to most patients.	S ⎤ (N_{1-2} only)	45	–	–
	N_{1-2}	50	38					S+RT ⎦	67	–	–

+ = range of radiation doses used during the study. All local and regional recurrences occurred with a dose of ≤5000 cGy (TDF 82). ++ = for the group with squamous cell carcinoma, there was no improvement of survival after postoperative radiation therapy. However, the following should be considered: in 27% (8/29) of S vs 52% (24/46) of S + RT group, the tumor was in N_2 or T_3 stage.

Postoperative Radiation Therapy as an Adjuvant Therapy after Pneumonectomy

The trial by Paterson and Russell (23) is unique in being the only study that was designed to evaluate the role of postoperative radiation therapy after pneumonectomy. Unfortunately, the stage of the tumor, the most important prognostic factor in carcinoma of the lung, was neither entered into the categories of randomization nor included in the analysis of the results. Another weakness of this study was that the target volume was too small to include most of the regional lymph nodes. Because there was no difference in survival statistics between the study and control groups at 3 years, one can state that there is no role for routine postoperative radiation therapy after pneumonectomy for patients with squamous cell or anaplastic carcinoma of the lung.

Postoperative Radiation Therapy for Patients with Resectable but Locally Advanced Carcinoma of the Lung (N_1, Unforeseen N_2, or T_3 Tumors)

The studies by Green et al. (14), Kirsh et al. (18), Choi et al. (9), and Lewin et al. (19) are important and interesting in that all four show significant improvement of survival by postoperative radiation therapy. The radiotherapeutic techniques used in these studies were different from others in that the target volume was large enough to include most of the mediastinal lymph nodes, including those at the thoracic inlet, and radiation doses were at ≥5000 cGy (TDF ≥ 82). Another significant aspect of these studies is the lack of serious pulmonary complications, attributable to the fact that most of the radiation doses were delivered by AP–PA

TABLE 3. *Performance status (Karnofsky scale) (16)*

Criteria of performance status (PS)		
Able to carry on normal activity; no special care is needed	100	Normal; no complaints; no evidence of disease
	90	Able to carry on normal activity; minor signs or symptoms of disease
	80	Normal activity with effort; some signs or symptoms of disease
Unable to work; able to live at home and care for most personal needs; a varying amount of assistance is needed	70	Cares for self; unable to carry on normal activity or to do active work
	60	Requires occasional assistance but is able to care for most of his needs
	50	Requires considerable assistance and frequent medical care
Unable to care for self; requires equivalent of institutional or hospital care; disease may be progressing rapidly	40	Disabled; requires special care and assistance
	30	Severely disabled; hospitalization is indicated although death not imminent
	20	Very sick; hospitalization necessary; active supportive treatment is necessary
	10	Moribund; fatal processes progressing rapidly
	0	Dead

TABLE 4. *Performance status (Zubrod scale) (33)*

Grade
0—Fully active, able to carry on all predisease activities without restriction (Karnofsky, 90–100)
1—Restricted in physically strenuous activity but ambulatory and able to carry out work of a light or sedentary nature. For example, light housework, office work (Karnofsky, 70–80)
2—Ambulatory and capable of all self-care but unable to carry out any work activities. Up and about more than 50% of waking hours (Karnofsky, 50–60)
3—Capable of only limited self-care, confined to bed or chair 50% or more of waking hours (Karnofsky, 30–40)
4—Completely disabled. Cannot carry on any self-care. Totally confined to bed or chair (Karnofsky, 10–20)

TABLE 5. *Guidelines of pulmonary functional reserve for postoperative radiation therapy (10)*

Parameters	Values[a]	
FEV_1	≥1.25 l	(≥45% predicted)
VC	≥1.75 l	(≥45% predicted)
MBC	≥45 l/min	(≥40% predicted)
PaO_2	≥70 mm Hg	
$PaCO_2$	≤42 mm Hg	

[a]These values are based on data of pulmonary-function studies obtained in 30 patients at 4 weeks after surgery.
FEV_1 = first-second vital capacity; VC = vital capacity; MBC = maximal breathing capacity; PaO_2 = partial pressure of oxygen of arterial blood; $PaCO_2$ = partial pressure of carbon dioxide of arterial blood; l = liter.

parallel opposing portals instead of an outright three-field approach (AP–RPO–LPO) or rotational techniques used by others (2,30) in the early stages of carcinoma of the lung associated with high rates of pulmonary complications. Histologic types of carcinoma of the lung also seem to play a role, inasmuch as the benefit of postoperative radiation therapy was larger for patients with adenocarcinoma than it was for those with squamous cell carcinoma (9,19,20).Unfortunately, all these studies suffer from the drawback of retrospective study, and there is an urgent need for prospective randomized studies for this particular group of patients.

In the preliminary report by Israel et al. (15) patients with positive lymph nodes (squamous cell carcinoma) who received adjuvant postoperative radiation therapy with or without chemotherapy and BCG also showed a tendency for improved relapse-free survival when compared with controls: at 60 weeks the relapse-free rate was 66% versus 45% for surgery with radiotherapy versus surgery alone. However, a follow-up study is necessary to draw any meaningful conclusions.

TABLE 6. *Pattern of failure in patients with squamous cell carcinoma (9)*

Sites of failure	Surgery	Surgery + RT
Reg. rec. only	11 (65%)	7 (32%)
Reg. rec. + distant mets.	0	3
Reg. rec. + brain	1	0
Reg. rec. + brain + distant mets.	1	0
Distant mets. only	3	6
Brain only	0	2
Other med. conditions	1	4
Total	17	22

RT = radiation therapy.
Reg. rec. = regional recurrence.

TABLE 7. *Pattern of failure in patients with adenocarcinoma (9)*

Sites of failure	Surgery		Surgery + RT	
Brain only	4 ⎫	(27%)	8 ⎫	(42%)
Brain + distant mets.	3 ⎬	(53%)	3 ⎬	(58%)
Brain + reg. rec.	1 ⎭		0 ⎭	
Reg. rec. only	2		0	
Reg. rec. + distant mets.	1		3	
Distant mets. only	3		4	
Other med. conditions	1		1	
Total	15		19	

RT = radiation therapy.
Reg. rec. = regional recurrence.

INDICATIONS

Postoperative radiation therapy is recommended for patients with positive regional lymph nodes (N_1, unforeseen N_2 lesions) or with incomplete resection of the tumor margins because of the invasion of the tumor beyond the pulmonary parenchyma and visceral pleura to the chest wall, mediastinal structures, carina, or diaphragm (T_3 lesions) (9,12,13,14,17–19,27). Because of the potential pulmonary injury associated with this treatment, patients should be carefully screened for their ability to tolerate the therapy and adequate pulmonary-function reserve before they are subjected to a course of 5.5 to 6 weeks of radiation therapy. Work-ups recommended for distant metastasis include radioisotope scans of the liver and bone, computed tomographic scan of the brain, liver-function studies, and carcinoembryonic antigen (CEA) (11), if these tests were not done before surgery. It is important that patients with a high risk of becoming pulmonary cripples after postoperative radiation therapy be identified and spared this treatment. General guidelines for selecting patients for postoperative radiation therapy are as follows:

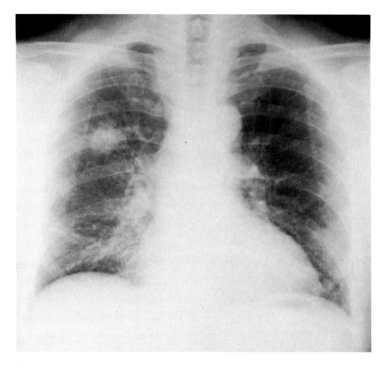

FIG. 1. A PA view of chest radiograph showing a 3 cm lesion at the right upper lobe that was found to be adenocarcinoma with metastases to hilar lymph nodes (N_1 lesion) by right upper lobectomy.

(a) The patient's performance status should be at $\geqslant 70$ on the Karnofsky scale and at grade 0–1 on the Zubrod scale (Tables 3,4) (16,33).

(b) Pulmonary-function reserve should be adequate for the additional insult by postoperative radiation therapy.

Based on the author's series of over 30 patients who had been followed with pulmonary-function studies before and 10 to 12 months after the postoperative radiation therapy, pulmonary-function guidelines for safe postoperative radiation therapy, obtained at 4 weeks after the curative surgical procedure, are shown in Table 5 (10).

RADIOTHERAPEUTIC TECHNIQUES

The importance of radiotherapeutic techniques cannot be overemphasized, inasmuch as the outcome of the treatment depends heavily on the success or failure of the sterilization of the residual tumor in the target volume and the relative frequency of serious complications associated with the adopted techniques.

Definition of Target Volume

The target volume for resectable but locally advanced carcinoma of the lung (N_1, unforeseen N_2, or T_3) lesions should include the tumor bed and the areas of entire

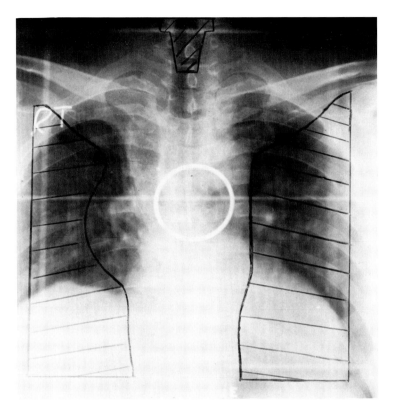

FIG. 2. An AP simulation film illustrating the target volume and cerrobend blocks for protection of normal tissue. The ipsilateral hilum, entire mediastinum, and both supraclavicular areas are included in the target volume for positive regional lymph nodes.

regional lymphatic drainage, which consist of the ipsilateral hilum including the bronchial stump with a 2 to 2.5 cm margin of uninvolved pulmonary tissue (as seen on the radiographs), the entire mediastinum, and the medial halves of both supraclavicular areas (Fig. 1–5) (9,14,18). Without adequate coverage of the entire mediastinum, including the lower mediastinum for the retrograde pathways (3,32) and both supraclavicular areas for the lymph nodes at the thoracic inlet, it is highly unlikely that one will succeed in sterilizing residual carcinoma in the target volume. When the tumor involves the chest wall or diaphragm, the tumor bed should be treated with a generous margin of 3 to 4 cm, including the regional lymphatic areas. The ipsilateral axilla should be included in the target volume when the primary lesion involves the lateral chest wall (T_3 lesion).

Optimum Dose and Fractionation Schedule

The optimum total dose for sterilization of microscopic residual carcinoma of the lung at the tumor bed or in the regional lymph nodes seems to be in the range

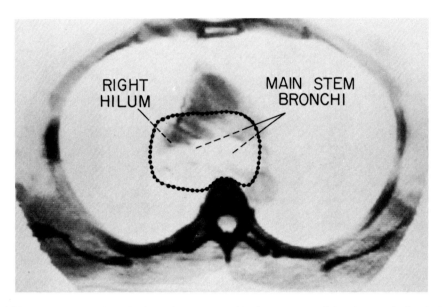

RIGHT
HILUM

MAIN STEM
BRONCHI

FIG. 3. A target volume is drawn in a computed body tomogram of the chest at the level of the central axis of the radiation-treatment field.

of 5200 to 6000 cGy, given by daily fractions of 180 to 200 cGy for five weekly treatments over a period of 5.5 to 6 weeks (TDF 86–99) (9,14,18). Analysis of the relation between the radiation dose and the rate of local or regional failure (9) showed that a radiation dose of ≥5200 cGy (TDF 86) is required to forestall a relapse of the tumor at the regional lymphatic areas or the tumor bed. In a study of preoperative radiation therapy, biopsy-proved metastatic carcinoma of the lung in the mediastinal lymph nodes was sterilized in 70% of patients by a radiation dose of 5500 to 6600 cGy (5,6). The radiation dose and fractionation schedule that have been used by the author are a total dose of 5600 cGy given by a daily dose of 180 to 200 cGy for five weekly treatments over a period of 5.6 to 6.2 weeks.

Radiation–Portal Arrangements

The primary objective for careful selection of radiotherapeutic techniques is to deliver a radiation dose of 5200 to 6000 cGy selectively to the regional lymphatic areas and the tumor bed to sterilize residual microscopic carcinoma of the lung, while the remaining pulmonary tissue, the heart, and the spinal cord are spared from excessive and damaging doses of radiation. The techniques used by the author give consideration to the amount of the remaining pulmonary tissue after lobectomy or pneumonectomy.

For patients who have had a lobectomy, a total tumor dose of 5600 cGy is delivered to the target volume by a sequential combination of AP–PA parallel opposing portals for the initial 3600 cGy and a three-field arrangement of AP–RPO–LPO for the additional 2000 cGy. With this technique, most of the remaining

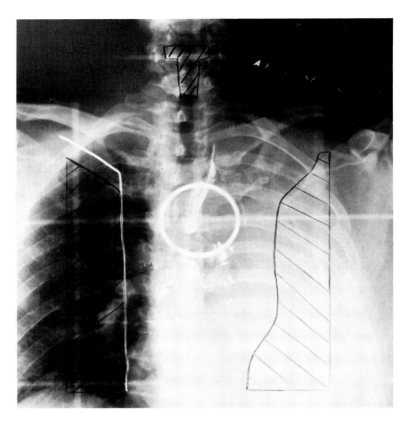

FIG. 4. An AP simulation film illustrating a target volume and cerrobend blocks for protection of normal tissue in a patient who had had a left pneumonectomy for squamous cell carcinoma of the left main-stem bronchus. There were unforeseen metastases to mediastinal lymph nodes ($T_2N_2M_0$).

pulmonary tissue and the spinal cord are spared from an excessive dose of radiation while the target volume is very well covered by an isodose line of ≥ 5200 cGy (Fig. 6).

For patients who had a pneumonectomy, a total tumor dose of 5600 cGy is delivered by a sequential combination of AP–PA parallel opposing portals for the initial 4200 to 4400 cGy and an arrangement of anterior and posterior oblique opposing portals for the additional 1200 to 1400 cGy: RAO–LPO (right anterior and left posterior oblique opposing portals) for the left-side lesion and LAO–RPO (left anterior and right posterior oblique opposing portals) for the right-side lesion (Fig. 7). With this approach, the bronchial stump and most of the mediastinum, except the posterior portion of the opposite mediastinum, are well covered by an isodose line of ≥ 5200 cGy (Fig. 8). The major advantage of this technique over the combination of AP–PA and AP–RPO–LPO is that less of the remaining pulmonary tissue is in harm's way.

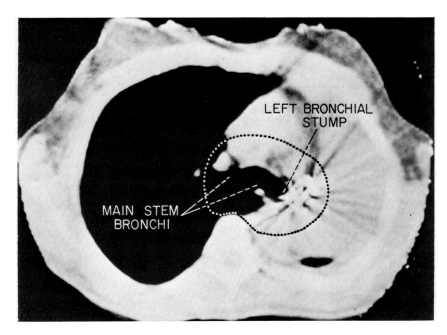

FIG. 5. A target volume, drawn in a computed body tomogram at the level of the central axis of the radiation-treatment field, encompasses the left bronchial stump, the carina, and the right main-stem bronchus.

Other techniques that have been associated with a high incidence of pulmonary complications are an outright three-field approach (AP–RPO–LPO) and rotational techniques (2,30). The amount of remaining pulmonary tissue within the zone of a significantly high radiation dose of ≥ 3000 cGy is quite considerable, and these techniques should be carefully tailored to the pulmonary-function reserve should they be chosen for the need.

RESULTS OF POSTOPERATIVE RADIATION THERAPY

The ultimate goal of postoperative radiation therapy is to improve the chance of cure for patients with a high risk of local and regional failures due to the probable residual tumor at the regional lymphatics and the tumor bed. However, the postoperative radiation therapy is a local and regional treatment, and its benefit may not be appreciated should there be pre-existing distant metastasis.

Survival in Relation to Stage and Histologic Type of Tumors

For patients with early stages of carcinoma of the lung ($T_1N_0M_0,T_2N_0M_0$ lesions), the cure rate by surgery alone is in the range of 30% to 40% (25,28,31), and the majority of failures are due to distant metastasis. As expected, there has been no significant improvement of survival for patients with early stages of carcinoma of the lung after treatment with postoperative irradiation (Fig. 9) (2,30). It is reasonable to expect that the cure rate of these patients can be improved when effective systemic

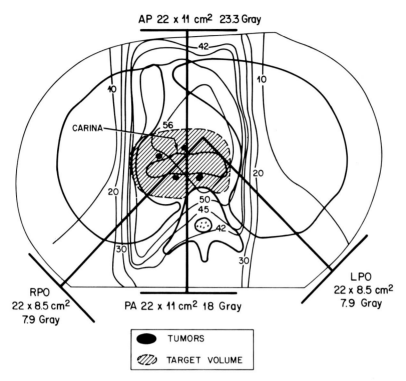

FIG. 6. A composite isodose for an approach that combines AP–PA parallel opposing portals (3600 cGy) with AP–RPO–LPO (2000 cGy) sequentially (10-MeV photon) for a planned total dose of 5600 cGy. The entire target volume is encompassed by an isodose line of ≥ 5200 cGy. For the dosimetry, a correction is made for the lung tissue in the path of the oblique beams.

treatments become available. Because of the occasional local and regional failures even in this group of patients, postoperative radiation therapy can be used selectively in combination with effective systemic treatments in the future.

For patients with locally advanced carcinoma of the lung (N_1, unforeseen N_2 or T_3 lesions), carefully administered postoperative radiation therapy has been able to improve survival. As shown in the author's series (9) and others (13,14,17,18,19,20), the cure rate of patients with N_2 lesions has been improved from 5% to 10% after treatment with just surgery to 10% to 30% after treatment with aggressive post-operative irradiation.

Contrary to expectation, the benefit of postoperative radiation therapy for patients with N_1, unforeseen N_2 or T_3 adenocarcinoma seems as conspicuous as or even better than that for patients with other histologic types (Fig. 10) (9,19,20). However, this should be clarified by further studies.

Patterns of Failure

It is interesting to note that the pattern of failure seems dependent on the histologic type of the tumor. Relapse at the tumor bed and the regional lymphatics is the most

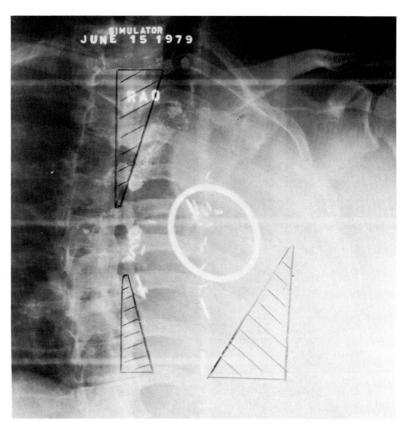

FIG. 7. A simulation film, right anterior oblique, of the anterior and posterior oblique opposing portals for the final 1200 to 1400 cGY after the initial 4200 to 4400 cGy by AP–PA parallel opposing portals, illustrating the adequate coverage of the left bronchial stump and most of the mediastinum.

common cause of failure for patients with N_1, unforeseen N_2 or T_3 stages of squamous cell carcinoma (Table 6) (9). Although the rate of regional recurrence was reduced from 65% (11/17) to 32% (7/22) by postoperative radiation therapy in the author's series, future trials should consider using radiation doses higher than 5200 cGy (TDF 86), probably in the range of 5600 to 5800 cGy (TDF 92–96), inasmuch as all patients who developed a local and regional recurrence had received a radiation dose of ≤5000 cGy (TDF 82). For patients with N_1, unforeseen N_2 or T_3 stages of adenocarcinoma, relapse at the brain seems the most common cause of failure (Table 7) (9), and elective whole-brain irradiation should be considered for this condition in future trials of this histologic type (8).

Morbidity and Complications

The risk of serious complications of normal vital structures in the thorax is real, and these potential complications have been described in the previous chapter.

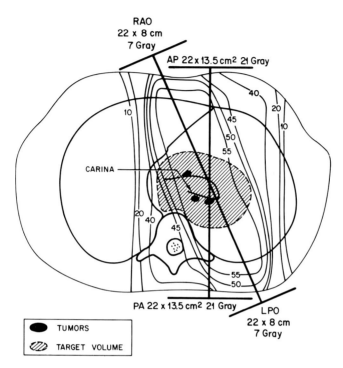

FIG. 8.   A composite isodose for an approach that combines AP–PA parallel opposing portals for the initial 4200 cGy with RAO–LPO for the final 1400 cGy for a planned total dose of 5600 cGy. Most of the target volume is encompassed by an isodose line of ≥ 5200 cGy. Most of the right lung is spared from a significant amount of radiation (≥2500 cGy).

Radiotherapeutic techniques should be tailored to individual patients' pulmonary and cardiovascular reserve. The incidence of serious pneumonitis induced by irradiation was 3.3% (3/92) in the author's series (9). It should be kept as low as possible by carefully evaluating the patient's cardio-respiratory reserve and by selecting proper postoperative radiotherapeutic techniques.

DISCUSSION

The role of postoperative radiation therapy for patients with resectable carcinoma of the lung should be evaluated separately according to the extent (stage) of the tumor. For patients with early stages ($T_1N_0M_0$, $T_2N_0M_0$) of carcinoma of the lung, the value of postoperative radiation therapy has not been demonstrated, although occasional local and regional failures have been the only site of failure until the patient's death. For patients with resectable but locally advanced stages (N_1, unforeseen N_2 or T_3 lesions) of carcinoma of the lung, improved survival has been demonstrated by several retrospective studies (9,13,14,18,19,20,24). There is, therefore, an urgent need to establish the value of postoperative radiation therapy by prospective randomized trials for these groups of patients (12,26). For these

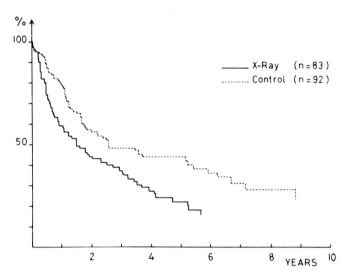

FIG. 9. Actuarial survival curves of patients with early stages (T₁N₀M₀, T₂N₀M₀) of carcinoma of the lung in the study by Van Houtte et al. No benefit was gained from postoperative radiation therapy when comparison was made with the control group (30).

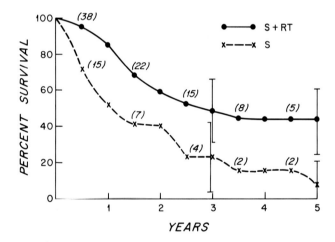

FIG.   10. Actuarial survival curves of patients with locally advanced adenocarcinoma of the lung (N₁, unforeseen N₂, T₃ lesions). Postoperative radiation therapy significantly influenced survival time (9).

trials, one should employ a radiation dose of ≥5600 cGy (TDF 92) to the tumor bed and the regional lymph nodes in the mediastinum and the thoracic inlet; an elective irradiation to the whole brain with a radiation dose of 3000 to 3600 cGy (TDF 49–59) should also be considered for patients with adenocarcinoma (8,9). It is very important that the gain of postoperative radiation therapy not be offset by serious pulmonary complications that can be prevented by carefully selecting radiotherapeutic techniques and carefully screening patients for adequate cardio-respiratory reserve.

REFERENCES

1. American Joint Committee for Cancer Staging and End-Results Reporting (1978): Staging of lung cancer, pp. 59–64, Chicago, Illinois.
2. Bangma, P. J. (1971): Post-operative radiotherapy. In: *Carcinoma of the Bronchus (Modern Radiotherapy)*, edited by T. J. Deeley, pp. 163–170. Appleton-Century-Crofts, New York.
3. Bell, J. W. (1965): Open abdominal biopsy before thoracotomy for lung cancer. *Geriatrics*, 20:715–727.
4. Bergh, N. P., and Schersten, T. (1965): Bronchogenic carcinoma. A follow-up study of a surgically treated series with special reference to the prognostic significance of lymph node metastases. *Acta Chir. Scand. Suppl.*, 347:1–42.
5. Bloedorn, F. G., Cowley, R. A., Cuccia, C. A., Mercado, R., Jr., Wizenberg, M. J., and Linberg, E. J. (1964): Preoperative irradiation in bronchogenic carcinoma. *Am. J. Roentgenol. Radium Ther. Nucl. Med.*, 92:77–87.
6. Bloedorn, F. G. (1966): Rationale and benefit of preoperative irradiation in lung cancer. *JAMA*, 196:128–129.
7. Bromley, L. L., and Szur, L. (1955): Combined radiotherapy and resection for carcinoma of the bronchus: Experiences with 66 patients. *Lancet*, 2:937–941.
8. Choi, C. H., and Carey, R. W. (1976): Small cell anaplastic carcinoma of lung. Reappraisal of current management. *Cancer*, 37:2651–2657.
9. Choi, N. C. H., Grillo, H. C., Gardiello, M., Scannell, J. G., and Wilkins, Jr., E. W. (1980): Basis for new strategies in postoperative radiotherapy of bronchogenic carcinoma. *Int. J. Radiat. Oncol. Biol. Phys.*, 6:31–35.
10. Choi, N. C. H., and Kazemi, H. (1980): Evaluation of pulmonary function changes by postoperative radiotherapy in patients with lung cancer. *Int. J. Radiat. Oncol. Biol. Phys.*, 6:1339.
11. Choi, N. C. H., and Bloch, K. J. (1980): Carcinoembryonic antigen (CEA) as a marker of radiation therapy in lung cancer. *Int. J. Radiat. Oncol. Biol. Phys.*, 6:1454–1455.
12. Choi, N. C. H. (1982): Reassessment of the role of postoperative radiation therapy in resected lung cancer [Editorial]. *Int. J. Radiat. Oncol. Biol. Phys.*, 8:2015–2018.
13. Chung, C. K., Stryker, J. A., O'Neill, M., Jr., and DeMuth, W. E., Jr. (1982): Evaluation of adjuvant postoperative radiotherapy for lung cancer. *Int. J. Radiat. Oncol. Biol. Phys.*, 8:1877–1880.
14. Green, N., Kurohara, S. S., George, III, F. W., Crews, Jr., Q. E. (1975): Postresection irradiation for primary lung cancer. *Radiology*, 116:405–407.
15. Israel, L., Bonadonna, G., Sylvester, R., and Members of the EORTC Lung Cancer Group (1979): Controlled study with adjuvant radiotherapy, chemotherapy, immunotherapy, and chemoimmunotherapy in operable squamous carcinoma of the lung. *Prog. Cancer Res. Ther.*, 11:443–452.
16. Karnofsky, D. A., Golbsy, R. B., and Pool, J. L. (1957): Preliminary studies on the natural history of lung cancer. *Radiology*, 69:477–487.
17. Kirsh, M. M., and Sloan, H. (1982): Mediastinal metastases in bronchogenic carcinoma: influence of postoperative irradiation, cell type, and location. *Ann. Thorac. Surg.*, 33:459–463.
18. Kirsh, M. M., Rotman, H., Argenta, L., Bove, E., Cimmino, V., Tashian, J., Ferguson, P., and Sloan, H. (1976): Carcinoma of the lung: Results of treatment over ten years. *Ann. Thorac. Surg.*, 21:371–377.
19. Lewin, A., Lavin, P., and Malcolm, A. (1981): Post-resection radiation therapy of bronchogenic carcinoma. *Int. J. Radiat. Oncol. Biol. Phys.*, 7:1224.
20. Martini, N., Flehinger, B. J., Zaman, M. B., and Beattie, E. J., Jr. (1981): Results of surgical treatment in N2 lung cancer. *World J. Surg.*, 5:663–666.
21. Matthews, M. J., Kanhouwa, S., Pickren, J., and Robinette, D. (1973): Frequency of residual tumor in patients undergoing curative surgical resection for lung cancer. *Cancer Treat. Rep.*, 4:63–67.
22. Mountain, C. F., McMurtrey, M. J., and Frazier, O. H. (1980): Regional extension of lung cancer. *Int. J. Radiat. Oncol. Biol. Phys.*, 6:1013–1020.
23. Paterson, R., and Russell, M. (1962): Clinical trials in malignant disease. Part IV, Lung cancer. Value of postoperative radiotherapy. *Clin. Radiol.*, 13:141–144.

24. Patterson, G. A., Ilves, R., Ginsberg, R. J., Cooper, J. D., Todd, T. R. J., and Pearson, F. G. (1982): The value of adjuvant radiotherapy in pulmonary and chest wall resection for bronchogenic carcinoma. *Ann. Thorac. Surg.*, 34:692–697.
25. Paulson, D. L., and Reisch, J. S. (1976): Long-term survival after resection for bronchogenic carcinoma. *Ann. Surg.*, 83:324–332.
26. Perez, C. A. (1982): Is postoperative irradiation indicated in carcinoma of the lung? [Editorial]. *Int. J. Radiat. Oncol. Biol. Phys.*, 8:2019–2022.
27. Sherman, D. M., Weichselbaum, R., and Hellman, S. (1981): The characteristics of long-term survivors of lung cancer treated with radiation. *Cancer*, 47:2575–2580.
28. Shields, T. W. (1980): Classification and prognosis of surgically treated patients with bronchial carcinoma: Analysis of VASOG studies. *Int. J. Radiat. Oncol. Biol. Phys.*, 6:1021–1027.
29. Spjut, H. J., and Mateo, L. E. (1965): Recurrent and metastatic carcinoma in surgically treated carcinoma of the lung. An autopsy survey. *Cancer*, 18:1462–1466.
30. Van Houtte, P., Rocmans, P., Smets, P., Goffin, J., Lustman-Maréchal, J., Vanderhoeft, P., and Henry, J. (1980): Postoperative radiation therapy in lung cancer: A controlled trial after resection of curative design. *Int. J. Radiat. Oncol. Biol. Phys.*, 6:983–986.
31. Wilkins, E. W., Jr., Scannell, J. G., and Craver, J. G. (1978): Four decades of experience with resections for bronchogenic carcinoma at the Massachusetts General Hospital. *J. Thorac. Cardiovasc. Surg.*, 76:364–368.
32. Zeidman, I. (1959): Experimental studies on the spread of cancer in the lymphatic system. IV. Retrograde spread. *Cancer Res.*, 19:1114–1117.
33. Zubrod, C. G., Schneiderman, M., Frei, E., Brindley, C., Gold, G. L., Shnider, B., Oviedo, R., Gorman, J., Jones, R., Jonsson, U., Colsky, J., Chalmers, T., Ferguson, B., Dederick, M., Holland, J., Selawry, O., Regelson, W., Lasagna, L., and Owens, A. H. (1960): Appraisal of methods for study of chemotherapy of cancer in man: Comparative therapeutic trial of nitrogen mustard and triethylene thiophosphoramide. *J. Chronic Dis.*, 11:7–33.

Thoracic Oncology, edited by N. C. Choi and
H. C. Grillo. Raven Press, New York © 1983.

Management of Superior Sulcus Carcinomas

Donald L. Paulson

*Department of Thoracic Surgery, Baylor University Medical Center, Dallas, Texas; and
Department of Thoracic and Cardiovascular Surgery, University of Texas Health Science
Center, Dallas, Texas 75246*

A tumor in the superior pulmonary sulcus usually is a carcinoma of the lung, producing a clinical pattern peculiar to its location. Other benign or malignant tumors, metastatic lesions, and inflammatory and infectious processes located in the apex of the lung or adjacent structures as tumors of bone or sympathetic ganglia or nerves, although less common than bronchogenic carcinoma, can produce the same clinical syndrome.

Hare (7) deserves credit for the first well-documented case report, which appeared in the *London Medical Gazette* in 1838, of the clinical pattern resulting from a cancer in the apex of the lung invading the sympathetic ganglia and brachial plexus. Tobias (22) presented a detailed description of the clinical syndrome produced by primary pulmonary cancer in this location and termed it the apico-costo-vertebral syndrome, but it was Pancoast for whom the syndrome was named, as a result of his description in a classic article, "Superior Pulmonary Sulcus Tumor," published in 1932 (18). According to Pancoast, such tumors always occurred "at a definite location at the thoracic inlet," producing "constant and characteristic clinical phenomena of pain in the eighth cervical and first and second thoracic trunk distribution... and Horner's syndrome." He described the roentgenographic findings as "a small homogeneous shadow at the extreme apex" associated with "more or less rib destruction and often vertebral infiltration."

Pancoast used the term *superior pulmonary sulcus* because it implied the approximate location of these tumors, presumably referring to the anatomic sulcus or groove made by the passage of the subclavian artery in the cupola of the pleura and apices of the upper lobes of the lungs, known as the subclavian sulcus or groove. In defining tumors in this precise location, Pancoast found it necessary to discard the term *apical chest tumor*, which he had originally used in an article (17) in 1924, "because it has proved to be confusing and has permitted the inclusion of other more common tumors in the upper part of the thorax."

Pancoast was of the opinion that tumors in the superior pulmonary sulcus were characterized not only by their location and symptoms but also by "a lack of origin from the lung, pleura, ribs or mediastinum." He considered tumors in this location atypical for carcinoma of the lung and suggested their origin possibly from some extrapulmonary structure as an embryonic epithelial rest of the fifth brachial pouch. He admitted that better knowledge of the histopathology of these tumors might change this interpretation, as indeed it has.

Pancoast further observed that "death occurred as a result of what seemed to be a comparatively trivial growth without detectable metastases roentgenologically" and that the growth "resisted all efforts at irradiation treatment: ... is obviously not subject to surgical removal although it is accessible, and it is rather rapidly fatal."

Although a variety of other tumors, including metastases, can produce the clinical pattern peculiar to their location at the thoracic inlet, it is generally accepted that the most common cause is a bronchogenic carcinoma arising in or near the superior pulmonary sulcus and invading the adjoining extrapulmonic structures by direct extension. It is the location of the tumor that is significant in producing the characteristic clinical pattern, not its pathologic structure or tissue of origin.

Confusion as to site of origin may well be due to the fact that characteristically the bulk of a true Pancoast tumor is extrapulmonary, beginning in an extreme peripheral location, with a plaquelike extension over the apex of the lung, involving principally the chest wall structures rather than the underlying parenchyma of the lung. It is well established that both adenomatous and squamous cell carcinomas can arise peripherally from scar tissue in the lung through a process of metaplasia. Apical pleural and subpleural scarring is common, having been found in 25% of postmortem examinations (9). Speculation may be justifiable, therefore, that at least some malignant tumors in the superior pulmonary sulcus are cancers arising in peripheral subpleural scars with early extrapulmonary extensions of growth. Apical pleural adhesions in the narrow confines of the apex of the chest facilitate extensions of the cancer to the lymphatics of the endothoracic fascia and adjoining structures of the thoracic inlet. Clinical findings of tumors largely separate from the lung support this thesis. Present-day knowledge, experience, and common usage justify the application of the term to lung cancers arising in the region of the superior pulmonary sulcus and producing the characteristic clinical pattern described by Pancoast.

BRONCHOGENIC CARCINOMA IN THE SUPERIOR PULMONARY SULCUS

Bronchogenic carcinomas developing peripherally in the apex of the lung and invading the superior pulmonary sulcus frequently are low-grade epidermoid carcinomas that grow slowly and metastasize late. Situated in the narrow confines of the thoracic inlet, they invade the lymphatics in the endothoracic fascia and involve, by direct extensions, the lower roots of the brachial plexus, the intercostal nerves, the stellate ganglion, the sympathetic chain, and adjacent ribs and vertebrae, producing severe pain and the Horner's syndrome (Pancoast's syndrome).

Symptoms and Diagnosis

The symptoms are characteristic of the location of the tumor in the superior pulmonary sulcus or thoracic inlet adjacent to the first and second thoracic and eighth cervical nerve roots, the sympathetic chain, and the stellate ganglion. Initially there is steady localized pain in the shoulder and the vertebral border of the scapula; later it extends down the ulnar distribution of the arm to the elbow (involvement of T1) and finally to the ulnar surface of the forearm and small and ring fingers of the hand (C8 dermatome) (Fig. 1). As the tumor extends by direct invasion to the sympathetic chain and stellate ganglion, Horner's syndrome and anhidrosis on the

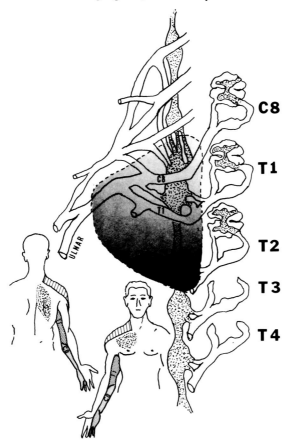

FIG. 1. Neural structures at the thoracic inlet involved by direct extension of a carcinoma in the superior pulmonary sulcus. The shaded area indicates the region of potential involvement, typically including C8, T1, and T2 nerve roots, the lower trunk of the brachial plexus, and the sympathetic chain. The dermatomes of C8 and T1 are illustrated, as well as the regions of referred pain in the scapular and pectoral regions (mediated through afferent pain fibers of the sympathetic trunk and ganglia). (From Paulson, D. L. (1975): Carcinomas in the superior pulmonary sulcus. *J. Thorac. Cardiovasc. Surg.*, 70:1095–1104. Reproduced with permission of C. V. Mosby.)

same side of the face and upper extremity develop. The pain is steady, severe, and unrelenting, often requiring opiates for relief. The patient soon discovers that support of the elbow of the affected arm by the opposite hand relieves the tension on the shoulder and upper arm. As involvement by the tumor progresses, weakness and atrophy of the muscles of the hand and absence of the triceps reflex are noted. Involvement of the posterior portions of the first or second ribs and the transverse processes or bodies of vertebrae occurs as the tumor advances, increasing the severity of the pain. The spinal canal and cord may be invaded or compressed, with symptoms of a spinal cord tumor resulting.

Pulmonary symptoms are notable by their absence and rarely constitute the presenting complaint; this explains the common history of initial consultation with an orthopedist or neurosurgeon.

The diagnosis of a tumor in the superior pulmonary sulcus is suspected from the characteristic history of pain along known nerve pathways of involvement and roentgen evidence of a shadow at the extreme apex of the chest or thoracic inlet. Horner's syndrome and bone involvement may be present or absent and are not necessary to alert the physician, but, when present, they support the diagnosis.

In most cases, roentgenograms of the thorax will disclose an obvious tumor involving the extreme apex of the lung (Fig. 2). In some cases, however, the

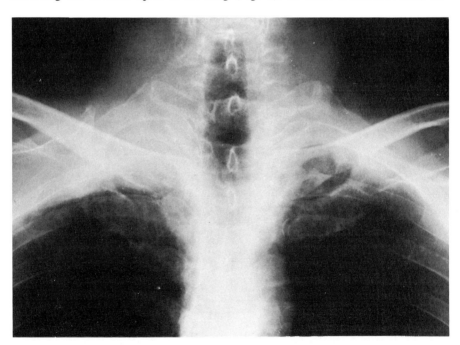

FIG. 2. Roentgenogram illustrating a tumor mass in the right apex of the chest with destruction of the right second rib. (From Paulson, D. L. (1976): Superior sulcus carcinomas. In: *Gibbon's Surgery of the Chest*, edited by Sabiston and Spencer. Reproduced with permission of W. B. Saunders.)

shadow appears as an apical pleural cap of thickening only, because of a plaquelike extension of the tumor, and may be considered a normal finding. If pain is present, more detailed roentgenographic studies, including planigraphy or films for bony detail, are more revealing. Bone destruction may not be obvious by ordinary radiologic techniques, and computed axial tomography is helpful to determine the extent of involvement.

Characteristically, most of the mass of a tumor in the superior pulmonary sulcus is an extension of the growth from the lung into and involving the surrounding structures in the cupola of the chest, including nerve roots, ganglia, and ribs posteriorly. In any patient with a tumor mass in the extreme apex of the chest and pain down the ulnar distribution of the arm in the areas innervated by the first thoracic and eighth cervical nerve roots (with or without Horner's syndrome) owing to involvement of the sympathetic chain and stellate ganglia, a presumptive diagnosis of bronchogenic carcinoma in the superior pulmonary sulcus is justified with an accuracy of better than 90%. Open biopsy of the cupola of the pleura may be made for pathologic proof through a supraclavicular scalenotomy incision (16), particularly in the case of inoperable or doubtful cases. The tumor may not be accessible to needle biopsy because of its size and location.

Standard bronchoscopic examination usually is unproductive of proof of malignancy owing to the extreme peripheral location of the tumor, although positive findings of malignant cells in the sputum have been reported in 16% of patients examined (9). It remains to be seen whether or not bronchoscopy and brush biopsies, particularly with flexible fiberoptic techniques, will be more productive. As is true for carcinomas in any location, the extent of the tumor and the stage of nodal involvement are the dominant factors in prognosis. Computed axial tomography (CAT scanning) is of great value in determining the location and extent of involvement of the ribs, the paraspinal region, and vertebrae. By definition, carcinomas in the superior pulmonary sulcus are T3 lesions, and if hilar or mediastinal nodes are involved they are N2 stage III lesions by the TNM classification for carcinomas of the lung. As is true for any location in the lung, patients with T3 N2 lesions do not survive over 2 years. Mediastinoscopy to determine the stage of nodal involvement is pertinent to the clinical pretreatment staging of the patient. Metastases to scalene or mediastinal nodes indicate survival of little more than 1 year, but palliative extended resection for relief of pain after irradiation may be justifiable in selected cases.

Involvement of the phrenic or recurrent laryngeal nerves or vena cava is a manifestation of a more extensive apical lung tumor arising in another location and is not characteristic of the true Pancoast tumor.

Pathology

Characteristically, most of the tumor is a gross extension of a tumor in the lung, at least 60% being outside the lung, involving chest wall, nerve roots, the lower trunk of the brachial plexus, sympathetic chain and ganglia, ribs, and bone (Fig. 3). Microscopically, squamous cell carcinomas predominate, although the large cell undifferentiated types are almost as common. Adenocarcinomas also are found in this location, but they are much less common and may be metastatic.

Characteristically, a true superior pulmonary sulcus tumor is relatively localized, except for local extensions, and does not metastasize to mediastinal or scalene lymph nodes until late in its course. Involvement of the hilar or mediastinal nodes, found in 25%, signifies a poor prognosis, with survival of only a little over 1 year.

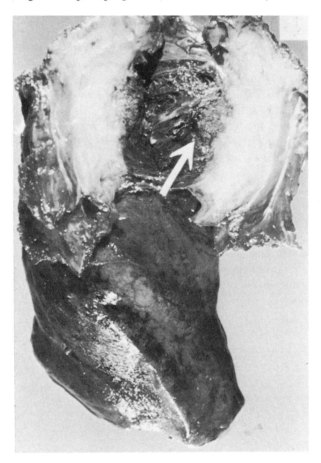

FIG. 3. Specimen of a superior sulcus tumor resected after preoperative irradiation. The intercostal nerves are visible in the cut section of the chest wall. Most of the tumor is extraordinary, presenting as an amorphous mass and viable carcinoma found only in the apex of the lung indicated by the arrow. (From Paulson, D. L. (1976): Superior sulcus carcinomas. In: *Gibbon's Surgery of the Chest*, edited by Sabiston and Spencer. Reproduced with permission of W. B. Saunders.)

Treatment

Generally, carcinomas in the superior pulmonary sulcus have been considered unsuitable for complete operative removal and cure; incomplete resection followed by irradiation has been done for palliation of pain only.

Irradiation therapy has been considered of little value by many observers, including Pancoast (18), Walker (23), and Herbut and Watson (10), although more recent reports have indicated prolongation of survival by this modality alone (4,6,9). Many of the earlier reports referred to irradiation of lesions diagnosed late or disturbed by a surgeon performing a thoracotomy for diagnosis. It is entirely possible that irradiation alone, given by modern techniques over undisturbed tumors in an early stage, may relieve pain, prolong survival, and produce a cure in some cases.

In the past, operative treatment has frequently been disappointing, and the lesion has been considered technically inoperable owing to the extent of involvement of adjacent structures. Irradiation therapy has been combined with incomplete resection, resulting in palliation of pain and prolonged survival in some cases. Dontas (3) reported incomplete resection followed by irradiation therapy for palliation of pain and concluded that the combination of surgical treatment and radiotherapy would give the best results in this type of carcinoma. Groves (5) reported 12 selected patients treated by incomplete resection and either interstitial irradiation (10 patients) or ^{60}Co teletherapy (2 patients), with prolonged survival for 4 patients and six deaths within 1 year. Hilaris et al. (11) reported 5-year survival for 6 of 38 patients treated by interstitial irradiation implanted for unresectable tumors at thoracotomy. The combination of resection of the parenchymal lesion and implantation of the unresected chest-wall residual cancer in 16 patients resulted in 3 of 9 patients surviving 5 years and 2 of 7 patients surviving 2.5 and 3.5 years, respectively.

Chardack and MacCallum (1,2) reported the first 5-year survival following complete en bloc resection of a superior pulmonary sulcus tumor followed by irradiation therapy of 6,528 rads in 54 days. It is probable that adequate resection of the tumor was responsible for the cure and that the subsequent irradiation therapy did not contribute to the final result.

Combined Preoperative Irradiation and Extended Resection

From 1956 to 1978, a total of 107 patients with primary carcinomas in the superior pulmonary sulcus were seen in a private practice of thoracic surgery (Table 1). Of these, 26 patients (24%) were considered inoperable at the time of diagnosis because

TABLE 1. *Carcinoma in the superior pulmonary sulcus in 107 patients (1956 to 1978)*

26 patients inoperable originally
9 patients became inoperable
3 patients refused operation
1 patient nonresectable
68 patients completed combined treatment

of distant metastases, local extent of the tumor, or age. Metastases that became obvious during the interval between diagnosis and operation rendered an additional 9 patients inoperable. Of 69 patients operated on after preoperative irradiation, 1 patient was judged to have a nonresectable lesion because of multiple areas of involvement by adenocarcinoma. Combined preoperative irradiation and extended resection were completed in 68 patients, with two operative deaths (3%).

Forty of 64 patients survived over 1 year after completion of combined treatment, 25 of 63 survived 2 years, 22 of 61 survived 3 years, 20 of 61 survived 4 years, and 19 of 59 survived more than 5 years. Thirteen of 46 patients eligible are alive and well 10 years or more after operation, including 7 of 25 patients who completed combined treatment 15 years ago or longer. There have been no deaths due to the superior sulcus carcinomas after 4 years. The causes of death for 3 patients who died after having survived more than 5 years after treatment of their superior sulcus tumors were leukemia, carcinoma of the stomach, and a heart attack.

Calculated by the actuarial method, there has been a 35% survival at 5 years and 26% at 10 years in a series of selected patients for whom combined preoperative irradiation and extended resection were done (64% of the total series). Forty-four percent in the group of patients without nodal involvement survived 5 years, and 33% survived 10 years (Fig. 4).

Rationale of Treatment

In this series, a histologic diagnosis was not obtained prior to the institution of combined treatment for bronchogenic carcinoma in the superior sulcus. It is believed

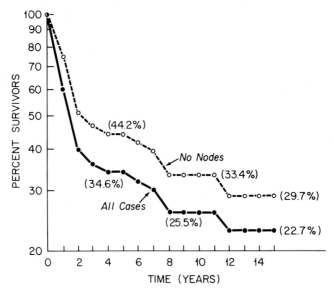

FIG. 4. Observed survival after combined preoperative irradiation and resection for carcinoma in the superior pulmonary sulcus in all cases and in those with no nodal involvement. After 4 years there have been no deaths due to bronchogenic carcinoma.

that, in general, the inaccessibility of the lesion, the risk of dissemination, and the increased morbidity through surgical interference, together with the adverse effect of biopsy on radiosensitivity of the tumor, contraindicate exploration for this purpose. Interference with or violation of the vascular bed of the tumor and its lymphatics, or the introduction of hematoma, low-grade infection, or inflammation, may lower the oxygen tension and decrease its sensitivity to irradiation, thus jeopardizing the opportunity for cure. Tissue proof is simply deferred to the time of resection, 3 to 4 weeks later.

The clinical syndrome of severe pain in the shoulder and along the ulnar distribution in the arm (due to involvement of nerve roots C8 and T1), together with roentgenographic evidence of a tumor in the apex of the chest, with or without bone destruction and Horner's syndrome, is diagnostic of a neoplastic process in the superior pulmonary sulcus invading the chest wall. Other lesions, including metastatic neoplasms and inflammatory lesions such as fibrosing pneumonitis and tuberculosis, may be confusing, but the severity and location of the pain, the radiologic appearance, and the statistical preponderance today emphasize the probability of bronchogenic carcinoma as a cause. Tuberculosis constitutes the most common error in diagnosis. When the clinical syndrome is atypical and the diagnosis doubtful, a calculated risk is taken, and antimicrobial therapy, as well as irradiation, is instituted in preparation for a thoracotomy. Open biopsy of the cupola of the pleura through a supraclavicular scalenotomy incision or needle biopsy is a useful procedure for inoperable or doubtful cases.

The purpose of presurgical irradiation is to modify the extent of the disease so that the lesion is better localized and thus more completely resectable with improved results, but without increased morbidity. The tumor dose used for bronchogenic carcinoma in the superior pulmonary sulcus is 3,000 rads given in 10 treatments over 12 elapsed days (15). It is approximately 75% of the cancericidal dose of 4,200 rads delivered in 2 weeks' time based on the Strandquist curve for squamous cell carcinoma of the skin. The aim of the subcancericidal dose is to localize the lesion and inhibit dissemination or implantation by destruction of the tumor cells at the periphery, to produce sclerosis of the vascular bed and the lymphatics, and to damage the viability and reproductive integrity of malignant cells not resected, implanted, or disseminated at the time of operation. Full cancericidal dosage carries the risk of increased radiologic and operative morbidity by sterilization or depopulation of normal tissue cells necessary for repair. The interval between radiation and operation has been shortened from the original 4 to 6 weeks to 3 to 4 weeks.

Although the optimum dosage and interval between radiation and surgery remain to be determined, clinical and experimental observations indicate that presurgical irradiation at doses that are not sufficient to completely sterilize or cause regression of the tumors treated decreases local recurrence, prevents the growth of tumor cells after dissemination, and increases survival, when compared with irradiation or surgery alone (8,12–14,20).

Pathology

Resection 3 to 6 weeks after completion of radiation therapy established the histologic diagnosis of presumably viable bronchogenic carcinoma in all but three cases included in this series. In these cases presenting with the classic Pancoast syndrome, irradiation is believed to have sterilized the tumors completely, so that viable cancer was not identifiable. Generally, pathologic examination of resected specimens has shown profound alterations in the neoplasms. Grossly, in the typical case, there is a peripheral pseudocapsule and central degeneration. The periphery of the tumor has been reduced to an amorphous fibrous mass, so that it is necessary to take sections deep within the lesion to find typical neoplastic cells. In the intermediate zone, necrosis with scattered cells featuring pyknotic nuclei can be seen as remains of damaged cancer cells. Pathologic findings indicate marked destruction, degeneration, giant cell formation, inflammation, fibrosis, and localization of the neoplastic mass by irradiation, so that it is possible to carry the line of resection much closer to the lesion without fear of dissemination or subsequent local recurrence (Fig. 5).

In general, the effects of irradiation can be correlated with survival after resection. In patients without nodal involvement, those with complete sterilization without residual viable tumor did well. Those with involvement of the chest wall by fibrosis, but with no evidence of viable tumor at that level, did well also, with one exception. On the other hand, those with extension of viable tumor into the chest wall, without irradiation effects, did poorly, with one exception.

Cell type was identifiable in 58 of 60 lesions resected after irradiation (1956 to 1974). There were 27 squamous cell carcinomas, 20 large cell undifferentiated carcinomas, 11 adenocarcinomas, and 2 undetermined cell types. Of the patients surviving 3 years or more, 11 had squamous cell carcinomas, 5 had undifferentiated large cell carcinomas, and 4 had adenocarcinomas; in 2 patients the cell type was undetermined (Table 2).

The stage of nodal involvement was found to be significant for prognosis, particularly if mediastinal nodes were found to be invaded. Twenty-two of 49 patients with either no nodes or intersegmental nodes survived 3 years, whereas none of those with hilar or mediastinal nodes survived much more than 1 year (Table 3).

Bone involvement carries a serious prognosis because it occurs late in the natural history of the lesion. Involvement of ribs or vertebrae was found in about one-half of all patients, but in one-fourth of 5-year survivors. Of patients with no nodal involvement, 23% of the patients with bone involvement survived over 5 years. In the absence of vascular as well as nodal involvement, 30% survived over 5 years. Bone destruction, if not too extensive, alone is not a sign of inoperability.There have been no complications attributable to the radiation therapy at the dosage recommended, such as radiation pneumonitis or bronchial fistula. Radiation neuritis has been observed in one patient receiving 4,500 rads preoperatively elsewhere.

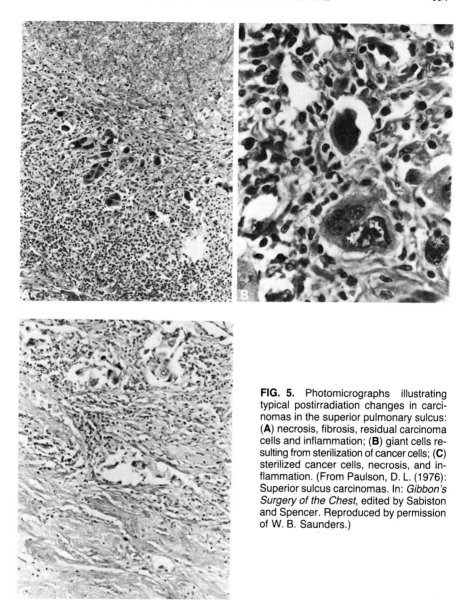

FIG. 5. Photomicrographs illustrating typical postirradiation changes in carcinomas in the superior pulmonary sulcus: (**A**) necrosis, fibrosis, residual carcinoma cells and inflammation; (**B**) giant cells resulting from sterilization of cancer cells; (**C**) sterilized cancer cells, necrosis, and inflammation. (From Paulson, D. L. (1976): Superior sulcus carcinomas. In: *Gibbon's Surgery of the Chest,* edited by Sabiston and Spencer. Reproduced by permission of W. B. Saunders.)

Surgical Technique

The surgical technique for resection of a superior sulcus tumor is an extended en bloc resection of the chest wall, usually including posterior portions of the first three ribs, portions of the upper thoracic vertebrae (including their transverse processes), the intercostal nerves, the lower trunk of the brachial plexus, the stellate

TABLE 2. *Cell types and survival for 60 patients with superior pulmonary sulcus carcinomas (1956 to 1975)*

Cell type	No. of patients	3-year survivors
Squamous cell	27	11
Large cell undifferentiated	20	5
Adenocarcinoma	11	4
Undetermined	2	2
Total	60	22

TABLE 3. *Nodal involvement and prognosis for superior pulmonary sulcus carcinomas (1956 to 1974)*

Stage of involvement	No. of patients	Survival	
		1 year	3 years
No nodes (T3 N0)	48	35	21
Intersegmental nodes (T3 N1)	1	1	1
Hilar or mediastinal nodes (Stages II and III) (T3, N1 or N2)	15	2	0
Total	64	38	22

ganglion, and a portion of the dorsal sympathetic chain, together with the involved lung, resected by means of either lobectomy or segmental resection (21).

The technique may vary to some degree, depending on the size and extent of the carcinoma, but in general the approach is uniform. A long parascapular incision should be used, starting just above the spine of the scapula and extending around the lower tip of the scapula and ending in the anterior axillary line. It is undesirable from the standpoint of function, and should not be necessary, to completely divide the upper portion of the trapezius and levator scapulae muscles, for they support the shoulder girdle. Almost complete section of the serratus anterior muscle attachments to the first three ribs will allow good elevation of the shoulder to expose the apex of the thoracic cage. The serratus posterior superior muscle is separated at its insertion on the ribs and preserved for later use in closing the thorax. The intrinsic dorsal musculature is separated by sharp dissection from the upper ribs and transverse processes to the laminae of the vertebrae. The chest cavity is entered through an incision in the third interspace, avoiding at first the posterior portion until the extent of the tumor is explored. The pleural cavity is opened sufficiently wide to allow appraisal of the extent of growth. The ribs and intercostal muscle bundles anterior to the growth are divided, allowing an adequate margin of normal tissue. After the first rib has been separated at the costochondral junction, the end of the rib to which the growth is attached is pulled downward to put under tension the cervical structures involved by the tumor. The scalene muscles are divided, and the subclavian artery and vein and lower trunk of the brachial plexus are identified (Fig. 6). Dissection along the subclavian artery may be tedious, but the artery is rarely invaded. It may be necessary to sacrifice one or more branches of the artery, including the internal mammary, the thyrocervical trunk, and, at times, the vertebral. Usually only that part of the plexus coming from the eighth cervical and first thoracic nerves that supplies the ulnar nerve is involved. In some cases of localized extent it will be possible to preserve the eighth cervical nerve, resecting only that portion of the lower brachial plexus trunk continuous with the first thoracic nerve root. The musculotendinous tissue is divided by sharp dissection above the first rib and transverse process down to the lamina of the vertebra, thus circumscribing the anterior and superior extent of the tumor. At this point there remains posteriorly a mass of bony attachment made up of ribs, transverse processes, and involved portions of the bodies of the vertebrae with included intercostal vessels and nerves and sympathetic chain. The transverse processes are cut with bone shears flush with the laminae, and the tubercle, neck, and head of the rib are elevated from their firm attachments to their sites on the sides of the bodies of the vertebrae. If

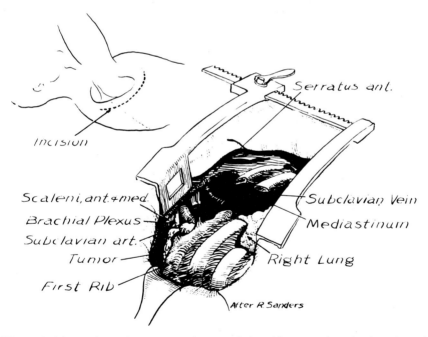

FIG. 6. Incision and anterior exposure for extended en bloc resection of a bronchogenic carcinoma in the right superior pulmonary sulcus. The first three ribs are divided anteriorly; the muscular attachments to the first rib are separated, and the subclavian vessels and brachial plexus are exposed. (From Paulson, D. L., and Shaw, R. R. (1971): Surgical treatment of bronchogenic carcinoma in the superior sulcus after preoperative irradiation. In: *The Craft of Surgery*, 2nd ed., edited by P. Cooper. Reproduced with permission of Little, Brown & Co.)

possible, it is desirable at this point to tense the intercostal nerves so that they can be divided behind the ganglion in the intervertebral foramen. The remaining bony attachments are dissected circumferentially around the fibrous capsule of the tumor mass, using a chisel, if necessary, to remove involved bone (Fig. 7). As much as one-fourth of the bodies of the involved vertebrae has been removed in this manner without disturbing the spinal support. The sympathetic nerves and ganglia, including a portion at least of the stellate ganglion, are resected with the tumor mass. A gauze pack temporarily controls bleeding from the prevertebral vessels and cancellous bone, but active bleeding points are controlled. If there is escape of cerebrospinal fluid from the divided dural cuff surrounding an intercostal nerve, it may be controlled by suturing an excised portion of muscle into the intervertebral foramen. The resection of the growth is then completed by upper lobectomy or segmental resection. Lymph nodes in the superior mediastinum and lower cervical region should be dissected and removed. Adequate pleural drainage is established by two tubes, one in the apex and another posteriorly. The preserved serratus posterior superior muscle may be used either to control oozing from the raw bony surfaces or to partially close the defect in the rib cage. Large defects in the chest wall involving more than portions of three ribs should be closed with plastic mesh to minimize paradoxical motion. Usually, however, the remaining defect can be covered adequately by closure of the muscles of the shoulder girdle, subcutaneous tissue, and skin.

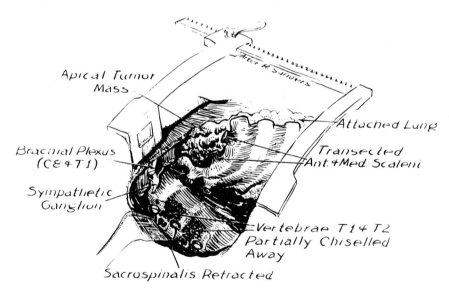

FIG. 7. Posterior aspect of resection en bloc of chest wall and tumor, together with the lower trunk of the brachial plexus, the sympathetic chain, intercostal nerves, and parts of the bodies of vertebrae. (From Paulson, D. L., and Shaw, R. R. (1971): Surgical treatment of bronchogenic carcinoma in the superior sulcus after preoperative irradiation. In: *The Craft of Surgery*, 2nd ed., edited by P. Cooper. Reproduced with permission of Little, Brown & Co.)

Extended radical lobectomy was done in 50 patients for carcinomas in the superior pulmonary sulcus to achieve adequate clearance of the regional lymphatics. Segmental resection was done in 18 patients as an adequate operation for the particular carcinoma involved or as a palliative procedure because of poor pulmonary function or extent of the tumor. Eight of 18 patients having segmental resections survived over 5 years.

Two operative deaths occurred, one due to a cerebral vascular stroke and the other to adrenal insufficiency and cardiac failure.

The subclavian artery was resected in 3 patients, and partial excision and endarterectomy were done in another. Grafts were used to reconstruct the artery in 2 patients, and 1 patient required an amputation of the arm later because of insufficient arterial circulation. None of the 4 patients in whom resection of the artery was necessary survived longer than 1 year.

Postoperative irradiation was given to 6 patients for residual or recurrent carcinoma. All died around 1 year or less following operation.

Permanent neurologic defects resulting from resection of the lower trunk of the brachial plexus involve the ulnar nerve but are not incapacitating. In cases in which the eighth cervical nerve root can be preserved, the defect secondary to resection of the first thoracic nerve root is not severe. Horner's syndrome and anhidrosis develop postoperatively secondary to the dorsal sympathectomy. The defects are not disabling, and for all patients who survived more than 3 years, the quality of life was excellent with complete relief of pain. In contrast, those who died before then had a poor quality of survival, primarily because of severe unremitting pain caused by persistence or local recurrence of carcinoma and also because of systemic effects of metastases.

Contraindications to operation include extensive invasion of the brachial plexus, subclavian artery, or vertebrae, mediastinal involvement (particularly perinodal), and distant metastases. Patients with ipsilateral intranodal involvement of the mediastinal or scalene nodes may be resected for palliation of severe pain, although generally the prognosis is poor in these cases.

CONCLUSION

Bronchogenic carcinomas in the superior pulmonary sulcus produce a characteristic clinical syndrome described by Pancoast. The relative inaccessibility of the tumor, with involvement of adjoining nerves, bone, and chest wall, has deterred surgeons from performing extended resections. Complete resections not uncommonly have been considered inadvisable or impossible. Irradiation therapy alone or in combination with incomplete resection has been advocated for palliation of pain, with prolonged survival in some cases.

Accuracy in defining the location of superior pulmonary sulcus tumors, as emphasized by Pancoast, is necessary to avoid confusion with other more extensive apical chest carcinomas. Differences in results of treatment often are due to confusion in definition and stage of involvement (19).

The results of preoperative irradiation of the undisturbed tumor combined with extended radical resection in selected patients with bronchogenic carcinoma in the superior pulmonary sulcus reveal an operability rate of 64% with 35% survival at 5 years and 26% at 10 years. In the group of patients without nodal involvement, 44% survived 5 years, and 33% survived 10 years.

REFERENCES

1. Chardack, W. M., and MacCallum, J. D. (1953): Pancoast syndrome due to bronchogenic carcinoma: Successful surgical removal and postoperative irradiation. *J. Thorac. Surg.*, 25:402.
2. Chardack, W. M., and MacCallum, J. D. (1956): Pancoast tumor (five year survival without recurrence or metastases following radical resection and postoperative irradiation). *J. Thorac. Surg.*, 31:535.
3. Dontas, N. S. (1957): The Pancoast syndrome. *Br. J. Tuberc.*, 51:246.
4. Fry, W. A., Carpender, J. W. J., and Adam, W. E. (1967): Superior sulcus tumor with 14-year survival. *Arch. Surg.*, 94:142.
5. Groves, L. K. (1962): Superior pulmonary sulcus tumor or Pancoast syndrome: Report of 12 patients treated with surgery and radiation. *Cleve. Clin. Q.*, 29:135.
6. Haas, L. L., Harvey, R. A., and Langer, S. S. (1954): Radiation management of otherwise hopeless thoracic neoplasms. *J. Am. Med. Assoc.*, 154:323.
7. Hare, E. S. (1838): Tumor involving certain nerves. *London Med. Gaz.*, 1:16.
8. Henschke, U. K., Frazell, E. L., Basaris, B. S., Nickson, J. J., Tollefsen, H. R., and Strong, E. W. (1964): Local recurrences after radical neck dissection with or without preoperative x-ray therapy. *Radiology*, 82:331.
9. Hepper, N. G. G., Herskovic, T., Witten, D. M., Mulder, D. W., and Woolner, L. B. (1966): Thoracic inlet tumors. *Ann. Intern. Med.*, 64:979.
10. Herbut, P. A., and Watson, J. S. (1964): Tumor of thoracic inlet producing Pancoast syndrome: Report of 17 cases and reviews of literature. *Arch. Pathol.*, 42:88.
11. Hilaris, B. S., Luomanen, R. K., and Beattie, E. J., Jr. (1971): Integrated irradiation and surgery in the treatment of apical lung cancer. *Cancer*, 27:1369.
12. Hoye, R. C., and Smith, R. R. (1961): Effect of small amounts of preoperative irradiation in preventing growth of tumor cells disseminated at surgery: Experimental study. *Cancer*, 14:284.
13. Inch, W. R., and McCredie, J. A. (1963): Effect of small dose of x-radiation on local recurrence of tumors in rats and mice. *Cancer*, 16:595.
14. Inch, W. R., and McCredie, J. A. (1964): Preoperative use of a single dose of x-rays: Local cancer recurrence. *Arch. Surg.*, 89:398.
15. Mallams, J. T., Paulson, D. L., Collier, R. E., and Shaw, R. R. (1964): Presurgical irradiation in bronchogenic carcinoma, superior sulcus type. *Radiology*, 82:1050.
16. McGoon, D. W. (1964): Transcervical technique for removal of specimen from superior sulcus tumor for pathologic study. *Ann. Surg.*, 159:407.
17. Pancoast, H. K. (1924): Importance of careful roentgen-ray investigations of apical chest tumors. *J. Am. Med. Assoc.*, 83:1407.
18. Pancoast, H. K. (1932): Superior pulmonary sulcus tumor: Tumor characterized by pain, Horner's syndrome, destruction of bone and atrophy of hand muscles. *J. Am. Med. Assoc.*, 99:1391.
19. Paulson, D. L. (1973): The importance of defining location and staging of superior pulmonary sulcus tumors (editorial). *Ann. Thorac. Surg.*, 15:549.
20. Powers, W. E., and Palmer, L. A. (1968): Biologic basis of preoperative radiation treatment. *Am. J. Roentgenol. Radium Ther. Nucl. Med.*, 102:176.
21. Shaw, R. R., Paulson, D. L., and Kee, J. L., Jr. (1961): Treatment of the superior sulcus tumor by irradiation followed by resection. *Ann. Surg.*, 154:29.
22. Tobias, J. W. (1932): Sincrome apico-costo-vertebral dolorosa por tumor, apexiano. Su valor diagnostico en el cancer primitivo pulmonar. *Rev. Med. Lat. Am.*, 17:1522.
23. Walker, J. E. (1964): Superior sulcus pulmonary tumor (Pancoast syndrome). *J. Med. Assoc. Ga.*, 35:364.

Thoracic Oncology, edited by N. C. Choi and H. C. Grillo. Raven Press, New York © 1983.

Curative Radiation Therapy for Unresectable Non-Small-Cell Carcinoma of the Lung: Indications, Techniques, Results

Noah C. Choi

Department of Radiation Therapy, Harvard Medical School; and Department of Radiation Medicine, Massachusetts General Hospital, Boston, Massachusetts 02114

Cancer of the lung is one of the major challenges to all professionals involved in health care because of the steadily rising incidence of over 135,000 new patients in the United States each year, without any relief in sight (6). Cancer of the lung, which has been the leading cause of death due to cancer in men, is now increasingly responsible for deaths among women. According to current knowledge, surgery seems to hold the best chance of a cure for the early stages of lung cancer (71). However, only 25% to 30% of all patients presenting with such tumors are suitable for either pneumonectomy or lobectomy (i.e., the tumor must be in stage I or II) (73,104,117). Of the many patients for whom curative surgery is not possible, only those with disease still limited to the chest are suitable for curative radiation therapy aimed at eradication of the tumor, a form of local and regional treatment capable of sterilizing both the primary tumor and the metastases in the regional lymph nodes (15,18,52,90).

When radiation therapy is carefully designed for each patient, it is feasible that an unresectable cancer of the lung that is still limited within the regional lymphatics can be sterilized by high doses of radiation delivered to the tumor-bearing areas while adjacent normal vital structures, such as the spinal cord, a large volume of the normal lung tissue, and the heart, are spared from excessive doses of radiation (28).

Patients referred for radiation therapy usually have conditions that are inoperable for one or more of the following reasons: advanced local tumors, insufficient respiratory reserve, advanced age, poor general condition, or refusal of an operation. When a patient is first seen, it is important to decide whether radiation therapy is to be curative or palliative. The survival curve for a group of patients with lung cancer who received curative radiation therapy becomes parallel to that for the normal population of the same age and sex from about the third to fourth year onward (36). Therefore, the rates for 3- to 4-year survival appear to provide a reasonable index for the effectiveness of the treatment in curing or controlling lung cancer. Use of curative high-dose radiation therapy (5,600–6,400 cGy) is indicated only when there is a chance of achieving long-term control. The candidates for

TABLE 1.

TNM Classification	Definitions[a]

Primary Tumor (T).

TX   Tumor proven by the presence of malignant cells in bronchopulmonary secretions but not visualized roentgenographically or bronchoscopically, or any tumor that cannot be assessed

T0   No evidence of primary tumor

TIS   Carcinoma *in situ*

T1   Tumor 3.0 cm or less in greatest diameter, surrounded by lung or visceral pleura, and without evidence of invasion proximal to a lobar bronchus at bronchoscopy

T2   Tumor more than 3.0 cm in greatest diameter, or a tumor of any size that either invades the visceral pleura or has associated atelectasis or obstructive pneumonitis extending to the hilar region. At bronchoscopy, the proximal extent of demonstrable tumor must be within a lobar bronchus or at least 2.0 cm distal to the carina. Any assoiated atelectasis or obstructive pneumonitis must involve less than an entire lung and there must be no pleural effusion

T3   Tumor of any size with direct extension into an adjacent structure such as the parietal pleura or the chest wall, the diaphragm, or the mediastinum and its contents; or a tumor demonstrable bronchoscopically to involve a main bronchus less than 2.0 cm distal to the carina; or any tumor associated with atelectasis or obstructive pneumonitis of an entire lung or pleural effusion

Nodal Involvement (N)

N0   No demonstrable metastasis to regional lymph nodes

N1   Metastasis to lymph nodes in the peribronchial or the ipsilateral hilar region, or both, including direct extension

N2   Metastasis to lymph nodes in the mediastinum

Distant Metastasis (M)

MX   Not assessed

M0   No (known) distant metastasis

M1   Distant metastasis present

Specify sites according to the following notations:

Pulmonary–PUL	Hepatic–HEP	Lymph Nodes–LYM	Skin–SKI	Eye–EYE
Osseous–OSS	Brain–BRA	Bone Marrow–MAR	Pleura–PLE	Other–OTH

Histopathology

Squamous cell carcinoma, adenocarcinoma, undifferentiated large cell, undifferentiated small cell (oat cell cancer)

curative radiation therapy should be as carefully selected as those for curative surgery. There is no justification for treating a dying patient with a high dose over a period of 5 to 6 weeks; such treatment only adds to a patient's terminal misery.

INDICATIONS: PROS AND CONS

Selection of Patients

Curative radiation therapy is indicated when (a) the cancer is locally advanced, but still limited within the chest (T3 or N2 tumor) without distant metastasis and (b) the cancer is in an early stage (T1–2N0M0 or T1–2N1M0) and is resectable

TABLE 1. *(continued)*

TNM Classification		Definitions[a]
Grade		
Well-differentiated, moderately well-differentiated, poorly to very differentiated, or numbers 1, 2, 3, 4		
Stage grouping		
Occult stage	TX N0 M0	Occult carcinoma with bronchopulmonary secretions containing malignant cells but without other evidence of the primary tumor or evidence of metastasis to the regional lymph nodes or distant metastasis
Stage I	TIS N0 M0	Carcinoma *in situ*
	T1 N0 M0 T1 N1 M0 T2 N0 M0[b]	Tumor that can be classified T1 without any metastasis or with metastasis to the lymph nodes in the peribronchial and/or ipsilateral hilar region only, or a tumor that can be classified T2 without any metastasis to nodes or distant metastasis
Stage II	T2 N1 M0	Tumor classified as T2 with metastasis to the lymph nodes in the peribronchial and/or ipsilateral hilar region only
Stage III	T3 with any N or M N2 with any T or M M1 with any T or N	Any tumor more extensive than T2, or any tumor with metastasis to the lymph nodes in the mediastinum, or any tumor with distant metastasis

[a]TNM classification system recommended by the American Joint Committee for Cancer Staging and End-Results Reporting (1).
[b]TX N1 M0 and T0 N1 M0 are also theoretically possible, but such a clinical diagnosis would be difficult if not impossible to make. If such a diagnosis is made, it should be included under stage I.

but is not operable because of medical contraindications (7) (Table 1). The patient's general condition should be good enough to tolerate a course of radiation therapy that lasts for 5.5 to 6.5 weeks: ≥70 on the Karnofsky scale (Table 2) and grade 0–1 on the Zubrod scale (Table 3) (61,122).

When there is malignant effusion in the pleura or pericardium, although it is still T3 tumor, radiation therapy should be considered palliative because of the difficulty of delivering an adequate curative dose to the entire unilateral pleural cavity or to the entire pericardial cavity without excessive damage to normal tissue. Also, when there is extensive involvement of supraclavicular lymph nodes (M1 tumor), which usually is a sign of widespread distant metastases, the radiation will not effect a cure and therefore should be considered palliative (7,43,73,104).

However, patients with minimal involvement (lymph node ≤ 2.5 cm) of the ipsilateral supraclavicular lymph node group can be saved with an aggressive high

TABLE 2. *Criteria for performance status (Karnofsky scale)*[a]

Able to carry on normal activity; no special care needed	100	Normal; no complaints; no evidence of disease
	90	Able to carry on normal activity; minor signs or symptoms of disease
	80	Normal activity with effort; some signs or symptoms of disease
Unable to work; able to live at home and care for most personal needs; varying amounts of assistance needed	70	Cares for self; unable to carry on normal activity or to do active work
	60	Requires occasional assistance but is able to care for most of needs
	50	Requires considerable assistance and frequent medical care
Unable to care for self; requires equivalent of institutional or hospital care; disease may be progressing rapidly	40	Disabled; requires special care and assistance
	30	Severely disabled; hospitalization is indicated although death not imminent
	20	Very sick; hospitalization necessary; active supportive treatment necessary
	10	Moribund; fatal processes progressing rapidly
	0	Dead

[a]From Karnofsky (61).

TABLE 3. *Performance status (Zubrod scale)*[b]

Grade	Description
0	Fully active, able to carry on all predisease activities without restriction (Karnofsky, 90–100)
1	Restricted in physically strenuous activity, but ambulatory and able to carry out work of a light or sedentary nature, e.g., light housework, office work (Karnofsky, 70–80)
2	Ambulatory and capable of all self-care, but unable to carry out any work activities; up and about more than 50% of waking hours (Karnofsky, 50–60)
3	Capable of only limited self-care; confined to bed or chair 50% or more of waking hours (Karnofsky, 30–40)
4	Completely disabled; cannot carry on any self-care; totally confined to bed or chair (Karnofsky, 10–20)

[b]From Zubrod (122).

dose of radiation therapy (28,36,57). Patients with severe chronic obstructive pulmonary disease, congestive heart failure, or recent myocardial infarction may be given radiation if it is carefully designed in terms of a dose fractionation schedule and target volume. The communication between radiation oncologists and internists must be close, of course, when curative radiation therapy is planned for these patients with such a high risk of potential complications. A pulmonary infection distal to the obstructive cancer is not a contraindication for radiation therapy, inasmuch as it is essential to open the occlusion to control the obstructive pneumonia. Patients with inactive pulmonary tuberculosis can be treated safely with radiation therapy if they have the proper antituberculosis medications. Superior vena cava syndrome alone, however, is not a contraindication for curative high-dose radiation therapy, unless there is evidence of distant metastasis (28,36,76).

Workup Procedures

Careful screening for distant metastases is necessary to save as many asymptomatic patients as possible from an unnecessary and prolonged course of 5.5 to 6.5 weeks of radiation therapy. Unfortunately, a screening test with a high specificity is not yet available. Radioisotope scans of the liver and bone and a computed tomographic scan of the brain, although nonspecific, are still recommended because gross asymptomatic metastases can be detected. Base-line studies of these frequently involved organs are also useful for future follow-up and managment. Laboratory examination of the blood cells and blood urea nitrogen and liver should be performed routinely. Patients with low hemoglobin concentrations (≤ 10 g/dl) require transfusion of packed red blood cells to increase the hemoglobin level to normal (≥ 12 g/dl). Low hemoglobin concentrations were found to be associated with a high rate of local recurrence after radiation therapy in carcinoma of the cervix (19). Leukopenia (WBC $\leq 2,500/mm^3$) and thrombocytopenia (platelets $\leq 100,000/mm^3$) should be carefully evaluated and corrected before radiation therapy begins. The condition of patients with hepatic or renal failure must be considered carefully, as they have limited tolerance to radiation therapy. A careful assessment of a patient's cardiopulmonary status is also an essential part of the general evaluation of the suitability of curative radiation therapy. Compromised radiation doses and target volumes are necessary for patients with either poor pulmonary reserve or poor cardiac reserve. The regional pulmonary function test is another useful way to assess pulmonary status (5,60,102), inasmuch as it predicts pulmonary functional status after either surgery or radiation therapy. Approximately 25% to 40% of patients who have been referred for radiation therapy because of cancer of the lung are eligible for curative radiation therapy after the currently available screening procedures (28,44).

General Supportive Care of Patients

The majority of patients receive radiation therapy on an outpatient basis, but in the hospital or out the social and psychological impacts of the diagnosis of cancer of the lung are so great that a counseling with involved physicians, social workers, and psychologists is invaluable, not only to the patient but also to the family. Of course, full cooperation of patients and their families is essential for the planned curative radiation therapy to be successful. Curative radiation therapy, which entails 5.5 to 6.5 weeks of treatment, is taxing to the patient, and therefore nutritional status must be optimally maintained by a balanced high-protein diet. With the help of proper nutrition, the usual weight changes during radiation therapy for patients with cancer of the lung are in the range of $\pm 5\%$ of the original weight before treatment. Almost all patients experience some degree of dysphagia as a result of radiation-induced esophagitis. The symptoms begin at the second or third week of treatment, reach a peak at the third or fourth week, and subside gradually over a period of 1.5 to 2 weeks after completion of the treatment. Patients should be advised not to take solids or other substances or liquids that may cause irritation to the esophagus during treatment, e.g., hot or very cold drinks, spices, alcohol, and rough foods. Protein supplements such as Sustacal are also recommended for patients with an excessive dysphagia. Topical anesthetics (lidocaine 2% viscous solution) and antacid preparations provide temporary relief of the symptom. When the esophagitis is severe, a reduction in the daily dose of radiation from 200 cGy to 180 cGy per treatment or a rest of 7 to 10 days is occasionally necessary. There may be monilial or herpes simplex viral infection of the oropharynx and esophagus that can mimic radiation-induced esophagitis. The moniliasis will respond to nystatin oral suspension.

Complexity of Radiation Therapy

Optimum radiation therapy for cure of a locally advanced carcinoma of the lung also requires a good support team, which should include physicists, dosimetrists, radiation therapy technologists, nurses, and machine-shop personnel. There also must be a computer to assist in the treatment planning, a simulator, and adequate treatment machines (10–25-MeV photon delivered by a linear accelerator). Last, but not least, there must be an experienced thoracic radiation oncologist. Large radiation therapy centers are better equipped to deal with this kind of complicated treatment than is a small community center.

RADIOTHERAPEUTIC TECHNIQUES

Definition of Target Volume

Carcinoma of the lung spreads through the lymphatics and the bloodstream and by direct invasion to the adjacent normal structures. The incidence of hilar and mediastinal lymph node involvement by metastatic deposits from cancer of the lung varies from 30% to 50% in surgically resectable cases (73,104,117). In the author's series (28) of 162 patients referred for curative radiation therapy because of cancer of the lung, 90% (147 patients) had metastatic involvement of either the mediastinal lymph nodes (131 patients) or the mediastinal lymph nodes plus the supraclavicular lymph nodes (16 patients) (Table 4). For a locally advanced unresectable cancer of the lung (T3 or N2 tumor), the target volume includes the primary tumor mass with a 2-cm margin of clinically uninvolved lung, the entire mediastinum, and the medial halves of both supraclavicular areas. The anatomic boundary for this volume is defined on the left by the lateral edge of the aortic arch, on the right by a line drawn 3 to 4 cm lateral to the right lateral wall of the trachea, inferiorly by 3.5 to 4 vertebral bodies below the carina, and superiorly by the cricoid cartilage (Fig. 1). Both supraclavicular areas are defined laterally by the midclavicular lines and inferiorly by a line drawn along the lower border of the first ribs (Fig. 2).

TABLE 4. *TNM stages for 162 patients[a]*

Stage	No. of patients
T3 N2 M0	53
T2 N2 M0	78
T3 N0 M0	9
T1–2 N0 M0	6
Supraclavicular lymph node (M1)	16

[a]Adapted from Choi and Doucette (28).
[b]The TNM staging system recommended by the American Joint Committee is used.

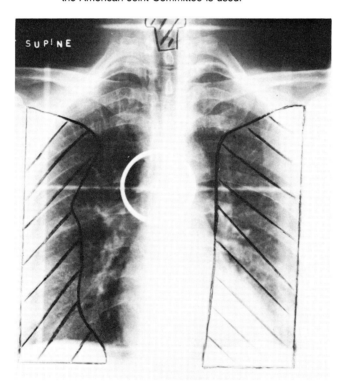

FIG. 1. An AP simulation film illustrates a target volume and cerrobend blocks for protection of normal tissues. This patient had a large squamous cell carcinoma of the right mainstem bronchus.

Target volumes described in the literature for unresectable cancer of the lung have varied from 10 × 8 cm² to 22 × 12 cm², excluding uninvolved normal lung protected by cerrobend blocks (28,33,34,40,81,96). The main reason for this large discrepancy is primarily the difference of the coverage for potentially involved lymph nodes in the mediastinum, including those at the thoracic inlet and the lower

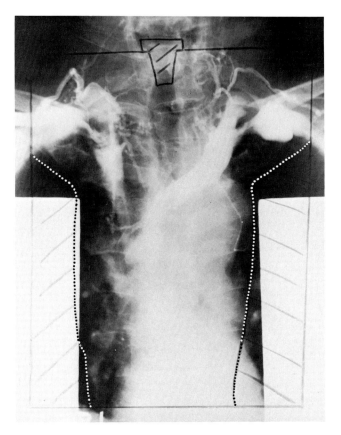

FIG. 2. Superior-vena-cavagram from a patient with superior vena cava obstruction by an underlying lung cancer. The target volume drawn in the film illustrates the need for a good margin below the clavicles to cover the involved lymph nodes at the junction of the innominate and subclavian veins.

mediastinum. A small lung cancer inoperable because of medical reasons can be treated with a small target volume. However, the majority of patients referred for curative radiation therapy because of surgically unresectable cancer of the lung require a large target volume that includes all potentially involved lymph nodes along the innominate vessels and at the junction of the innominate and subclavian vessels at the upper mediastinum and both supraclavicular areas (as illustrated by the superior-vena-cavagram of Fig. 2) and along the lower thoracic esophagus and descending thoracic aorta at the lower mediastinum.

The main emphasis for radiotherapeutic coverage of the routes of lymphatic spread by cancer of the lung has been on the antegrade routes toward cephalad direction. However, the retrograde route toward the upper abdomen seems to be another important direction of the spread that has received inadequate attention from radiation oncologists. In experiments with transplantable V_2 carcinoma in rabbits,

Zeidman (120) demonstrated that retrograde metastases occurred via collateral lymphatics when the lymph nodes at the antegrade routes were involved by the tumor. Bell (11) emphasized the importance of the retrograde pathway to the upper abdomen even in the clinically resectable early stages of cancer of the lung by demonstrating 12% incidence of metastatic involvement of the celiac, gastric, and upper abdominal aortic lymph nodes when patients with resectable cancer of the lung were subjected to upper abdominal exploration before thoracotomy. The retrograde pathway was also supported by autopsy studies in which the incidences of metastatic involvement of the upper abdominal lymph nodes were 26% to 30%, which were more frequent than that of any nodal group other than the mediastinal lymph nodes (70,78). These are the reasons that the target volume we use includes the entire lower mediastinum extending down to the diaphragm to cover the retrograde route. Typical examples of target volumes we use are shown in Figs. 1 through 5.

Optimum Dose and Fractionation Schedules

There are several different fractionation schedules that have similar biological effects on both normal and malignant tissues. Nominal standard dose (NSD) and time-dose and fractionation (TDF) factor have been advocated as a reference dose when different fractionation schedules of radiation therapy are compared for their effects on normal as well as tumor tissues (79,106).

In experimental tumor models, control of localized tumor is a function of radiation dose, tumor size, immunological status of the host, and the like (26). An optimum fractionation schedule for cancer of the lung is a radiation therapy schedule that

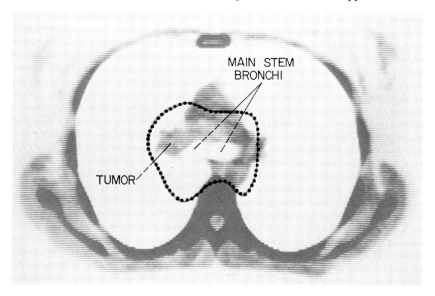

FIG. 3. Target volume drawn on a computed body tomogram at the level of the central axis of the radiation treatment field.

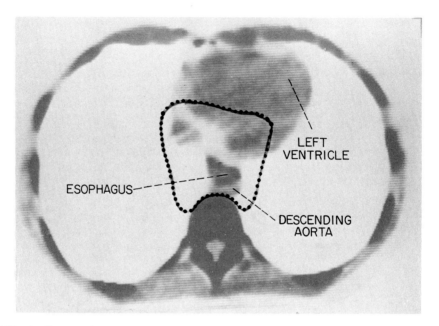

FIG. 4. Target volume drawn on a computed body tomogram at the lower aspect of the mediastinum encompasses lymphatics along the descending aorta, esophagus, and pulmonary ligaments.

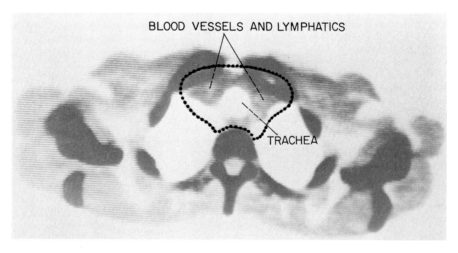

FIG. 5. Target volume drawn on a computed body tomogram at the level of the sternal notch encompasses lymphatics at the thoracic inlet.

gives the best control of localized tumor with the least complication rate. Survival rate alone probably is not a fair yardstick when different fractionation schedules are compared for cancer of the lung. Many patients die with distant metastatic tumors that were outside the thorax before radiation therapy was started, even when there has been no microscopic evidence of residual tumor at the primary site and regional lymph nodes. In preoperative radiation therapy studies, no evidence of microscopic residual tumor was found in 29% to 54% of patients with total radiation doses of 4,700 to 6,000 cGy, with a daily dose of 180 to 200 cGy (15,18,52). Metastatic tumors in the mediastinal lymph nodes were just as sensitive to radiation as were the primary lesions (15). Clinical studies of the relationship between radiation doses and control rates for localized tumors have demonstrated that there is a reasonable correlation between dose and response in lung cancer (28,82). Other important factors for control of localized tumor, in addition to radiation doses, are the tumor stage and, possibly, the histologic type of the tumor and the patient's general condition (28,81). The benefit of improved control of localized tumor by higher radiation doses (5,600–6,400 cGy) rather than lower-to-moderate radiation doses (4,000–4,900 cGy) may not become apparent until 1.5 years or more after treatment (28). This implies that low-to-moderate doses of radiation (4,000–4,900 cGy) will achieve a relatively good short-term rate of control of localized tumor ($\simeq$70%) up to 1 year after treatment by delaying active tumor growth. However, the long-term ($\geq$18 months) rates of control of localized tumor are 76% with high-dose therapy (5,600–6,400 cGy) versus 29% with low-dose (4,000–4,900 cGy) radiation therapy. This difference is also reflected in survival rates. Radiation therapy delivered in a split course, in which a rest period of 2 to 3 weeks is given at the halfway point of the entire course of the treatment (5–6 weeks), has been extensively studied (4,9,44,51,55,64,65,81,96). Patients' reactions up to this point provide a convenient way of selecting patients who will tolerate high-dose curative radiation therapy (21). However, there is no clear evidence that a split course of radiation therapy does any better than continuous treatments. With the currently available data, an optimum schedule of radiation therapy seems to be in the range of a total dose of 5,600 to 6,400 cGy, given as a daily dose of 180 to 200 cGy per treatment for five treatments weekly over a period of 5.6 to 7 weeks (28,82,96).

Radiation Portal Arrangements

The arrangement of the radiation portals is dependent on the planned total dose, the types of radiation, and the shape of the target volume. Because of the scatter radiation of low-energy beams and the large penumbra of a ^{60}Co unit, high-energy beams (10–25-MeV photon) seem to be the choice for curative radiation therapy, with a targeted total dose of 5,600 to 6,400 cGy. An arrangement of two parallel opposing portals (POP) applied anteriorly (AP) and posteriorly (PA) to the chest is simple and accurate, with the least risk of a geographic miss. However, the maximum dose that can be delivered with this technique is in the range of 4,400 to 4,600 cGy because of the tolerance of the spinal cord. A posterior spinal cord block has been used to limit the spinal cord dose to 5,000 cGy or less while a total dose 6,000 cGy is delivered at the midplane (81). Unfortunately, a zone of a low tumor dose that is generated at the posterior mediastinum along the vertebral column can also protect the tumor (Fig. 6). An outright three-field arrangement of an

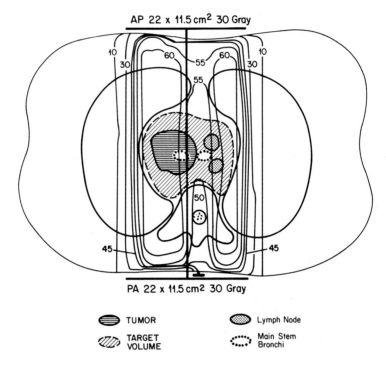

AP 22 x 11.5 cm² 30 Gray

PA 22 x 11.5 cm2 30 Gray

⬭ TUMOR   ⬭ Lymph Node

▨ TARGET VOLUME   ⠿ Main Stem Bronchi

FIG. 6. A composite isodose for AP and PA POP with a posterior cord block. A large portion of the target volume, including the tumor and lymph nodes, is underdosed when a posterior spinal cord block is placed to protect the spinal cord (total dose 6,000 cGy by 10-MeV photon).

anteroposterior (AP), right posterior oblique (RPO), and left posterior oblique (LPO) is a reasonable technique to deliver the dose to a small target volume located centrally. The drawbacks of this technique are a relatively high radiation dose (50% of total dose) to the pulmonary tissue in the path of the oblique beams, the potential risk of a geographic miss along the paravertebral areas, and the difficulty of dealing with a large target volume ($\geq 1,400$ cm³) because of the poor pulmonary tolerance (Fig. 7). The rotational technique is undesirable as an outright approach for the same reasons. However, it can be used as a method to boost a radiation dose to the main tumor mass. A treatment technique that we have developed is a combination of AP–PA POP with a three-field AP, RPO, and LPO arrangement, with which one can deliver a high radiation dose (5,600–6,000 cGy) to the target volume while normal vital structures are kept below the threshold dose that would cause permanent radiation injuries (spinal cord dose $\leq 4,400$ cGy and pulmonary dose in the path of the oblique beams $\leq 1,200-1,400$ cGy) (Fig. 8). With this technique, the total dose of 6,000 cGy is delivered by an arrangement of AP–PA POP for the initial 3,600 cGy and by the three-field (AP, RPO, and LPO) arrangement for the additional 2,400 cGy, using a daily dose of 180 to 200 cGy. Any target volume away from the mainstem bronchus and mediastinum requires a supplemental dose of 600 to 800 cGy to increase the minimum dose to the tumor to 6,000 to 6,400 cGy,

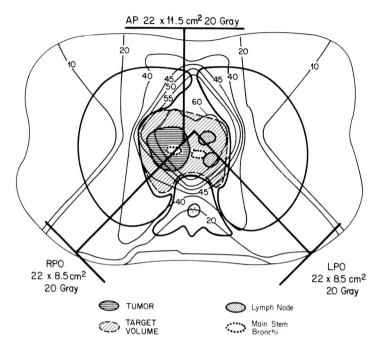

FIG. 7. A composite isodose for an outright three-field approach by AP, RPO, and LPO (total dose 6,000 cGy by 10-MeV photon).

depending on the composite isodose plan (Fig. 9). For this technique to be successful, individually tailored cerrobend blocks are essential for protection of the uninvolved pulmonary tissue from the AP–PA portals and protection of the spinal cord from the oblique beams (Fig. 10).

Dose Distribution in the Target Volume

Because of the increased transmission of photons through the low-density lung tissue, the actual dose received, without correction by the tumor, from supervoltage units such as a ^{60}Co or an 18-MeV linear accelerator is 15% to 30% higher than that calculated on the assumption that the tissue is of homogeneous unit density. As computed body tomography (CBT) becomes increasingly available to radiation oncologists, radiation dosimetry is expected to improve, because there will be accurate body contours at different levels of the target volume, improved definition of tumor size and location relative to other normal vital structures, and precise measurement of the thickness of the pulmonary tissue in the path of the radiation, for which a correction is necessary for the increased transmission (Fig. 8). It is essential to have a target volume and tumor mass drawn in a contour with a composite isodose plan from which one can estimate the maximum and minimum tumor doses. Every effort should be made to achieve the ideal treatment plan, which would give the least variation of the radiation doses within the target volume, with the maximum

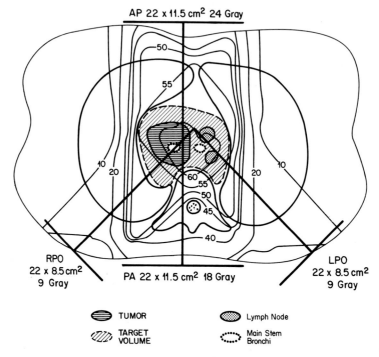

FIG. 8. A composite isodose for an approach that combines AP–PA POP (3,600 cGy) with AP–RPO–LPO (2,400 cGy) sequentially (10-MeV photon). The advantages of this approach over the outright three-field approach (Fig. 7) include less lung volume within the zone of the radiation dose ($\geq$ 2,000 cGy) and better coverage of the target volume along the paravertebral regions.

differential of radiation dose between the tumor and the surrounding normal tissue. CBT has been relatively inaccurate in defining metastatic tumors in hilar and mediastinal lymph nodes (115). However, it is probably the best method to define a tumor extension to the parietal pleura or to the chest wall (Fig. 11) (42, 103).

RESULTS OF HIGH-DOSE RADIATION THERAPY

Cure is the primary goal of high-dose radiation therapy for unresectable cancer of the lung. However, the radiation therapy is a local and regional treatment that cannot alter the course of the disease if there is preexisting distant metastasis. Other goals for high-dose radiation therapy include control of the local tumor and relief of symptoms. The rate of control of the local and regional tumor is a good criterion for the effectiveness of the local and regional treatment, i.e., high-dose radiation therapy (28,82,96).

Survival in Relation to Radiation Doses, Target Volumes, and Stages of Tumors

The actuarial method for data concerning survival rates is to be favored because it makes use of all the information available without waiting until a specified time

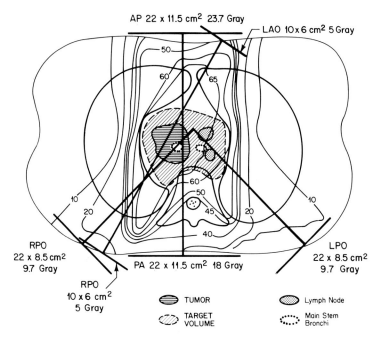

FIG. 9. Final composite isodose for AP–PA POP (3,600 cGy) and AP–RPO–LPO (2,400 cGy) with a supplement of 1,000 cGy to the main tumor by LAO and RPO. The entire target volume is encompassed by an isodose line of ≥ 6,000 cGy, with the main tumor being at the line of ≥ 6,500 cGy. For the dosimetry, a correction is made for the lung tissue in the path of the oblique beams.

has elapsed for the whole group (10,29). The rates of survival at 3 to 4 years are very close to the rates of actual clinical cure, inasmuch as the survival curve for patients with cancer of the lung treated by curative radiation therapy becomes parallel to that for the normal population of the same age and sex at 3 to 4 years (36). For patients with unresectable cancer of the lung subjected to high-dose radiation therapy, the cure rates are in the range of 5% to 15% at 5 years, depending on the selection of patients and treatment techniques (21,33,44). Some of the reported results are shown in Table 5. It is interesting to note that median survival and short-term survival, up to 1.5 years, of patients who received curative radiation therapy for unresectable cancer of the lung are independent of the ranges of radiation doses (4,000–6,400 cGy) and target volumes (16 × 10 cm² to 22 × 16 cm²) (Fig. 12) (28). A trend for improved survival after high-dose large-volume radiation therapy did not become apparent until 1.5 to 2 years after this treatment. It is suggested that data for long-term survival at 2 years or more would be preferable to data for median or short-term survival at 1.5 years or less when results of curative radiation therapy for unresectable cancer of the lung are compared for the different radiation doses and target volumes. From the survival data in Fig. 12 and the results reported by others (9,36,50,55) it is postulated that the slopes of the survival curves during the first 1.5 years, which are initially steep, represent the fate of patients according to the outcome of the preexisting distant metastases, whereas the slopes of the

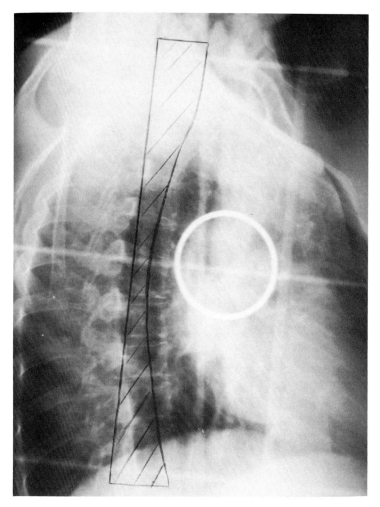

FIG. 10. A simulation film, RPO, of the three-field arrangement. A cerrobend block is designed to shield the spinal cord from the beam.

survival curves at 1.5 years and later, which are well leveled off and dependent on radiation doses, represent the fate of patients according to the outcome of the primary and regional tumors. Considerable effort has been made in studying the effectiveness of a split course of radiation therapy in cancer of the lung (4,9,21,28,44,51). The results reported thus far do not show that it has any significant benefit over continuous radiation therapy (Table 6). However, the split-course regimen is a good way to select patients who should have palliative versus curative radiation therapy.

Control Rates for Local and Regional Tumors

The rate of control of local and regional tumors is probably the best criterion for the effectiveness of various radiotherapeutic approaches using different dose levels

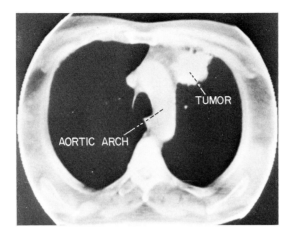

FIG. 11. The extension of the tumor at the left upper lobe to the chest wall and the aortic arch is well demonstrated by this computed body tomogram at the level of the aortic arch. This is not clear on regular chest radiographs.

and target volumes. This rate is a function of radiation dose, tumor size (stage of tumor), and other less well understood systemic factors (28,82). Clinical criteria described in the literature in an attempt to measure the effectiveness of radiotherapeutic approaches include early resolution of the tumor 1 month after radiation therapy and a degree of local tumor clearance within a relatively short time after treatment (81,96,101). However, one should be aware of pitfalls in such approaches. During the early period after radiation therapy, we are measuring the diameter of a mass of nonviable tumor cells, and this measurement describes only the rate of removal of lysed tumor cells and tumor stroma. In experimental studies using easily measurable transplants of spontaneous mammary carcinoma and radiation-induced osteogenic sarcoma in C3H mice and a benzpyrene-induced fibrosarcoma in rats, no correlation was found between the rate of early regression of the tumor and the eventual control of the localized tumor (26,110,114). An explanation for these findings may be that for permanant control of a localized tumor the radiation dose must be sufficient to give lethal injuries to all tumor cells. Therefore, even radiation doses that are quite ineffective in terms of achieving sterilization of a tumor would be expected to damage lethally almost all tumor cells (99.99%). Certainly, over short periods of observation, gross measurements of tumor size would not enable one to discriminate survival fractions of 10^{-4} and 10^{-7}, which would indicate a low and a high probability of tumor control (110). The time needed for residual viable tumor cells to repopulate to a size that is detectable clinically and radiographically after high-dose radiation therapy in lung cancer is 18 to 24 months (28). An additional factor that makes it difficult to measure an irradiated tumor mass in the lung are radiation-induced injuries to the lung, which, as shown by radiography, become stabilized 9 to 12 months after the irradiation (52). According to our series, the rate of control of localized tumors at 18 months and longer is well correlated with survival (Table 7, Fig. 12). Further studies are needed to define

TABLE 5. Results of definitive radiation therapy for unresectable non-small-cell lung cancer

Authors	Year	Type of radiation	Total dose (cGy)	No. of patients	Survival rate (%)				
					1 yr	2 yr	3 yr	4 yr	5 yr
Schulz (97)	1957	280-kV X-rays	3,000–4,500	385	15	5	3	1	1
Guttman (50)	1965	2-MeV photon	5,000/25 F/5 wk	95[a]	58	27	18	11.5	7.4
Pierquin et al. (86)	1965	22-MeV photon	4,000–7,000	324	30	—	10	—	—
Deeley & Singh (35)	1967	8-MeV photon	4,500/20 F/4 wk	266	—	—	10	—	—
Roswit et al. (91)	1968	200–260-kV X-rays or ^{60}Co	4,000–5,000/20–25 F/4–5 wk	308	22	—	—	—	—
Petrovich et al. (83)	1978	Megavoltage	5,000–6,000/4–6 wk	171	—	15	—	—	—
Perez et al. (81)	1980	^{60}Co or higher-energy photon	4,000–6,000/20–30 F/4–6 wk	272	45	25	—	—	—
Holsti & Mattson (55)	1980	^{60}Co or 33-MeV photon	5,000/25 F/5 wk	158	27	12	7	—	6
Choi (28)	1981	2–10-MeV photon	5,000–6,400/25–34 F/5–7 wk	108	48	24	19	7	7

[a]All patients were found to have unresectable tumors at thoracotomy.

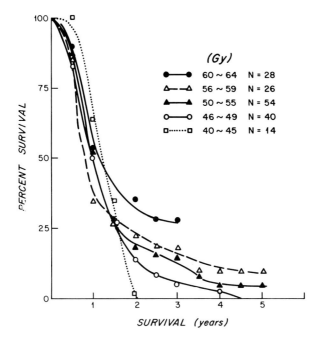

FIG. 12. Actuarial survival rates for patients treated with various radiation doses and target volumes with minimum follow-up of 2 years (28). N = number of patients.

optimum criteria to be used in evaluation of various radiotherapeutic approaches. There is also an urgent need for an optimum radiotherapeutic approach that would play an important role in the future when effective systemic therapies such as chemotherapy or immunotherapy become available.

Most physicians will recommend irradiation for alleviation of presenting symptoms, but in the absence of symptoms and in the absence of good screening methods for distant microscopic metastases, physicians occasionally do not anticipate the need for the therapy until it is too late (12). It must be emphasized that a cure by radiation therapy can be achieved only when the tumor is still limited within the primary site and the regional lymphatics, without distant metastases (28,36,50, 81,96,97).

Relief of Distressing Symptoms

Some of the symptoms and their susceptibilities to alleviation by radiation therapy are as follows:

Hemoptysis, which is alarming to patients and their families, is well relieved in over 90% of patients with a moderate dose (3,000–4,000 cGy) of radiation (66,69,98).

Dyspnea associated with obstruction of the trachea, carina, or mainstem or lobar bronchi is also well relieved in over 80% of patients by radiation therapy. The radiation dose required to achieve prolonged palliation of the dyspnea is in the

TABLE 6. *Comparison of split-course vs. continuous radiation therapy for unresectable non-small-cell lung cancer*

Authors	Treatment schedules and total dose[a] (cGy)	No. of patients	Randomization of study	Outcome	Median survival	Survival (%) 1 yr	2 yr	3 yr	5 yr
Levitt et al. (65)	6,000/30 F/6 wk vs. 1,800/3 F/3 D—4 wk off—1,800/3 F/3 D	29	Yes	N.S.[b]	—	10	—	—	—
Abramson & Cavanaugh (4)	6,000/30 F/6 wk vs. 2,000/5 F/1 wk—3 wk off—2,000/5 F/1 wk	233	No	N.S.	—	25	—	—	—
Johnson et al. (58)	4,800/20 F/4 wk vs. 2,800/4 F/11 D	100	Yes	N.S.	—	35 / 30	9	9	6
Lee et al. (64)	5,000/25 F/5 wk vs. 2,600/13 F/2.6 wk—3–4 wk off—2,400/12 F/2.4 wk	188	Yes	N.S.	—	33 / 40 / 40	9	6	6
Salazar et al. (96)	4,000–6,000/20–30 F/4–6 wk vs. 4,000–6,000/10–25 F/4–9 wk with 2 wk off at halfway	160	No	Better with split course	7.7 M[c] / 11.5 M	35 / 46	—	—	—
Holsti & Mattson (55)	5,000/25 F/5 wk vs. 5,500/28 F/7–8 wk with 2–3 wk off at halfway	363	Yes	N.S.	—	27 / 29	12 / 11	7 / 7	6 / 2
Perez et al. (81)	4,000–6,000/20–30 F/4–6 wk vs. 2,000/5 F/1 wk—2 wk off—2,000/5 F/1 wk	365	Yes	N.S.	41–47 wk / 37 wk	45 / 45	25 / 10	—	—
Choi (28)	5,000–5,500/25–28 F/5–5.6 wk vs. 2,400/8 F/1.6 wk—2–3 wk off—2100/7 F/1.4 wk	54	No	N.S.	12 M / 13 M	48 / 50	18 / 19	15	4.8
Sealy et al. (101)	3,000/15 F/3 wk—2 wk off—2,000/10 F/2 wk vs. 2,000/5 F/1 wk—3 wk off—2,000/5 F/1 wk	269	Yes	N.S.	37 wk / 31 wk	—	—	—	—

[a]F = fraction, D = day.
[b]N.S. = not significant.
[c]M = month.

TABLE 7. *Local tumor control in relation to radiation doses*

Radiation doses (Gray)	Local tumor control	
	12 Months	≥18 Months
56–64	23/29 (79%)	13/17 (76%)
50–55	23/30 (76%)	8/16 (50%)
40–49	22/32 (69%)	4/14 (29%)

From Choi and Doucette (28).

range of 4,500 to 5,000 cGy. However, diffuse pulmonary involvement by the tumor and lymphangitic carcinomatosis, which also present with severe dyspnea, are most unlikely to be relieved by radiation therapy.

Cough, another distressing symptom, can be relieved by irradiation, although not as dramatically as hemoptysis or dyspnea. Cough associated with tumors located in the mainstem bronchus or carina is more likely to be relieved and is more easily relieved than that associated with a peripheral tumor of the lung. Radiation therapy itself induces dry cough as a result of dryness and irritation of the tracheal and bronchial mucosa. Most patients feel quite comfortable 4 to 5 months after completion of radiation therapy, when the response of normal tissue to irradiation has progressed beyond the acute and subacute stages.

Local pain associated with direct spread of the tumor to the surrounding normal structures, such as the chest wall, vertebral bodies, brachial plexus, and mediastinum, has also been well relieved by irradiation. The duration of the symptomatic relief is a function of the extent of the tumor and the radiation dose, which itself is limited by the tolerance of normal tissues in the target volume. With a moderate dose of radiation (4,000–4,600 cGy), good symptomatic palliation has been achieved in the majority of patients.

Superior vena cava syndrome, as mentioned earlier, is a common complication of locally advanced cancer of the lung. The more recent the onset of the symptoms caused by the obstruction of venous drainage, the faster the relief of the distressing symptoms by irradiation. A superior-vena-cavagram is useful for the design of radiation portals (Fig. 2). For rapid decompression, a schedule of radiation therapy by either (a) 180 to 200 cGy per treatment, two to three treatments daily for the first 4 to 5 days, followed by the regular 200 cGy per treatment daily to a total dose of 4,500 to 5,000 cGy (an approach we use) or (b) a large fraction, 400 cGy per treatment, daily for the first 3 to 4 days, followed by the regular 200 cGy per treatment daily to the same total dose, has been very effective, with ≥80% relief of the presenting symptoms (94). As mentioned earlier, patients presenting with superior vena cava syndrome without evidence of distant metastasis should be given a full course of high-dose radiation therapy, because some of them could survive many years (28,36,76).

Hoarseness is another common presenting symptom of cancer of the lung. Paralysis of the left, rather than the right, recurrent laryngeal nerve is more common because of its long anatomic course into the thorax. Relief of the hoarseness by irradiation depends on the degree of injury to the recurrent laryngeal nerve by the tumor and its duration. Hoarseness alone without distant metastasis should not preclude high-dose radiation therapy, because some of these patients can survive for many useful years.

Bone pain, neurological deficit due to a cord compression, and symptoms of increased intracranial pressure and neurological deficit due to metastatic lesions in the brain are other distressing symptoms. Short-term palliation of these conditions by irradiation has been satisfactory. A patient with a distant metastasis as a single site of relapse deserves carefully planned radiation therapy in which a moderate-to-high radiation dose of 4,500 to 5,000 cGy is used, because such patients occasionally are long-term survivors.

Patterns of Failure after Curative Radiation Therapy

Common patterns of failure after high-dose curative radiation therapy are failure only at distant sites, local or regional failure plus distant metastasis, and local and regional failure only without distant metastasis. With high-dose large-volume radiation therapy, rates of control of local and regional tumor have reached over 60% to 70% (28,81). To develop a comprehensive program to deal not only with the local or regional tumor but also with the metastatic deposit at distant sites, it is important to review patterns of failure after high-dose radiation therapy. According to the results from our series and reports by others, the most frequent sites of distant failure are brain, bone, liver, and the opposite lung (Table 8) (1,28,32,40,63). The pattern of failure seems to be related to the histologic type of tumor. With squamous cell carcinoma and large cell carcinoma there is an association of failure at the local and regional areas more often than at the distant sites. On the other hand, with adenocarcinoma, the association of failure is at the brain or bone more often than at other locations (28,105). The role of elective irradiation to the brain has been

TABLE 8. *Patterns of failure after curative irradiation*

Histologic type (no. of patients)	Primary site or regional areas	Brain	Bone	Liver	Opposite lung
Squamous cell carcinoma (63)	43% (29%)[a]	16% (6.3%)	32% (16%)	16%	11%
Adenocarcinoma (24)	21% (8%)	38% (17%)	37% (17%)	29% (8%)	12.5%
Large cell carcinoma (17)	65% (47%)	35% (12%)	17%	6%	12%
Undifferentiated carcinoma (7)	12%	57% (43%)	57%		14%

From Choi and Doucette (28).
[a]Numbers in parentheses represent failure rates at the specific site as the only site of failure until the patient's death.

under investigation in stage III carcinoma of the lung, with a preliminary suggestion of some benefit (31). There is a need for further studies with respect to the role of elective irradiation to the sites of frequent failure, such as the brain and liver, in the management of carcinoma of the lung.

Morbidity and Complications: Normal Tissue Tolerance to Radiation Therapy

The responses of normal tissue in the thorax to radiation therapy can be categorized as early, intermediate, and late. There also are early systemic effects that include transient mild nausea during the first week of treatment, some anorexia, and fatigue during the latter half of the course of treatment (third to sixth weeks).

Radiation-induced esophagitis characterized by a mild-to-moderate degree of retrosternal discomfort associated with dysphagia usually begins at the third week of irradiation (threshold dose, 2,500–3,000 cGy) and reaches its peak at the fourth week. Esophagograms taken at the peak of the acute reaction reveal the margins of the barium column to be serrated. They usually are amenable to medications such as prochlorperazine for nausea and topical analgesics such as lidocaine 2% viscous solution for retrosternal discomfort. The course of the radiation-induced esophagitis is self-limited, lasting 10 to 14 days after the completion of radiation therapy. Later sequelae such as stenosis, ulceration, and fistula formation of the esophagus are very rare. Without direct invasion of this normal structure by the underlying cancer of the lung, there was no incidence of fistula formation in our series of 162 cases (28).

The use of certain chemotherapeutic agents (e.g., doxorubicin and daunorubicin) has been associated with potentiation and recall of radiation-induced esophagitis (47,56,74). Even with relatively low radiation doses, e.g., 500 to 2,500 cGy, which are below the esophageal tolerance dose, these potentiation and recall phenomena have been observed. Omission of doxorubicin from a few cycles of a combination chemotherapy program immediately before and after radiation therapy has reduced the frequency and severity of this complication. Frequent recalls of severe radiation-induced esophagitis could lead to a stricture. As more and more patients are likely to be subjected to doxorubicin because of its effectiveness in small cell carcinoma of the lung and in breast cancer and other tumors that appear less frequently, it is important for us to be aware of this potential complication and to plan in advance the use of both radiation therapy and doxorubicin in such a way that this undesirable side effect can be avoided.

Irradiation-induced injuries to normal tissue that appear after an intermediate latent period of 1 to 4 months include radiation pneumonitis and radiation carditis. Radiation-induced myelopathy has a long latent period of 1 to 2 years.

Radiation pneumonitis is a serious but controllable complication. The cancericidal dose for cancer of the lung is in the range of 5,600 to 6,400 cGy, whereas the threshold dose for radiation pneumonitis is 2,000 to 2,500 cGy (75,85,92,93). Factors that influence the incidence and degree of radiation pneumonitis include exposed lung volume, total dose to the tissue, size of fractions, fractionation schedule, radiation energy, and inhomogeneity factor. Among these factors, the exposed lung volume is probably the most important and critical in curative radiation therapy for cancer of the lung. The maximum lung volume that can be included in the high-dose zone (>5,000 cGy) without the likelihood of significant clinical symptoms is in the range of 25% to 30% of the total lung volume (93). With the currently available regional pulmonary function studies, this volume factor can be defined more clearly than before in terms of ventilation, perfusion, and volume (Fig. 13) (60). In our series, 4 of 80 patients (5%) treated with high doses (≥5,000 cGy) and large volumes (18 × 13 cm² to 22 × 16 cm² for AP–PA, and 18 × 8.5 cm² to 22 × 8.5 cm² for RPO and LPO) of radiation therapy with individually tailored cerrobend blocks developed symptomatic pneumonitis for which they were treated conservatively with bed rest and corticosteroids (28). This pulmonary injury was a contributing factor to the death of one patient who had severe underlying chronic obstructive pulmonary disease. Common presenting symptoms for acute radiation pneumonitis are cough, dyspnea, congestion, fullness of the chest, and a mild-to-moderate degree of fever (99–101°F). Chest radiograms may be negative at early stages. However, patchy consolidation and diffuse haziness in the area of the previous radiation therapy are the common early radiographic changes that follow the pattern of radiation portals later. Treatment of this acute radiation pneumonitis includes absolute bed rest, bronchodilators, oxygen therapy, and corticosteroids (49,72,92,93). In our experience, the acute symptoms of radiation pneumonitis have been well relieved by prednisone, 40 to 60 mg/day for 10 to 14 days. After control of the acute symptoms, the prednisone can be tapered over a period of

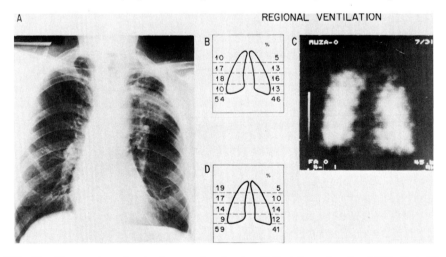

FIG. 13. Changes in regional pulmonary function (ventilation) 4 months after 4,800 cGy in 22 fractions over 49 days to a target volume that included the left hilum and the entire mediastinum in addition to the primary tumor (squamous cell carcinoma) at the left upper lobe. The decrease in the regional ventilation at the left upper region is compensated by the right lung. **B** and **D** show regional ventilation data before and after radiation therapy, respectively.

several weeks. One should be aware of the possibility of subclinical radiation injuries in the lung activated by rapid withdrawal of the high doses of corticosteroids (23). Antibiotics are given only for positive sputum culture. The late sequela of the acute radiation pneumonitis is pulmonary fibrosis, which usually is asymptomatic and is demonstrable radiographically only along the hilar and the paramediastinal areas where the previous radiation therapy was given. Safety guides for thoracic radiation therapy for the underlying lung cancer include careful selection of patients by exclusion of those with very large tumors or with severe underlying pulmonary disease, frequent redesigns of the radiation portals primarily along the periphery of the primary tumor mass at 2,000 to 2,500 cGy and again at 3,400 to 3,600 cGy as the atelectatic lung reexpands or a significant degree of tumor regression occurs in a patient with a large tumor mass (28), use of individually tailored cerrobend blocks to shield uninvolved pulmonary tissue, use of a regular size of fraction in the range of 180 to 200 cGy per day, corrections for lung inhomogeneity in the radiation dosimetry, and the use of high-energy beams. Split-course radiation therapy is a good and safe approach for patients at high risk for radiation pneumonitis (55,101). When total thoracic irradiation is judged necessary for palliation of metastatic tumors, the threshold dose for radiation pneumonitis is in the range of 2,000 to 2,500 cGy delivered at a rate of 150 cGy per day in adults (75). For young children, a total dose of 1,400 to 1,500 cGy delivered at daily fractions of 150 cGy is near the limit of tolerance (119). When adjuvant chemotherapeutic agents are used, notably actinomycin D, there should be a reduction in the tolerance dose of radiation by at least 10% to 15% (85). Tests of regional pulmonary function have been helpful in selecting patients at high risk among those with underlying chronic obstructive pulmonary disease (60).

Radiation-induced injuries to the heart have been rare in patients treated for cancer of the lung. Radiation pericarditis is the most common of the clinical cardiac damages induced by irradiation. Except when cancer of the lung arises in the left lower lobe behind the heart, an average target volume for high-dose curative radiation therapy for cancer of the lung includes most of both atria and a small portion of the right ventricle at the base (Fig. 14). In our series of 162 cases of cancer of the lung, there was only 1 patient whose symptoms were suggestive of pericarditis, and they responded well to conservative measures. Common presenting symptoms for acute pericarditis induced by irradiation are fever, tachycardia, substernal pain, and dyspnea. Pericardial friction rub and effusion are frequent. Other objective findings include a widened cardiac silhouette and changes on the electrocardiogram that consist of elevation of the ST segment, decrease of the QRS voltage, and inversion of T waves. Carcinomatous pericarditis is a more common entity that should be at the top of the list for differential diagnosis. Conservative management with bed rest and other supportive measures usually is adequate. The course of acute pericarditis is self-limited. However, it can lead to a chronic constrictive pericarditis when a large portion of the heart is included in the target volume. The threshold dose for radiation-induced cardiac damage is 4,000 cGy in 4 weeks to a major portion of the heart (108). Extreme caution is required when adjuvant chem-

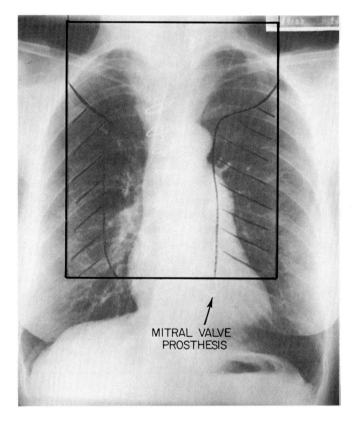

MITRAL VALVE
PROSTHESIS

FIG. 14. A target volume and cerrobend blocks for protection of uninvolved lung are drawn on a radiograph of the chest, AP view, of a patient with a carcinoma of the right upper lobe bronchus. Both ventricles are without the target volume.

otherapeutic agents, such as doxorubicin, are used with irradiation because of their synergistic cardiotoxicity (68). However, the risk of synergistic cardiotoxicity can be minimized by a well-prepared plan in which doxorubicin is omitted from a few cycles of combination chemotherapy before and after radiation therapy. Efforts should also be made so that the amount of the heart in the high-dose zone can be reduced as much as possible by use of supplemental lateral or oblique beams in addition to the AP–PA POP. Acute exacerbation of subclinical radiation-induced injuries to the heart has also been reported following sudden withdrawal of high doses of corticosteroids (23).

Myelopathy induced by irradiation is another rather serious but preventable complication. There are two distinct types of radiation injury to the spinal cord that include an early transient myelopathy and a late irreversible injury leading to paresis or paralysis. The early transient myelopathy (Lhermitte's sign) is characterized by a complaint of electric-shock sensation radiating down the back and over the extremities on flexion of the neck. It occurs a few months after the completion of radiation therapy and persists for 2 to 3 months without any sequelae. Temporary demyelination of the spinal cord due to the radiation-induced inhibition of myelin production by the oligodendroglia has been postulated as the underlying mechanism for this phenomenon (59). There is no good correlation between the early transient myelopathy and the late irreversible myelitis. The threshold dose for Lhermitte's sign is approximately 4,000 cGy in 4 weeks (TDF 66).

Late irreversible radiation-induced myelitis is a serious complication that should be prevented at all costs, because there is no effective treatment for it. It is characterized by a long (10–24 months) latent period and its resemblance to a clinical presentation of a partial or complete transection of the spinal cord (Brown-Séquard syndrome) (16,84). Diagnosis of this condition is made by exclusion of other conditions such as a metastatic tumor compressing the spinal cord. The threshold dose for radiation myelitis is in the range of 4,400 to 4,600 cGy in 22 to 23 fractions over 4.4 to 4.6 weeks (TDF 73–76) for large-field radiation therapy (16,28). It is, of course, imperative that there be careful planning of curative radiation therapy for malignant tumors in the chest. By use of a combination of AP–PA POP with an AP, RPO, and LPO (3 fields) or multiple fields, this serious late complication can be avoided.

PROGNOSTIC FACTORS IN CANCER OF THE LUNG

It is important to review the prognostic factors for patients with cancer of the lung, because the decisions of management depend on these variables.

Extent of Tumor

The stage of the tumor is one of the most important prognostic factors in cancer of the lung (73,104,117). As we are very familiar with the good correlation between the cure rate and the stage of cancer of the lung, complete workups to define the extent of the tumor are essential before decisions regarding managment are made. Within the unresectable T3 or N2 cancer of the lung, the rate of control of localized tumor is closely related to the size of the tumor by the curative radiation therapy (82). Without good control of the local tumor, one cannot expect a cure. There have been several studies that have demonstrated a clear correlation between survival rate and rate of control of the local tumor (28,32,81,96). For technically operable, but medically inoperable, cancer of the lung, Smart and Hilton achieved a 22.5% 5-year survival rate by curative radiation therapy, which is not much lower than average surgical results (73,107).

Performance Status

The patient's functional status is closely related to the patient's tolerance to surgery, radiation therapy, and chemotherapy. Definitive radiation therapy is well tolerated by patients who are ambulatory and able to provide self-care (≥70 on the Karnofsky scale) (28,61,121). Poor performance status with 50 or lower on the

Karnofsky scale implies that the patient's condition is too poor to tolerate radical radiation therapy, either because of the presence of clinically undetectable widespread microscopic distant metastases or because of poor medical condition unrelated to the tumor. The radiation dose that can be tolerated reasonably well by those with poor performance status ($\leq$50 on the Karnofsky scale) is in the range of 3,500 to 4,000 cGy (TDF 58–66), which is too low to be cancericidal for large unresectable tumors.

Histologic Types of Tumors

The biological aggressiveness of cancer of the lung may be correlated with the degree of differentiation in the early stage of squamous cell carcinoma (62). However, histologic grading has relatively little effect in patients with advanced cancers. Histologic types alone do not have any significant impacts on 5-year cure rates (62, 104). There is no difference of the rates of control of local tumors among different types of cancer of the lung at 18 months or more after definitive radiation therapy (28).

Weight Loss

A good correlation has been observed between survival and a significant weight loss (>10 lb or >5 kg) in the 6 months preceding treatment (101,121). The significant weight loss usually is a systemic manifestation of an advanced stage of the underlying cancer of the lung.

Age

Age alone probably does not have a significant impact on prognosis for patients with cancer of the lung. Sealy et al. (101) reported that older patients ($\geq$60 years) tend to fail as a result of local progression of the tumor or death without progression, whereas younger patients tend to die from metastatic causes after curative radiation therapy. There is a need for further studies on this aspect of the age factor, which may have a therapeutic implication in future protocol studies.

Sex

The sexual factor alone probably does not have any significant bearing on prognosis. Adenocarcinoma is the most common histologic type among female patients. This tumor has a predilection at the periphery of the lung in 60% to 70% of all cases, and the cure rate for the peripheral tumor is better than that for the central tumor after surgical resection (62). However, there may be an unknown systemic factor among female patients, inasmuch as better survival has been reported for female patients than for male patients, even after radiation therapy for unresectable carcinoma of the lung (101).

Location of Tumor

The location of the tumor probably has some bearing on a patient's tolerance to curative radiation therapy. The functioning volume of the lung is much less at the upper lobe than at the lower lobe, according to regional pulmonary function studies (5,60). This anatomic configuration offers a safety margin for tumors of the upper lobe that is much better than that for the lower lobe for either curative radiation therapy or surgery. It may be that Pancoast tumor has less aggressiveness than tumors that are not situated at the apex of the lung, inasmuch as the cure rate for tumors in the apex is far better than that for tumors of the same stage at other locations (14,80).

Carcinoembryonic Antigen

The concentration of carcinoembryonic antigen (CEA) is elevated (≥ 6 ng/ml) in 40% to 50% of patients with stage II through stage IV cancer of the lung (17, 27). Its frequencies of elevation relative to tumor stages were 43% (42/97) and 46% (12/26) for tumors in stages III and IV (27). Relative frequencies of elevated CEA in relation to histologic types in stage III tumors were 33% (11/33) for squamous cell carcinoma, 65% (15/23) for adenocarcinoma, 22% (5/22) for oat cell carcinoma, and 56% (9/16) for large cell carcinoma. According to the results from our series of 144 patients with bronchogenic carcinoma and reports by others (17,27,48), the initial CEA value for a stage III tumor before radiation therapy is closely related to the patient's survival. For example, survival rates of 6 months or more without relapse were observed in 46% (17/37), 58% (17/29), and 14% (2/14) for patients with initial CEA values of 1 to 5.8 ng/ml, 6 to 20 ng/ml, and 21 to 600 ng/ml, respectively. A good correlation has also been observed between the clinical courses of patients and the serial changes in CEA values with the treatment (30). Plasma CEA values before radiation therapy and the serial changes after treatment are of prognostic importance for patients with stage III cancer of the lung.

NEW TRENDS IN PROSPECT

For improvement in the results from current radiation treatment for stage III cancer of the lung, new approaches are needed to improve the rate of control of local and regional tumors and to deal with microscopic distant metastases of the tumor. Despite the reasonably good rate (50%–76%) of local tumor control by high-dose radiation therapy, the majority of these patients with T3 or N2 cancer still die with distant metastases that were present before the start of radiation therapy (15,28,81,95). Local failure after high-dose radiation therapy has been attributed mainly to the presence of hypoxic tumor cells, which constitute approximately 1% of all tumor cells (89). Thorough investigations have revealed that for the same rate of control of local tumor, hypoxic tumor cells require a much higher radiation dose (2.3–3.0 times higher) than well-oxygenated tumor cells (46). Therefore, attempts have been made to improve the rate of local tumor control and to deal with distant metastases as follows:

1. Attempts aimed at reducing the potential impact of hypoxic tumor cells have included radiation therapy under a hyperbaric condition (20,111), trials of high-LET beams such as neutrons (39), trials of modified fractionation schedules (2,58), trials of electron-affinic compounds such as misonidazole (37,116), and trials of hyperthermia (109). All these studies are still in experimental stages.

2. Attempts to improve differential dose distribution between the tumor volume and normal tissue have included interstitial implants of radioactive seeds such as [198]Au, radon, and [125]I (53,54) and the use of intraoperative ^{60}Co or electron beam (3). The intraoperative radiation therapy, which is an attractive way of supplementing the radiation dose to the main mass, is under clinical investigation. Results of the interstitial implants of radioactive seeds are encouraging for the apical tumors, perhaps as good as the results from combined external preoperative radiation therapy followed by surgery (14,80).

3. Systemic treatments in combination with radiation therapy have not been studied extensively. Results of radiation therapy plus either single-agent or multidrug chemotherapy have been disappointing (Table 9) (13,22,38,83,99,100). However, there is a need for further trials using more effective systemic agents and a high radiation dose in the range of 5,600 to 6,400 cGy, which would achieve a rate of ≥70% for local tumor control (28,82). Immunotherapy is another systemic treatment that could be fruitful in stage III cancer of the lung when it is used in combination with effective radiation therapy. Intrapleural BCG and oral levamisole have been effective for stage I cancer of the lung when they have been used after curative surgical procedures (8,67). A few representative trials of adjuvant immunotherapy in stage III cancer of the lung are shown in Table 10 (87,88,113). Tumor burden seems to be a key factor for the effectiveness of the immunotherapy. To establish the value of adjuvant immunotherapy in stage III cancer of the lung, additional trials are needed in which an optimum radiation therapy schedule is used that will reduce the tumor burden to the minimum.

4. Superfractionated radiation therapy is an attractive approach for cancer of the lung (112,118). Repair of sublethal radiation damage in aerobic mammalian cells is essentially complete within 2 to 4 hr (41,45,111). When a rapidly proliferating tumor cell population such as cancer of the lung is growing in normal tissue whose cells are nonproliferative or slowly proliferating, an advantage accrues to the tumor cells if the intertreatment interval is greater than 4 hr. In such a situation, greater therapeutic efficacy is expected with the use of two or three treatment sessions per day, with an essentially normal dose per fraction, total dose levels, and 4-hr intervals or longer between the fractions. A clinical study to evaluate the response of normal human skin to a superfractionation schedule of 200-kV deep X-rays, on two or three fractions daily with approximately 4 hr between treatments, demonstrated that the radiation dose needed to yield a constant acute skin response was reduced by 8% to 10% (24). Tolerance to a superfractionation schedule of radiation therapy has been good when a small fraction (100–200 cGy) has been delivered three times daily to the chest (25). In Burkitt's lymphoma, a response rate of 74% (25/34) was obtained by a superfractionation schedule (120 cGy three times daily), which was

TABLE 9. *Radiotherapy vs. radiotherapy plus chemotherapy for unresectable non-small-cell carcinoma of the lung*

Authors	Radiotherapy[a]	Chemotherapy[b]	Histologic types	Median survival (M)		Survival rate (%) at 1 year	
				RT	RT+Chemo	RT	RT+Chemo
Carr et al. (22)	4,500–5,000 in 23–29 F over 4–9 wk	5-FU, 10 mg/kg first 5 days of RT	Squamous cell	—	—	42	60
			Adenocarcinoma	—	—	32	36
			Large cell	—	—	31	28
Petrovich et al. (83)	5,000–6,000 over 4–6 wk	CCNU, hydroxyurea	All types	6.3	7.2	15	7
Sealy (100) (St. 53)	5,000 in 25 F over 5 wk	CTX/HN₂, MTX	Squamous cell	8	4.8	—	—
			Adenocarcinoma	9.5	6.7	—	—
			Large cell	6	4	—	—
Sealy (100) (WPL)[c]	5,000 in 25 F over 5 wk	CTX, MTX, CCNU	Adenocarcinoma	6.7	6.7	—	—
			Large cell				
Eagan et al. (38)	4,000 in 10 F over 5 wk	CAP	Adenocarcinoma	—	16.8	—	—
			Large cell				
		CAD	Large cell	—	7.2	—	—

[a]Unit of radiation dose is cGy (rad). F = fraction.

[b]5-FU = 5-fluorouracil; CTX = cyclophosphamide; HN₂ = nitrogen mustard; MTX = methotrexate; CAP = cyclophosphamide, Adriamycin, and cis-platinum; CAD = cyclophosphamide, Adriamycin, and DTIC.

[c]WPL = working party for lung cancer.

TABLE 10. *Adjuvant immunotherapy in lung cancer*

Authors	Stages of tumors	Treatments	Median survival	Survival rate (%)				
				1 yr	2 yr	3 yr	4 yr	5 yr
McKeally et al. (67)	I	Surgery (36 pt)	—	77	60	55		
		vs.						
		Surgery + intrapleural BCG[a] + INH (30 pt)		95	90	90		
Amery (8)	I and II	Surgery (96 pt)	[b]					
		vs.						
		Surgery + levamisole (82 pt)						
Takita et al. (113)	III	Surgery ± postop. RT[c]	12 M	—	—	—		
		vs.						
		Surgery + postop. RT + autologous-tumor-cell vaccine (30 pt)	35 M	—	—	—		
Pines (87)	III SCC[d]	RT (4,600–5,000 cGy) (23 pt)	—	47		4	—	0
		vs.						
		RT + BCG (weekly/monthly) (25 pt)		76		12	—	12
Pines (88)	III SCC	RT	—	55	33	11		
		vs.						
		RT + levamisole + BCG (monthly)		50	—	—		
		vs.						
		RT + levamisole + BCG (bimonthly)		94	76	23		

[a]BCG = bacillus Calmette-Guérin.
[b]The benefit of adjuvant levamisole was found in patients weighing ≤70 kg.
[c]RT = radiation therapy.
[d]SCC = squamous cell carcinoma.

a dramatic improvement over the rate of 11% (1/9) obtained from a conventional schedule (220 cGy once per day) (77). Clinical trials are needed to assess the value of superfractionation schedules in cancer of the lung.

REFERENCES

1. Abadir, R., and Muggia, F. M. (1975): Irradiated lung cancer: An autopsy analysis of spread pattern. *Radiology*, 114:427–430.
2. Abe, M., Yabumoto, E., Nishidai, T., and Takashi, M. (1977): Trials of new forms of radiotherapy for locally advanced bronchogenic carcinoma. *Strahlentherapie*, 153:149–158.
3. Abe, M., Takahashi, M., Yabumoto, E., Adachi, H., Yoshii, M., and Mori, K. (1980): Clinical experiences with intraoperative radiotherapy of locally advanced cancers. *Cancer*, 45:40–48.
4. Abramson, N., and Cavanaugh, P. J. (1973): Short-course radiation therapy in carcinoma of the lung: A second look. *Radiology*, 108:685–687.
5. Ali, M. K., and Ewer, M. S. (1980): Preoperative cardiopulmonary evaluation of patients undergoing surgery for lung cancer. *Cancer Bulletin*, 32:100–104.
6. American Cancer Society (1983): Cancer statistics, 1983. *CA*, 33:9–25.
7. American Joint Committee for Cancer Staging and End-Results Reporting (1978): *Staging of Lung Cancer*, pp. 59–64. AJCCSERR, Chicago.
8. Amery, W. K. (1978): A placebo-controlled levamisole study in resectable lung cancer. *Prog. Cancer Res. Ther.*, 6:191–201.
9. Aristizabal, S. A., and Caldwell, W. L. (1976): Radical irradiation with the split-course technique in carcinoma of the lung. *Cancer*, 37:2630–2635.
10. Armitage, P. (1971): *Statistical Methods in Medical Research*, pp. 408–414. John Wiley & Sons, New York.
11. Bell, J. W. (1965): Open abdominal biopsy before thoracotomy for lung cancer. *Geriatrics*, 20:715–727.
12. Berry, R. J., and Laing, A. H. (1977): The role of radiotherapy in treatment of inoperable lung cancer. *Int. J. Rad. Oncol. Biol. Phys.* 2:433–439.
13. Bleehen, N. M. (1980): The treatment of inoperable lung cancer by radiotherapy and chemotherapy. *Int. J. Rad. Oncol. Biol. Phys.*, 6:1007–1012.
14. Blitzer, P. H., Dosoretz, D. D., Wilkins, E. W., Jr., Grillo, H. C., and Choi, N. C.: The treatment and prognosis of apical lung cancer. *Int. J. Rad. Oncol. Biol. Phys.* (*in press*).
15. Bloedorn, F. G., Cowley, R. A., Cuccia, C. A., Mercado, R., Jr., Wizenberg, M. J., and Linberg, E. J. (1964): Preoperative irradiation in bronchogenic carcinoma. *Am. J. Roentgenol. Radium Ther. Nucl. Med.*, 92:77–87.
16. Boden, G. (1948): Radiation myelitis of the cervical spinal cord. *Br. J. Radiol.*, 21:464–469.
17. Bolla, M., Vrousos, C., Agnus-Delord, C., Kolodie, H., and Paramelle, B. (1980): One year survival rate in patients with carcinoma of the lung treated with split course irradiation: Correlation with serum value of carcinoembryonic antigen. *Int. J. Rad. Oncol. Biol. Phys.*, 6:1055–1056.
18. Bromley, L. L., and Szur, L. (1955): Combined radiotherapy and resection for carcinoma of the bronchus: Experiences with 66 patients. *Lancet*, 2:937–941.
19. Bush, R. S., Jenkin, D. T., Allt, W. E. C., Beale, F. A., Bean, H., Dembo, A. J., and Pringle, J. F. (1978): Definitive evidence for hypoxic cells influencing cure in cancer therapy. *Br. J. Cancer [Suppl. III]*, 37:302–306.
20. Cade, I. S., and McEwen, J. B. (1978): Clinical trials of radiotherapy in hyperbaric oxygen at Portsmouth, 1964–1976. *Clin. Radiol.*, 29:333–338.
21. Caldwell, W. L., and Bagshaw, M. A. (1968): Indications for and results of irradiation of carcinoma of the lung. *Cancer*, 22:999–1004.
22. Carr, D. T., Childs, D. S., Jr., and Lee, R. E. (1972): Radiotherapy plus 5-FU compared to radiotherapy alone for inoperable and unresectable bronchogenic carcinoma. *Cancer*, 29:375–380.
23. Castellino, R. A., Glatstein, E., Turbow, M. M., Rosenberg, S., and Kaplan, H. S. (1974): Latent radiation injury of lungs or heart activated by steroid withdrawal. *Ann. Intern. Med.*, 80:593–599.
24. Choi, C. H., and Suit, H. D. (1975): Evaluation of rapid radiation treatment schedules utilizing two treatment sessions per day. *Radiology*, 116:703–707.
25. Choi, C. H., and Carey, R. W. (1976): Small cell anaplastic carcinoma of lung: Reappraisal of current management. *Cancer*, 37:2651–2657.

26. Choi, C. H., Sedlacek, R. S., and Suit, H. D. (1979): Radiation-induced osteogenic sarcoma of the C3H mouse: Effects of *Corynebacterium parvum* and WBI on its natural history and response to irradiation. *Eur. J. Cancer*, 15:433–442.
27. Choi, N. C. H., and Bloch, K. J. (1980): Carcinoembryonic antigen (CEA) as a marker of radiation therapy in lung cancer. *Int. J. Rad. Oncol. Biol. Phys.*, 6:1454–1455.
28. Choi, N. C. H., and Doucette, J. A. (1981): Improved survival of patients with unresectable non-small-cell bronchogenic carcinoma by an innovated high-dose en-bloc radiotherapeutic approach. *Cancer*, 48:101–109.
29. Colton, T. (1974): *Statistics in Medicine*, pp. 237–250. Little, Brown, and Co., Boston.
30. Concannon, J. P., Dalbow, M. H., Hodgson, S. E., Headings, J. J., Markopoulos, E., Mitchell, J., Cushing, W. J., and Liebler, G. A. (1978): Prognostic value of preoperative carcinoembryonic antigen (CEA) plasma levels in patients with bronchogenic carcinoma. *Cancer*, 42:1477–1483.
31. Cox, J. D., Stanley, K., Petrovich, Z., Paig, C., and Yesner, R. (1981): Cranial irradiation in cancer of the lung of all cell types. *J. Am. Med. Assoc.*, 245:469–472.
32. Cox, J. D., Eisert, D. R., Komaki, R., Mietlowski, W., and Petrovich, Z. (1979): Patterns of failure following treatment of apparently localized carcinoma of the lung. *Prog. Cancer Res. Ther.*, 11:279–288.
33. Coy, P., and Kennelly, G. M. (1980): The role of curative radiotherapy in the the treatment of lung cancer. *Cancer*, 45:698–702.
34. Deeley, T. J. (1966): A clinical trial to compare two different tumor dose levels in the treatment of advanced carcinoma of the bronchus. *Clin. Radiol.*, 17:299–301.
35. Deeley, T. J., and Singh, S. P. (1967): Treatment of inoperable carcinoma of the bronchus by megavoltage x-rays. *Thorax*, 22:562–566.
36. Deeley, T. J. (1967): The treatment of carcinoma of the bronchus. *Br. J. Radiol.*, 40:801–822.
37. Dische, S., Saunders, M. I., Flockhart, I. R., Lee, M. E., and Anderson, P. (1979): Misonidazole—A drug for trial in radiotherapy and oncology. *Int. J. Rad. Oncol. Biol. Phys.*, 5:851–860.
38. Eagan, R. T., Lee, R. E., Frytak, S., Fleming, T. R., Creagan, E. T., Ingle, J. N., and Kvols, L. K. (1979): Randomized trial of thoracic irradiation plus combination chemotherapy for unresectable adenocarcinoma and large cell carcinoma of the lung. *Int. J. Rad. Oncol. Biol. Phys.*, 6:1401–1406.
39. Eichhorn, H. J., and Lessel, A. (1976): A comparison between combined neutron- and telecobalt-therapy with telecobalt-therapy alone for cancer of the bronchus. *Br. J. Radiol.*, 49:880–882.
40. Eisert, D. R., Cox, J. D., and Komaki, R. (1976): Irradiation for bronchial carcinoma: Reasons for failure. *Cancer*, 37:2665–2670.
41. Elkind, M. M., and Sutton, H. (1960): Radiation response of mammalian cells grown in culture. I. Repair of x-ray damage in surviving Chinese hamster cells. *Radiat. Res.*, 13:556–593.
42. Emami, B., Melo, A., Carter, B. L., Munzenrider, J. E., and Piro, A. (1978): Value of computed tomography in radiotherapy of lung cancer. *Am. J. Roentgenol. Radium Ther. Nucl. Med.*, 131:63–67.
43. Emami, B., Lee, D. J., and Munzenrider, J. E. (1978): The value of supraclavicular area treatment in radiotherapeutic management of lung cancer. *Cancer*, 41:124–129.
44. Emami, B., Munzenrider, J. E., Lee, D. J., and Rene, J. B. (1979): Radical radiation therapy of advanced lung cancer. *Cancer*, 44:446–456.
45. Fowler, J. F., Bewley, D. K., Morgan, R. L., and Silvester, J. A. (1965): Experiments with fractionated x-irradiation of the skin of pigs. II. Fractionation up to five days. *Br. J. Radiol.*, 38:278–284.
46. Gray, L. H. (1961): Radiobiologic basis of oxygen as a modifying factor in radiation therapy. *Am. J. Roentgenol. Radium Ther. Nucl. Med.*, 85:803–815.
47. Greco, F. A., Brereton, H. D., Kent, H., Zimbler, H., Merrill, J., and Johnson, R. E. (1976): Adriamycin and enhanced radiation reaction in normal esophagus and skin. *Ann. Intern. Med.*, 85:294–298.
48. Gropp, C., Havemann, K., and Scheuer, A. (1980): The use of carcinoembryonic antigen and peptide hormones to stage and monitor patients with lung cancer. *Int. J. Rad. Oncol. Biol. Phys.*, 6:1047–1053.
49. Gross, N. J. (1977): Pulmonary effects of radiation therapy. *Ann. Intern. Med.*, 86:81–92.
50. Guttman, R. (1971): Radical supervoltage therapy in inoperable carcinoma of the lung. In: *Modern Radiotherapy—Carcinoma of the Bronchus*, edited by T. J. Deeley, pp. 181–195. Appleton-Century-Crofts, New York.

51. Hazra, T. A., Chandrasekaran, M. S., Colman, M., Prempree, T., and Inalsingh, A. (1974): Survival in carcinoma of the lung after a split course of radiotherapy. *Br. J. Radiol.*, 47:464–466.

52. Hellman, S., Kligerman, M. M., von Essen, C. F., and Scibetta, M. P. (1964): Sequelae of radical radiotherapy of carcinoma of the lung. *Radiology*, 82:1055–1061.

53. Hilaris, B. S., Luomanen, R. K., and Beattie, E. J., Jr. (1971): Integrated irradiation and surgery in the treatment of apical lung cancer. *Cancer*, 27:1369–1373.

54. Hilaris, B. S., and Martini, H. (1979): Interstitial brachytherapy in cancer of the lung: A 20 year experience. *Int. J. Rad. Oncol. Biol. Phys.*, 5:1951–1956.

55. Holsti, L. R., and Mattson, K. (1980): A randomized study of split-course radiotherapy of lung cancer: Long term results. *Int. J. Rad. Oncol. Biol. Phys.*, 6:977–981.

56. Horwich, A., Lokich, J. J., and Bloomer, W. D. (1975): Doxorubicin, radiotherapy and esophageal stricture. *Lancet*, 2:561–562.

57. Huber, C. M., DeGiorgi, L. S., Levitt, S. H., and King, E. R. (1972): Carcinoma of the lung: An evaluation of the scalene node biopsy in relation to radiation therapy of the supraclavicular region. *Cancer*, 29:84–89.

58. Johnson, R. J. R., Walton, R. J., Lim, M. L., Zylak, C. J., and Painchand, L. A. (1973): A randomized study on survival of bronchogenic carcinoma treated with conventional or short fractionation radiation. *Clin. Radiol.*, 24:494–497.

59. Jones, A. (1964): Transient radiation myelopathy (with reference to Lhermitte's sign of electrical paraesthesia). *Br. J. Radiol.*, 37:727–744.

60. Kanarek, D. J., Choi, C. H., Ahluwahlia, B., Latty, A., and Kazemi, H. (1977): The effect of radiation therapy for lung cancer on pulmonary function in patients with severe obstructive lung disease. *Am. Rev. Respir. Dis.*, 115:128.

61. Karnofsky, D. A., Golbsy, R. B., and Pool, J. L. (1957): Preliminary studies on the natural history of lung cancer. *Radiology*, 69:477–487.

62. Katlic, M., and Carter, D. (1979): Prognostic implications of histology, size, and location of primary tumors. *Prog. Cancer Res. Ther.*, 11:143–150.

63. Komake, R., Cox, J. D., and Eisert, D. R. (1977): Irradiation of bronchial carcinoma. II. Pattern of spread and potential for prophylactic irradiation. *Int. J. Rad. Oncol. Biol. Phys.*, 2:441–446.

64. Lee, R. E., Carr, D. T., and Childs, D. S., Jr. (1976): Comparison of split-course radiotherapy and continuous radiotherapy for unresectable bronchogenic carcinoma: 5-year results. *Am. J. Roentgenol. Radium Ther. Nucl. Med.*, 126:116–123.

65. Levitt, S. H., Bogardus, C. R., and Ladd, G. (1967): Split-course radiation therapy in the treatment of advanced lung cancer. *Radiology*, 88:1159–1161.

66. Line, D., and Deeley, T. J. (1971): Palliative therapy. In: *Modern Radiotherapy—Carcinoma of the Bronchus*, edited by T. J. Deeley, pp. 298–306. Appleton-Century-Crofts, New York.

67. McKeally, M. F., Maver, C. M., Alley, R. D., Kausel, H. W., Older, T. M., Foster, E. D., and Lininger, L. (1979): Regional immunotherapy of lung cancer using intrapleural BCG: Summary of a four year randomized study. *Prog. Cancer Res. Ther.*, 11:471–476.

68. Merrill, J., Greco, F. A., Zimbler, H., Brereton, H. D., Lamberg, J. D., and Pomeroy, T. C. (1975): Adriamycin and radiation: Synergistic cardiotoxicity. *Ann. Intern. Med.*, 82:122–123.

69. Mohiuddin, M., Rouby, E., and Kramer, S. (1979): Results of a pilot study with extended fractionation in the treatment of lung cancer. *Int. J. Rad. Oncol. Biol. Phys.*, 5:2039–2042.

70. Moore, S. W., and Cole, D. R. (1955): Primary malignant neoplasms of the lung. *Ann. Surg.*, 141:457–468.

71. Morrison, R., Deeley, T. J., and Cleland, W. P. (1963): The treatment of carcinoma of the bronchus: A clinical trial to compare surgery and supervoltage radiotherapy. *Lancet*, 1:683–684.

72. Moss, W. T., Haddy, F. J., and Sweany, S. K. (1960): Some factors altering severity of acute radiation pneumonitis: Irradiation with cortisone, heparin, and antibiotics. *Radiology*, 75:50–54.

73. Mountain, C. F., McMurtrey, M. J., and Frazier, O. H. (1980): Regional extension of lung cancer. *Int. J. Rad. Oncol. Biol. Phys.*, 6:1013–1020.

74. Newburger, P. E., Cassady, J. R., and Jaffe, N. (1978): Esophagitis due to adriamycin and radiation therapy for childhood malignancy. *Cancer*, 42:417–423.

75. Newton, K. A., and Spittle, M. F. (1969): Analysis of 40 cases treated by total thoracic irradiation. *Clin. Radiol.*, 20:19–22.

76. Nogeire, C., Mincer, F., and Botstein, C. (1979): Long survival in patients with bronchogenic carcinoma complicated by superior vena caval obstruction. *Chest*, 75:325–329.

77. Noron, T., and Onyango, J. (1977): Radiotherapy in Burkett's lymphoma: Conventional vs. su-
    perfractionated regime—early results. *Int. J. Rad. Oncol. Biol. Phys.*, 2:399–406.
78. Ochsner, A., and DeBakey, M. (1942): Significance of metastases in primary carcinoma of lungs.
    J. Thorac. Surg., 11:357–387.
79. Orton, C. G., and Ellis, F. (1973): A simplification in the use of the NSD concept in practical
    radiotherapy. *Br. J. Radiol.*, 46:529–537.
80. Paulson, D. L. (1975): Carcinomas in the superior pulmonary sulcus. *J. Thorac. Cardiovasc.
    Surg.*, 70:1095–1104.
81. Perez, C. A., Stanley, K., Rubin, P., Kramer, S., Brady, L., Perez-Tamayo, R., Brown, S.,
    Concannon, J., Rotman, M., and Seydel, H. G. (1980): A prospective randomized study of various
    rradiation doses and fractionation schedules in the treatment of inoperable non-oat-cell carcinoma
    of the lung. Preliminary report by the Radiation Therapy Oncology Group. *Cancer*, 45:2744–
    2753.
82. Perez, C. A., Stanley, K., Grundy, G., Hanson, W., Rubin, P., Kramer, S., Brady, L. W.,
    Marks, J. E., Perez-Tamayo, R., Brown, G. S., Concannon, J. P., and Rotman, M. (1982): Impact
    of irradiation technique and tumor extent in tumor control and survival of patients with unresectable
    non-oat cell carcinoma of the lung. *Cancer*, 50:1091–1099.
83. Petrovich, Z., Ohanian, M., and Cox, J. (1978): Clinical research on the treatment of locally
    advanced lung cancer. *Cancer*, 42:1129–1134.
84. Phillips, T. L., and Buschke, F. (1969): Radiation tolerance of the thoracic spinal cord. *Am. J.
    Roentgenol. Radium Ther. Nucl. Med.*, 104:659–664.
85. Phillips, T., and Margolis, L. (1972): Radiation pathology and the clinical response of lung and
    esophagus. In: *Frontiers of Radiation Therapy and Oncology, Vol. 6*, edited by J. M. Vaeth, pp.
    254–273. University Park Press, Baltimore.
86. Pierquin, B., Gravis, P., and Gelle, X. (1965): Étude de 688 cas de cancers bronchiques traités
    par téléradiothérapie (200 Kv et 22 Mv). *J. Radiol. Electrol.*, 46:201–216.
87. Pines, A. (1976): A 5-year controlled study of B.C.G. and radiotherapy for inoperable lung cancer.
    Lancet, 1:380–381.
88. Pines, A. (1980): BCG plus levamisole following irradiation of advanced squamous bronchial
    carcinoma. *Int. J. Rad. Oncol. Biol. Phys.*, 6:1041–1042.
89. Powers, W. E., and Tolmach, L. J. (1963): A multicomponent x-ray survival curve for mouse
    lymphosarcoma cells irradiated in vivo. *Nature*, 197:710.
90. Rissanen, P. M., Tikka, U., and Holsti, L. R. (1968): Autopsy findings in lung cancer treated
    with megavoltage radiotherapy. *Acta Radiol. Ther. (Stockh.)*, 7:433–442.
91. Roswit, B., Patno, M. E., Rapp, R., Vienbergs, A., Feder, B., Stuhlbarg, J., and Reid, C. B.
    (1968): The survival of patients with inoperable lung cancer: A large scale randomized study of
    radiation therapy versus placebo. *Radiology*, 90:688–697.
92. Roswit, B., and White, D. C. (1977): Severe radiation injuries of the lung. *Am. J. Roentgenol.
    Radium Ther. Nucl. Med.*, 129:127–136.
93. Rubin, P., and Casarett, G. W. (1968): *Clinical Radiation Pathology, Vol. I*, pp. 460–461. W. B.
    Saunders, Philadelphia.
94. Rubin, P., and Ciccio, S. (1971): High daily dose for rapid decompression in superior mediastinal
    obstruction. In: *Modern Radiotherapy—Carcinoma of the Bronchus*, edited by T. L. Deeley, pp.
    276–297. Appleton-Century-Crofts, New York.
95. Rubin, P. (1979): The radiotherapeutic approach: Reappraisal and prospects. *Prog. Cancer Res.
    Ther.*, 11:333–340.
96. Salazar, O. M., Rubin, P., Brown, J. C., Feldstein, M. L., and Keller, B. E. (1976): Predictors
    of radiation response in lung cancer—A clinico-pathological analysis. *Cancer*, 37:2636–2650.
97. Schulz, M. D. (1957): The results of radiotherapy in cancer of the lung. *Radiology*, 69:494–498.
98. Schulz, M. D. (1966): Palliation by radiotherapy in bronchogenic carcinoma. *J. Am. Med. Assoc.*,
    196:850.
99. Schultz, H. P., Overgaard, M., and Sell, A. (1980): Inoperable lung cancer treated by x-ray
    therapy and combination chemotherapy with CCNU, adriamycin and vinblastine. *Int. J. Rad.
    Oncol. Biol. Phys.*, 6:1071–1074.
100. Sealy, R. (1979): Combined radiotherapy and chemotherapy in non-small cell carcinoma of the
    lung. *Prog. Cancer Res. Ther.*, 11:315–323.

101. Sealy, R., Lagakos, S., Barkley, T., Ryall, R., Tucker, R. D., Lee, R. E., and Ehlers, G. (1982): Radiotherapy of regional epidermoid carcinoma of the lung: A study in fractionation. *Cancer*, 49:1338–1345.
102. Secker Walker, R. H., Provan, J. L., Jackson, J. A., and Goodwin, J. (1971): Lung scanning in carcinoma of the bronchus. *Thorax*, 26:23–32.
103. Seydel, H. G., Kutcher, G. J., Steiner, R. M., Mohiuddin, M., and Goldberg, B. (1980): Computed tomography in planning radiation therapy for bronchogenic carcinoma. *Int. J. Rad. Oncol. Biol. Phys.*, 6:601–606.
104. Shields, T. W. (1980): Classification and prognosis of surgically treated patients with bronchial carcinoma: Analysis of VASOG studies. *Int. J. Rad. Oncol. Biol. Phys.*, 6:1021–1027.
105. Shin, K. H., Birdsell, J., Geggie, P. H. S., and Brown, I. S. (1980): Adenocarcinoma of the lung: Ten years' experience in Southern Alberta Cancer Center. *Int. J. Rad. Oncol. Biol. Phys.*, 6:835–840.
106. Shukovsky, L. J. (1970): Dose, time, volume relationships in squamous cell carcinoma of the supraglottic larynx. *Am. J. Roentgenol. Radium Ther. Nucl. Med.*, 108:27–29.
107. Smart, J. (1966): Can lung cancer be cured by irradiation alone? *J. Am. Med. Assoc.*, 195:1034–1035.
108. Stewart, J. R., Cohn, K. E., Fajardo, L. F., Hancock, E. W., and Kaplan, H. S. (1967): Radiation induced heart disease. *Radiology*, 89:302–310.
109. Sugaar, S., and LeVeen, H. H. (1979): A histopathologic study on the effects of radiofrequency thermotherapy on malignant tumors of the lung. *Cancer*, 43:767–783.
110. Suit, H. D. (1973): Radiation biology: A basis for radiotherapy. In: *Textbook of Radiotherapy*, edited by G. H. Fletcher, pp. 95–96. Lea & Febiger, Philadelphia.
111. Suit, H. D., and Urano, M. (1969): Repair of sublethal radiation injury in hypoxic cells of a C3H mouse mammary carcinoma. *Radiat. Res.*, 37:423–434.
112. Suit, H. D. (1977): Superfractionation (editorial). *Int. J. Rad. Oncol. Biol. Phys.*, 2:591–592.
113. Takita, H., Takada, M., Minowada, J., Han, T., and Edgerton, F. (1978): Adjuvant immunotherapy of stage III lung carcinoma. *Prog. Cancer Res. Ther.*, 6:217–223.
114. Thomlinson, R. H., and Craddock, E. A. (1967): Response of experimental tumor to x-rays. *Br. J. Cancer*, 21:108.
115. Underwood, G., Hooper, R., Axelbaum, S., and Goodwin, D. (1979): Computed tomography scanning of the thorax in the staging of bronchogenic carcinoma. *N. Engl. J. Med.*, 300:777–778.
116. Wasserman, T. H., Phillips, T. L., Johnson, R. J., Gomer, C. J., Lawrence, G. A., Sadee, W., Marques, R. A., Levin, V. A., and Van Raalte, G. (1979): Initial United States clinical and pharmacologic evaluation of misonidazole (RO-07–0582), a hypoxic cell radiosensitizer. *Int. J. Rad. Oncol. Biol. Phys.*, 5:775–786.
117. Wilkins, E. W., Jr., Scannell, J. G., and Craver, J. G. (1978): Four decades of experience with resections for bronchogenic carcinoma at the Massachusetts General Hospital. *J. Thorac. Cardiovasc. Surg.*, 76:364–368.
118. Withers, H. R., and Peters, L. J. (1980): Biologic aspects of radiation therapy. In: *Textbook of Radiotherapy*, edited by G. H. Fletcher, pp. 150–153. Lea & Febiger, Philadelphia.
119. Wohl, M. E. B., Griscom, N. T., Traggis, D. G., and Jaffee, N. (1975): The effects of therapeutic radiation delivered in early childhood upon subsequent lung function. *Pediatrics*, 4:507–516.
120. Zeidman, I. (1959): Experimental studies on the spread of cancer in the lymphatic system. IV. Retrograde spread. *Cancer Res.*, 19:1114–1117.
121. Zelen, M. (1973): Keynote address on biostatistics. *Cancer Chemother. Rep.*, 4:31–42.
122. Zubrod, C. G., Schneiderman, M., Frei, E., Brindley, C., Gold, G. L., Shnider, B., Oviedo, R., Gorman, J., Jones, R., Jonsson, U., Colsky, J., Chalmers, T., Ferguson, B., Dederick, M., Holland, J., Selawry, O., Regelson, W., Lasagna, L., and Owens, A. H. (1960): Appraisal of methods for study of chemotherapy of cancer in man: Comparative therapeutic trial of nitrogen mustard and triethylene thiophosphoramide. *J. Chronic Dis.*, 11:7–33.

Thoracic Oncology, edited by N. C. Choi and
H. C. Grillo. Raven Press, New York © 1983.

Immunotherapy for Lung Cancer

Martin F. McKneally and James A. Bennett

Albany Medical College, ME 514, Albany, New York 12208

There is a reasonable biological basis for exploring stimulation of the immune response as a component of the treatment of lung cancer. In animal tumor systems it has been well documented that viruses and chemical carcinogens induce the growth of tumors whose cell surface configurations are antigenic. The surface biochemistry of the normal cell that undergoes malignant transformation is altered in a way that is recognizable by components of the host immunological defenses. If an immune response can then be initiated against the altered tumor cell, an exquisitely sensitive, nontoxic, and reasonably efficient system composed of a variety of cells and cell products can be brought to bear on the specifically targeted tumor cells. A distinction should be made between a tumor cell which is *antigenic*, one that bears recognizable cell surface antigens capable of interacting with products of an immune response, and one which is *immunogenic*, one whose cell surface antigens are sufficiently discordant that they elicit an immune response. Highly immunogenic tumors in animals tend to be easily eliminated by the immune system. The same is probably true in humans. A highly immunogenic diploid choriocarcinoma, metastatic to the lungs at multiple sites from a malignantly transformed focus of placental tissue, is readily controllable with single-drug chemotherapy using methotrexate (38,42). The completeness of this response probably depends in part on the fact that paternal antigens are present in the chorionic tumor tissue (rendering the tumor immunogenic in the maternal host) and in part on the reversion of the maternal host to a more normal immunological state following termination of pregnancy (1,35). Unfortunately, most spontaneously arising tumors in animals and humans are not as immunogenic as choriocarcinoma, and the activation of an immune response against them is problematical.

However, there is substantial evidence *in vivo* and *in vitro* to indicate that human tumor cells express unique antigens and that the immune system can play a role in inhibiting their progressive growth. Concomitant immunity to subcutaneous autografts of viable human cancer cells has been demonstrated in many tumor-bearing patients (18,32,89). The simultaneous rejection of these subcutaneous implants of tumor cells and progressive growth of the endogenous tumor suggests that there are immunological components directed against the tumor but that these components are somehow blocked from controlling the growth of endogenous tumor. Infiltration of tumors by lymphocytes, macrophages, and plasma cells has been associated with a favorable prognosis in gastric (12), breast (13), and lung (23) cancers. There have been some reports of spontaneously regressing cancers (74), including lung cancer (27). Although the overall incidence of such spontaneous regression is low, it has occurred most frequently (5–10%) in patients with hypernephroma, neuroblastoma, retinoblastoma, choriocarcinoma, and malignant melanoma. There have also been occasional reports describing regression of metastases after surgical resection of primary tumors, particularly hypernephroma. The incidence of cancer is much higher in individuals with deficient or declining immunological function. In genetic immunodeficiency diseases such as ataxia-telangiectasia and Wiskott-Aldrich syndrome, 10% to 13% of all patients die of malignancy (46). Between 6% and 10% of kidney transplant recipients receiving intensive immunosuppressive therapy develop malignant tumors (40,76). This is 100 times the expected incidence for age-matched normal cohorts. Several explanations have been proposed, such as simultaneous stimulation and suppression of the lymphoid system, but it is noteworthy that more than half the tumors are not lymphoid. Skin cancers predominate, but a variety of other epithelial tumors occur, which indicates that something more than an adverse effect restricted to lymphoid tissue has been produced by prolonged immunosuppression. Further circumstantial evidence of a role for the immune response in cancer is the fact that cancer is primarily a disease of old age (24), a time when immunological function seems to be less adequately controlled and cell-mediated immunity has been documented to be decreased (82).

In vitro, antigens specific to human tumor cells have been demonstrated in serological studies by Old et al. (20,79). These workers identified antigens that are unique to individual tumors and antigens that are found only on tumors of a specific histologic type. This pattern of antigenicity has been found in melanoma, acute leukemia, brain tumors, and renal cell carcinoma. Hellström et al. have recently isolated antibodies from cultured hybrid cells that are uniquely reactive against melanoma cells (105). The hybrid cells were produced by immunizing mice with a human melanoma, then fusing spleen cells from these mice with a mouse myeloma in order to produce a specifically immune hybrid cell with deregulated antibody production. This hybrid cell was cultured, and then cells from selected cultures were cloned for the production of antibody. This group presently has three hybrid cell lines that produce monoclonal antibodies reactive against melanoma. The reactivity is greatest against the melanoma cells used for immunization and very weak against allogeneic melanomas. There is no reactivity against fibroblasts from the patient from whom the immunizing melanoma was obtained, against human tumors of different histologic types, or against normal human cell lines. This work provides important evidence of unique tumor-specific antigens in man which are distinct from normal cell surface antigens, and it parallels the observations in animal tumor systems on which the field of tumor immunology is based.

Another cogent and interesting demonstration of tumor-specific antigens in human cancers has been made by studying leukocyte adherence to glass in the presence of tumor extract. By this technique, antigens common to tumors of the breast (29), colon (95), and lung (96) have been identified. Thomson et al. (96) have shown that the leukocytes from patients with lung cancer recognize extracts from lung cancers of the same histologic type. It is intriguing that they also cross-react with extracts from other histologic types of lung cancer, but not with other cancers. This work may prove extremely useful in immunodiagnosis of early lung cancers. Whether or not these antigens can be exploited to elicit a therapeutic immune response is a challenging problem. Although distinctive lung cancer antigens are demonstrable, it is uncertain whether or not they can be used effectively to reduce or control lung cancer growth.

Unrealistic hopes for the conquest of cancer by stimulation of the immune response were based in part on our historical knowledge of the dramatic effect of immune stimulation in eliminating smallpox from the world and significantly reducing the incidence of paralytic poliomyelitis, diphtheria, and other infectious diseases. It is important to emphasize that control of these epidemic diseases was brought about not by immunotherapy but by *immunoprophylaxis*, i.e., exposure of the host to the immunogen *before* the challenge dose of organisms. Smallpox, once the scourge of the world, has been eliminated as an infectious problem exclusively by the use of immunoprophylaxis, introduced by a country doctor in Gloucestershire in 1798. Because the cow pox virus caused a relatively mild disease and shared antigenic determinants with smallpox, those immunized with cow pox prior to exposure to the smallpox virus enjoyed lifelong immunity to this deforming and often lethal disease. *Immunotherapy* has never been a component of the treatment of smallpox. It is possible to create equally dramatic immunological control of many transplantable tumors in genetically identical laboratory animals. If the host animal is first exposed to a small dose of tumor cells or extracts of tumor-specific antigens, that animal will be resistant to subsequent challenge with large doses of viable tumor cells. Stimulation of the immune response in this setting is an example of *immunoprophylaxis*. Unfortunately, cross-reacting immunogenic tumor cells or tumor cell extracts have not been regularly found among human tumors. Hence, at this time immunoprophylaxis is not a feasible method of treating human cancer.

Lobar pneumonia and rabies are two human infections in which there are reliable data from controlled trials demonstrating the effectiveness of *immunotherapy*. In lobar pneumonia, Finland and his colleagues (28), using the alternate-case method of assignment, examined the mortality among patients treated with type-specific antiserum for pneumococcal pneumonia in the interval from 1924 to 1929. Mortality was significantly reduced among patients treated with type-specific antiserum; 22.7% of patients in the treated group and 32.5% in the control group died of pneumonia. Among patients with early disease (i.e., those presenting to the hospital within 3 days of the onset of symptoms) the improvement in survival was more evident; 14.4% of patients with early cases treated with immunotherapy died, whereas 27.9% of comparable patients who were not treated with antiserum died. Other studies by Cecil (21) in New York City confirmed the therapeutic efficacy of antibody treatment in patients with established pneumococcal pneumonia.

An unplanned clinical immunotherapy experiment occurred in Iran (10), where there are many rabid wolves and wild dogs. A massive attack by these animals occurred in a community in 1975. Almost half of those bitten refused to be transported to the World Health Organization vaccination center in Teheran for administration of rabies vaccine. Of the 45 patients who were treated with daily rabies vaccinations, none died. Of 32 who refused treatment, 15 died. This study confirms the clinical impression that vaccination, that is, active stimulation of the host immune response, can be helpful in reducing the mortality from rabies even though vaccination is initiated after the onset of rabies infection. In this sense rabies vaccination represents a true form of immunotherapy. There are, however, some elements of immunoprophylaxis, in that the host's immunity is being stimulated during a latent interval, during which the virus particles are migrating toward the central nervous system and establishing growth there. This latent interval in rabies is in many ways similar to the situation following surgical removal of a carcinoma of the lung without clinical evidence of disseminated metastases. It is well established from the excellent postmortem studies of Matthews (60), carried out on patients who died of causes unrelated to cancer within the first 30 days after putatively curative resection, that over 30% of patients resected for cure have residual microscopic disease demonstrable within the thorax or at distant sites. Presumably a further fraction have microscopic metastases that are not detectable by the conventional postmortem examination. When these two fractions are combined, the total relapsing fraction of approximately 70% for resected lung cancer patients is accounted for. We postulate that the use of stimulation of the immune response against these micrometastatic cells during the dormant or latent interval is a form of therapy analogous to immunotherapy for rabies.

In the laboratory, there are only a handful of transplantable animal tumors that can be influenced by immunotherapy, and investigators who are keenly interested in immunotherapy transport these tumors and their host animals from laboratory to laboratory in order to have an experimental model which will conform to their hopes and expectations for cancer control in man. This is pointed out not to derogate the importance of this experimental work but to put it into perspective. In fact, several useful clinical protocols have arisen from the study of these animal tumors. These models have also led to the classification of immunotherapy into three categories: active, adoptive, and passive. Active immunotherapy refers to a direct stimulation of the immune response. This can be done nonspecifically with microbes or microbial products in the hope that a generalized activation of the lymphoreticular system will spill over and interfere with the growth of tumor cells. Active specific immunotherapy is the administration of the targeted tumor cells themselves or membrane extracts from these tumor cells. Passive or adoptive immunotherapy refers to the addition of immunological components to a putatively inadequate immune system.

There have been some early successes using immunotherapy for treatment of human cancers. Most of these human trials have employed some form of active immunotherapy. Klein (47) has reported on the eradication of multiple superficial basal cell or squamous cell carcinomas after sensitizing patients to an antigen they had never seen before, dinitrochlorobenzene. He then elicited a delayed hypersensitivity reaction at the site of the tumor by painting it with minute doses of the sensitizing antigen. Morton (72) has described the regression of cutaneous lesions of malignant melanoma after injecting them with BCG, an attenuated strain of *Mycobacterium bovis*. Mathé (57) has shown that patients who were in remission from acute lymphoblastic leukemia benefited from further treatment with subcutaneous inoculations of BCG and/or allogeneic leukemia cells. In spite of these outstanding successes, most trials of immunotherapy have not significantly prolonged the life spans of cancer patients. Probably the biggest obstacle hindering the efficacy of immunotherapy is that it is effective only against relatively small and localized tumors. Mathé (58) has shown that cure of mouse leukemia is obtained with immunotherapy only in those animals in which the number of transplanted leukemia cells is less than 10^5. Similarly, direct injection of BCG into solid tumors in the guinea pig can successfully cause regression of the primary tumor, eradication of proven metastases in the draining lymph nodes, and prolonged immunity to rechallenge with tumor cells (88), but the treatment is effective only if the total number of tumor cells is less than 10^6 in the primary tumor and less than 10^5 in the draining node (36); 10^6 cells would occupy a volume of approximately 0.1 cc, smaller than the volume of the smallest biopsy forceps for the fiberoptic bronchoscope. The usual patient with lung cancer presents to a physician with 10^{10} or 10^{11} malignant cells. In 75% of cases, some of these cells have disseminated, and many of them have successfully colonized distant organs as microscopic or clinically evident metastases. It is clear from these calculations that immunotherapy is not justifiable in the treatment of advanced cancer and that its successful adjunctive use is dependent on reduction of the tumor by the primary treatments (surgery, radiation, and chemotherapy) to a very small fraction of its initial size.

We have outlined in Table 1 a list of clinical trials that have employed immunotherapy in the treatment of lung cancer. Only those trials that had survival data available in the literature at the time of preparation of this chapter are listed, but a large number of additional trials are underway. About half of the trials listed in this table have described a clinical benefit from immunotherapy. However, this is a misleadingly optimistic account of the usefulness of immunotherapy in lung cancer. Most immunotherapy trials in lung cancer have not demonstrated significant clinical benefit. Many negative trials either are not reported or are not continued long enough to obtain meaningful data. This may be due to a breakdown in clinical organization, accumulation of insufficient numbers of patients for meaningful statistical analysis, or early signs of toxicity from immunotherapy precluding its further use. Some of the trials described in this table were based on small numbers of patients followed for a relatively short period of time, and their significance will be more clearly defined at a later date. In spite of these reservations, it seems reasonable to conclude from these trials that immunotherapy can play a role in improving the survival of patients with lung cancer, although its role is limited.

A natural experiment in humans suggested that postoperative empyema improved the survival fraction of lung cancer patients treated at the affiliated hospitals of the Albany Medical College (84). For completeness, it should be recorded that other observers have reported beneficial (92), indifferent (17,68), and even negative

TABLE 1. *Clinical studies in immunotherapy for lung cancer*

		Therapy	Patient status	Clinical effect of immunotherapy	Comments	References
Active nonspecific						
1. Surgery	±	Tice BCG, 10^7 live organisms, i.pl. after surgery	Surgically resectable non-small-cell cancer of the lung	Significant increase in survival ($p = .02$) and disease-free interval ($p = .003$) in stage I patients	Randomized trial (169 patients) begun 1973	64,65
2. Surgery	±	Glaxo BCG, 10^7 live organisms, i.pl. after surgery	Surgically resectable nonanaplastic bronchogenic carcinoma	No effect on survival in stage I patients	Randomized trial (92 patients) begun May 1976	43
3. Surgery	±	Levamisole, 2.5 mg/m² orally 3 consecutive days before surgery, twice a week for 18 months after surgery, and Tice BCG, 10^7 live organisms, i.pl. 4th day after surgery	Surgically resectable non-small-cell cancer of the lung	No effect on survival	Randomized trial (52 patients) begun March 1976	99,100
4. Surgery	±	Connaught BCG, 120 mg/3 ml orally, weekly × 4, twice a month ×3, every 3 months × 5; begun 5 days after surgery	Surgically resectable bronchogenic carcinoma	No effect on survival or disease-free interval	Randomized trial (308 patients) begun 1973; 2-year follow-up on all patients	67
5. Surgery	±	Levamisole, 50 mg orally t.i.d. 3 consecutive days before surgery; after surgery, same regimen every 2 weeks	Surgically resectable bronchogenic carcinoma	Significant increase in disease-free interval in patients <70 kg ($p < .05$)	Randomized trial (178 patients); 1-year follow-up	2,4
6. Surgery	±	Pasteur BCG, 75 mg scarified once a week	Surgically resectable squamous cell carcinoma of lung	Significant increase in survival	Randomized trial (43 patients); 18-month analysis	81

Treatment		Immunotherapy	Disease	Result	Trial	Ref.
7. Surgery	±	Glaxo BCG, 5 × 10⁸ live organisms, s.d. 10 days after surgery; single dose	Surgically resectable lung carcinoma	No effect on survival	Randomized trial (120 patients); 5-year follow-up	25
8. Surgery	±	Tice BCG, i.d., Tine multiple puncture	Surgically resectable bronchogenic carcinoma	Significant increase in disease-free interval ($p = .05$) after 1 year	Nonrandomized trial (78 patients); mean follow-up 20 months; 30% of patients who received BCG also received autologous tumor cells	106
9. Surgery	±	Chemotherapy or *C. parvum* or Chemotherapy + *C. parvum*, 3–4 mg s.c. weekly for 1st year, twice a month for 2nd year	Stage I non-small-cell lung cancer	At 3 years no difference in survival between groups	Nonrandomized trial; majority of patients received surgery alone	56
10. Surgery or radiotherapy	±	Tice BCG, 10⁸ live organisms, multipuncture with Tine technique, once a week ×4, then twice a month ×2, then once a month ×9	Stages II, III, IV bronchogenic carcinoma	Significant increase in survival ($p = .01$)	Randomized trial (55 patients); 2-year follow-up	98
11. Surgery or radiotherapy	±	Pasteur BCG cell wall skeleton, 300 µg i.d. 7–10 days after surgery, then 200 µg biweekly for 30 weeks, then 200 µg monthly	All stages of lung carcinoma	Significant increase in survival ($p < .0001$)	455 patients treated, 380 historical controls; 2-year update; some patients also received BCG-CWS i.l.	103,104
12. Surgery or radiotherapy	±	Glaxo BCG, 0.1 ml i.d. monthly ×7	Lung carcinoma in patients with no metastatic symptoms on diagnosis	No effect on survival	Randomized trial (75 patients); data collected 1971–1974	6

TABLE 1. *(continued)*

	Therapy	Patient status	Clinical effect of immunotherapy	Comments	References
13. Radiotherapy ±	Glaxo BCG, 25–125 × 10⁸ live organisms; Heaf gun, weekly for 1st year, then every 2 weeks	Advanced squamous cell lung carcinoma	Significant increase in disease-free interval ($p = .02$)	Randomized trial (48 patients); data collected 1970–1973	80
(400 + rads)					
14. Surgery, then chemotherapy	BCG i.d., Tine plate 2–4 × 10⁸ organisms given once before surgery and then once a month ×4 after surgery	Surgically resectable lung carcinoma	Significant increase in survival ($p < .05$)	Randomized trial (126 patients); follow-up 10–28 months	70,71
15. Chemotherapy or Chemotherapy ±	*C. parvum*, 2.5 gm/m² i.v. weekly Tice BCG, 10⁸ live organisms scarified weekly ×12, then biweekly	Unresectable, metastatic, or recurrent bronchogenic carcinoma	No effect on survival or hematologic tolerance of chemotherapy	Randomized trial (79 patients); *C. parvum* discontinued after 19 patient entries because of toxicity; median follow-up 30 weeks	87
16. Chemotherapy ±	*C. parvum*, 4.2 mg s.c. once a week ×8	Stage III inoperable lung carcinoma	No effect on survival	Randomized trial (66 patients); 12-month analysis	22
17. Chemotherapy ±	*C. parvum* (Merieux strain), 4 mg s.c. weekly	Advanced squamous or oat cell bronchogenic carcinoma	Significant increase in survival (squamous $p < .001$; oat cell $p < .05$)	Randomized trial (143 patients); 3-year analysis	44
18. Chemotherapy ±	Thymosin, 60 mg/m² or 20 mg/m² s.c.	Small cell carcinoma of the lung	Significant increase in survival in thymosin 60 group that had low pretreatment levels of total T cells and α_2 HS	Randomized trial (50 patients); patients entered between Feb. 1976 and Jan. 1977	50

	Treatment	Regimen	Disease	Result	Trial	Ref.
19.	Chemotherapy ± and radiotherapy	BCG, scarification, multiple doses	Small cell carcinoma of the lung	Significant decrease in long-term survival in BCG group ($p = .019$)	Randomized trial (417 patients entered as of 3/14/79)	62
20.	Chemotherapy ± and radiotherapy	BCG-MER, 100 µg i.d. in 4 sites every 6 weeks	Small cell carcinoma of the lung	Significant increase in median survival by MER in patients with extensive disease at diagnosis	Randomized trial (99 patients); 1-year analysis	45

Active specific

	Treatment	Regimen	Disease	Result	Trial	Ref.
21.	Surgery ±	Autologous tumor cells treated with con-A and neuraminidase given i.d. (5×10^7 cells) in CFA on day of surgery, then every 2 weeks ×3, and Glaxo BCG i.d. once a month beginning 1 month after surgery	Surgically resectable stage III lung carcinoma	Significant increase in survival ($p = .05$)	Randomized trial, historical controls also compared (30 patients); follow-up 5–51 months	93
22.	Surgery ±	Chemotherapy ± allogeneic lung-cancer-associated antigen in CFA i.d. monthly ×3 beginning 17 days after surgery	Surgically resectable lung carcinoma	Significant increase in disease-free interval in stage I patients ($p = .001$)	Randomized trial (69 patients); mean follow-up 24 months	90
23.	Primary therapy: surgery, radiation, chemotherapy ±	Pasteur BCG, $3–5 \times 10^8$ live organisms scarified every 2 weeks, begun 3 weeks after surgery ± killed (5000 R) allogeneic lung carcinoma, $5–10 \times 10^7$ cells s.c. and i.d. every 2 weeks	All stages of lung carcinoma	Significant increase in disease-free interval in stage I & II patients; no difference between BCG and BCG + cells	Randomized trial (74 patients); data collected 1973–1975	37,77

glycoprotein ($p = .006$, $p = .036$, respectively)

effects (19) of empyema on survival. Based on our own experience and on the observations of Klein (47), Morton (72), and Zbar (88) that regional or local administration of BCG is capable of controlling progressive neoplastic growth, our group initiated a trial of regional immunotherapy in lung cancer. After putatively complete surgical resection, 117 patients were randomized either to receive a single intrapleural inoculation of Tice BCG, 10⁷ colony-forming units, or to enter into the control group. The details of this trial have been published elsewhere (63,65). In 66 patients with stage I lung cancer, control patients had a high incidence of recurrent cancer, both early and late, whereas patients treated with BCG tended to have later recurrences, and there was a considerably smaller number of recurrences (Fig. 1A). Patients with stage II or stage III lung cancer derived no additional benefit from intrapleural BCG as adjuvant therapy following surgery (Fig. 1B). Intrapleural BCG

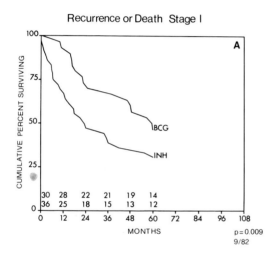

FIG. 1. Results of BCG treatment for patients with stage 1 *(top)* and stage 2 and 3 *(bottom)* lung cancer.

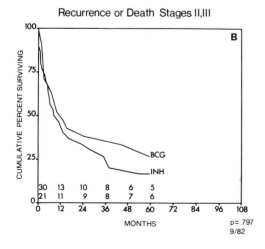

was of no benefit and may have been harmful to patients with unresectable lung cancer who were treated with radiation and chemotherapy (85). There are several cooperative groups retesting our protocol of intrapleural BCG in surgically resected stage I lung cancer patients in an effort to confirm or refute its efficacy. Preliminary analyses of their data show no therapeutic benefit. Interestingly, Wright and Hill and their colleagues in Seattle have been able to show a therapeutic benefit from intrapleural BCG, but this therapeutic advantage is enjoyed only by those patients who were PPD-negative prior to treatment (102).

Reviewing our statistics in light of the Seattle experience, we found that the therapeutic benefit of BCG could be explained almost entirely by the patients who were PPD-negative. Patients who were PPD-positive had approximately the same survival curve as the control patients (Fig. 2). These recent observations support the hypothesis that a primary response to the adjuvant agent is necessary to achieve a therapeutic antitumor effect.

A confounding variable in these trials, and in our own later trials, has been a fluctuation in the antitumor effectiveness of the biological agent BCG (11). This problem emphasizes the importance of identifying the compound in the BCG organism that is responsible for its effect on tumor growth. Comprehensive studies by Ribi et al. (83) have indicated that essential elements are trehalose dimycolate and muramyl dipeptide, components of the BCG cell wall that are also found in the cell walls of *Corynebacterium parvum* and *Nocardia rubra*. Until the pharmacology of their use as an antitumor agent is worked out, it seems reasonable to continue to use the living organisms or crude cell wall preparations.

Yamamura and his colleagues have employed BCG cell walls in lung cancer patients intrapleurally and intracutaneously. Their conclusion from comparisons

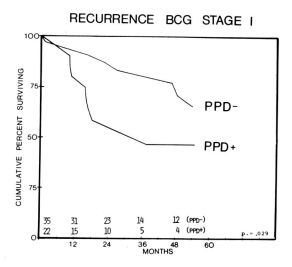

FIG. 2. Therapeutic benefit of BCG for PPD-negative stage 1 lung cancer patients.

with historical control patients is that this form of immunotherapy has been beneficial to their patients (104).

In a trial using Glaxo BCG, Baldwin and his colleagues found that stage I lung cancer patients did not benefit from intrapleural administration of this agent, when compared with randomized control patients (51). The pretreatment tuberculin status of these patients was not reported, but it is likely that most of them were tuberculin-positive. Based on our data, and that of Wright et al. (102), this should reduce the effectiveness of BCG in this population.

BCG administered by the cutaneous route, at a site remote from the resected primary tumor, has been reported to be unhelpful (26), beneficial at a marginal level of significance (81), and distinctly beneficial (33) in a variety of studies.

Cutaneous administration of complete Freund's adjuvant, an immunostimulant analogous to BCG, has been evaluated with and without the addition of isolated lung tumor antigens in an interesting study initiated by Stewart, Hollinshead, and their colleagues (90). In the original study, the results of treatment with extracted lung tumor antigens given in combination with complete Freund's adjuvant were compared with the outcome in patients treated by surgery alone. The control group was a contemporaneous and nonrandomized one, but these preliminary data suggested that there was some benefit from this form of immunotherapy in stage I patients. It is especially interesting and important that patients developed positive skin tests to the tumor antigens that persisted in some instances for as long as 4 years. The investigators in this trial deserve great credit for the effort required to complete this trial. The tumors were excised by surgeons in Ottawa, and tumor tissue was transported by commercial airline pilots to Washington, where it was delivered to Dr. Ariel Hollinshead, a biochemist at George Washington University. The tumor antigens from the lung cancer cells were extracted by Dr. Hollinshead, and the sterile extracts were then returned by the same technique to Dr. Stewart, who administered them to the patients. The trial was predicated on the notion that there are cross-reacting antigens between individual human lung cancers, a premise supported by the studies of Old, Hellström, and Thomson described earlier. This Ottawa trial was enlarged to a multiinstitutional cooperative trial that enlisted over 100 patients in 1979 (94). At present, some therapeutic benefit is evident in the subgroup treated with complete Freund's adjuvant and the subgroup treated with complete Freund's adjuvant admixed with tumor cell extracts. If it proves true that adding homologous tumor cells to BCG has an additional benefit, it will be extremely useful to be able to use tumor cells from one patient to immunize another. In our own experience using a patient's autologous tumor cells as the source of the vaccine (61) there has been a problem securing enough tumor tissue to make an adequate vaccine when the lesions are small.

Another similar randomized trial using tumor antigen and BCG as the adjuvant has been carried out at the Naval Medical Center (Walter Reed Army Hospital) coordinated by Dr. Ronald Herberman of the Immunology Branch of the National Cancer Institute and Dr. Robert Oldham of Vanderbilt University (37). This small trial in resectable lung cancer patients again suggested a therapeutic benefit in those patients treated in the two immunotherapy arms of the trial. These patients were given BCG by the cutaneous route or BCG plus irradiated tumor cells. It is uncertain from this study whether or not any additional advantage was achieved by the use of the tumor cells, and further follow-up with expansion of the study is required.

In a study by Israel (44), subcutaneous administration of *C. parvum* was shown to prolong the survival of patients receiving chemotherapy for advanced lung cancer. A preliminary study carried out using *C. parvum* in surgically resectable lung cancer patients demonstrated the safety and feasibility of administering this agent by the intrapleural route (52). This provided the basis for a large randomized trial of intrapleural *C. parvum* for adjuvant treatment of surgically resectable stage I lung cancer patients. To date, intrapleural *C. parvum* has not improved the recurrence rate or survival in these patients (53,54).

Nocardia rubra and *N. rubra* cell wall skeletons have been administered to lung cancer patients at all stages in clinical trials directed by Yamamura (104). This organism, like *C. parvum*, shares the trehalose dimycolate moiety in its cell wall with BCG. Favorable initial experience with this agent in Japan merits further evaluation in controlled trials.

Amery and co-workers have reported their experience with levamisole, an antihelminthic drug that inadvertently was found to potentiate immunological reactivity in animals. It was the initial impression of these workers that levamisole reduced the recurrence rate of lung cancer in treated patients, as compared with randomized controls (2). An especially intriguing aspect of this study was the apparent reduction in the number of recurrences at distant sites (5). In the ensuing 4 years, the status of this study has changed. There have been changes within the data base, and data from other workers, suggesting that levamisole is not helpful at the dosage and schedule used in the original study. At the present time, analysis of the levamisole-treated and control patients shows no difference (3). However, a therapeutic benefit seems to have occurred in those patients with body weights less than 70 kg, who therefore received greater dosages of levamisole on a per kilogram basis.

There are two other studies which suggest that levamisole is not helpful to patients with resectable lung cancer. An important study by Anthony et al. (7) indicated an unexpected increase in non-cancer-related deaths in the levamisole group, with an unusually high incidence of cardiorespiratory failure among the patients treated with this agent. Hill's cooperative group in Seattle has found that the addition of levamisole to intrapleural BCG treatment in stage I lung cancer patients delays the time to conversion of the tuberculin test and reduces the efficacy of intrapleural BCG as an adjuvant (101).

Thymosin is a soluble polypeptide isolated from calf thymus by Goldstein in 1966. In preclinical studies (31), thymosin seems to restore rather than augment immune function. This has proved unequivocally beneficial to children with congenital immunodeficiency (97). Because patients receiving chemotherapy usually are in need of immunological restoration, Lipson and his colleagues (50) studied the immunotherapeutic effect of thymosin in patients with small cell bronchogenic carcinoma receiving combination chemotherapy for their disease. Patients were randomized to receive, in addition to their chemotherapy, thymosin 60 mg/m^2, thymosin 20 mg/m^2, or placebo. Thymosin was given subcutaneously twice a week during the first 6 weeks of chemotherapy. Patients receiving the higher dose of thymosin had a significantly longer ($p = 0.044$) median survival time. The benefit from thymosin appeared to be greatest ($p = 0.006$) in patients with low T-lymphocyte levels before the initiation of therapy.

There are interesting pieces of immunological and pharmacological information to be learned from all of these studies. This information adds to our understanding of the host immune system in its interactions with immunopotentiator and tumor. In reviewing these studies, one is left with the feeling that we are gaining insights into the manipulation of this interrelationship to the therapeutic advantage of the host.

An immunotherapeutic agent that has recently been introduced for evaluation is interferon. There have been no controlled clinical trials using interferon for the treatment of lung cancer, partly because of the insufficient supply of interferon, which is an endogenous protein found in leukocytes, fibroblasts, and other mammalian cells; interferon must be extracted and purified by a very expensive process that produces relatively small amounts of this agent. Mammalian cells increase their production of interferon in response to viral infection. It has the ability to alter mammalian cells in a way that prevents their colonization by viruses, and it derives its name from this interference. Its mechanism of action involves activation of at least two intracellular enzymes, a cyclic-AMP-independent protein kinase (86) and 2'5'-oligoadenylate synthetase (69), which together inhibit protein synthesis at the level of translating RNA-encoded messages into the construction of proteins. In addition to inhibiting the replication of viruses, it also inhibits the growth of mammalian cells, including tumor cells (41,49).

There are suggestive but poorly controlled data from therapeutic trials with interferon in Europe that have led the American Cancer Society and the National Cancer Institute to provide funds for controlled clinical trials with interferon in this country. The great expense of interferon results from the large supplies of human cells necessary for its production. A major breakthrough in this area was announced recently when Swiss workers reported the ability to synthesize active human interferon-producing bacterial cultures by recombinant DNA experiments wherein a portion of the human genome responsible for producing interferon was successfully introduced into the genome of bacteria (55,73). Production of large supplies of interferon will be greatly facilitated by this potentially important contribution from recombinant DNA research.

Preliminary data from a noncontrolled trial of interferon for treatment of lung cancer by Krown and her colleagues (48) at New York Memorial Sloan-Kettering Cancer Center showed no therapeutic benefit from interferon and moderate toxicity in terms of fever, anorexia, and bone marrow depression. However, in other small noncontrolled trials, some improvement from interferon treatment has been reported in osteogenic sarcoma (91), myeloma (75), lymphoma (66), and breast cancer (14), as well as laryngeal papillomatosis (34).

Several aspects of immunotherapy need to be refined to make it a more acceptable modality of cancer treatment. Further study of the pharmacology of immunopotentiators is required in order to work out their appropriate dose, route, and schedule of administration. This can be done at the preclinical level in experimental animals, following the models that have been used for chemotherapy. The development of tests to monitor responses to immunopotentiators in humans would be helpful in titrating their dose and schedule. In cases in which microbes like BCG or microbial products are used, standardization of these agents is required to assure that their activity will be the same from one day to the next. Finally, a better understanding of the regulation of the immune response is needed. Overstimulation of the immune system can sometimes lead to suppression rather than augmentation of immunity, because of the activation of suppressor cells (30). When one is initially dealing with weakly antigenic human tumors, overstimulation could subvert attempts to convert this weak antigenicity into immunogenicity (15,16).

It is disappointing to report that immunotherapy, at the present state of knowledge of the art, is not yet ready for widespread use in clinical practice as an adjunct to the standard methods of surgery and radiation therapy. It is reasonable to expect progress in the testing of immunotherapy in lung cancer because of the development of several excellent cooperative surgical study groups and the initiation of new modes of therapy, including direct intralesional injection of BCG into lung tumors by transthoracic fine-needle technique or by transbronchoscopic injection. Studies using these techniques are under way at the Universtiy of California at Los Angeles under Carmack Holmes (39) and at Yale University under Richard Matthay and his colleagues (59). The next 5 years will be a period of careful documentation in well-controlled cooperative surgical trials. These trials should provide useful information about the pharmacology of immunostimulants in the setting of minimal residual disease that may allow the addition of immunotherapy to the armamentarium of proven effective remedies against lung cancer.

ACKNOWLEDGMENTS

Portions of the work represented above were supported by NCI Contract NO1-CB-53940, PHS General Clinical Research Center Grant MO1-RR-00749, and the Center for Laboratories and Research of the New York State Department of Health.

REFERENCES

1. Adcock E. W., III, Teasdale, F., August, C. S., Cox, S., Meschia, G., Battaglia, F. C., and Naughton, M. A. (1973): *Science*, 181:845–847.
2. Amery, W. K. (1975): *Br. Med. J.*, 3:461–464.
3. Amery, W. K., et al. (1982): Four-Year Results from Double-Blind Study of Adjuvant Levamisole Treatment in Resectable Lung Cancer. In: *Immunotherapy of Human Cancer,* edited by W. D. Terry and S. A. Rosenberg, pp.123–133. Excerpta Medica, New York.
4. Amery, W. K. (1978): A placebo-controlled Levamisole study in resectable lung cancer. In: *Immunotherapy of Cancer: Present Status of Trials in Man,* edited by W. D. Terry and D. Windhorst, pp. 191–202. Raven Press, New York.

5. Amery, W. K., Cosemans, J., Gooszen, H. C., Cardozo, E. L., Louwagie, A., Stam, J., Swier-enga, J., Vanderschueren, R. G., and Veldhuizen, R. W. (1979): *Cancer Immunol. Immunother.*, 7:191–198.

6. Anthony, H. M., et al. (1978): *Cancer*, 42:1784–1792.

7. Anthony, H. M., Mearns, A. J., Mason, M. K., Scott, D. G., Moghissi, K., Deverall, P. B., Rozycki, Z. J., and Watson, D. A. (1979): *Thorax*, 34:4–12.

8. Azuma, I., Yamawaki, M., and Yamamura, Y. (1978): *Cancer Immunol. Immunother.*, 4:95–100.

9. Baglioni, C. (1979): *Cell*, 17:255–264.

10. Bahmanyar, M., Fayaz, A., Nour-Saleki, S., Mohammadi, M., and Koprowski, H. (1976): *JAMA*, 236:2751–2754.

11. Bennett, J. A. and McKneally, M. F. (1980): *Proc. Am. Assoc. Cancer Res.*, 21:249.

12. Black, M. M., Opler, S. R., and Speer, F. D. (1954): *Surg. Gynecol. Obstet.*, 98:725–734.

13. Black, M. M., Speer, F. D., and Opler, S. R. (1956): *Am. J. Clin. Path.*, 26:250–265.

14. Borden, E., Dao, T., Holland, J., Gutterman, J., and Merigan, T. (1980): *Proc. Am. Assoc. Cancer Res.*, 21:187.

15. Broder, S., and Waldmann, T. A. (1978): *N. Engl. J. Med.*, 299:1281–1284.

16. Broder, S., and Waldmann, T. A. (1978): *N. Engl. J. Med.*, 299:1335–1341.

17. Brohee, D., Vanderhoeft, P., and Smets, P. (1977): *Eur. J. Cancer*, 13:1429–1436.

18. Brunschwig, A., Southam, C. M., and Levin, A. G. (1965): *Ann. Surg.*, 162:416–425.

19. Cady, B. and Clifton, E. E. (1967): *J. Thorac. Cardiovasc. Surg.*, 53:102–108.

20. Carey, T. E., Takahashi, T., Resnick, L. A., Oettgen, H. F., and Old, L. J. (1976): *Proc. Natl. Acad. Sci. USA*, 73:3278–3282.

21. Cecil, R. L., and Plummer, N. (1930): *JAMA*, 95:1547–1553.

22. Dimitrov, N. V., et al. (1978): Combination therapy with corynebacterium parvum and doxorubicin hydrochloride in patients with lung cancer. In: *Immunotherapy of Cancer: Present Status of Trials in Man*, edited by W. D. Terry and D. Windhorst, pp. 181–190. Raven Press, New York.

23. DiPaola, M., Bertolotti, A., Colizza, S., and Coli, M. (1977): *J. Thorac. Cardiovasc. Surg.*, 73:531–537.

24. Dorn, H. F. and Cutler, S. J. (1958): *Public Health Monograph No. 56.*

25. Edwards, F. R., et al. (1978): *Thorax*, 33:250–252.

26. Edwards, F. R. (1979): *Thorax*, 34:801–806.

27. Emerson, G. L., Emerson, M. S., and Sherwood, C. E. (1968): *J. Thorac. Cardiovasc. Surg.*, 55:225–230.

28. Finland, M. (1930): *N. Engl. J. Med.*, 202:1244–1247.

29. Flores, M., Marti, J. H., Grosser, N., MacFarlane, J. K., and Thomson, D. M. P. (1977): *Cancer*, 39:494–505.

30. Gershon, R. K., and Metzler, C. M. (1979): Regulation of the immune response. In: *The Immunopathology of Lymphoreticular Neoplasms*, edited by J. J. Twomey and R. A. Good, pp. 23–51. Plenum Press, New York.

31. Goldstein, A. L., Low, T. L. K., Rossio, J. L., Ulrich, J. T., Naylor, P. H., and Thurman, G. B. (1978): Recent developments in the chemistry and biology of thymosin. In: *Immune Modulation and Control of Neoplasia by Adjuvant Therapy*, edited by M. A. Chirigos, pp. 281–291. Raven Press, New York.

32. Grace, J. T., Perese, D. M., Metzgar, R. S., Sasabe, S., and Holdridge, B. (1961): *J. Neurosurg.*, 18:159–167.

33. Hadziev, S., Kavaklieva-Dimitrova, J., Mandulova, P., Madzarova, S., and Spassova, M. (1980): *Neoplasma*, 27:83–94.

34. Haglund, S., Lundquist, S., Ingimarsson, S., Cantell, K., and Strander, H. (1982): Interferon therapy in juvenile laryngeal papillomatosis. In: *Immunotherapy of Human Cancer*, edited by W. D. Terry and S. A. Rosenberg, pp.407–409. Excerpta Medica, New York.

35. Han, T. (1974): *Clin. Exp. Immunol.*, 18:529–535.

36. Hanna, M. G., and Peters, L. C. (1975): *Cancer*, 36:1298–1304.

37. Herberman, R. B., Weese, J. L., Oldham, R. K., Bonnard, G. D., Perlin, E., Heim, W., Miller, C., Reid, J., and Connor, R. J. (1979): Prospects for immunotherapy of lung cancer with specific immunoadjuvants. In: *Lung Cancer: Progress in Therapeutic Research*, edited by F. M. Muggia and M. Rozencweig, pp. 521–530. Raven Press, New York.

38. Holland, J. F., Hreshchyshyn, M. M., and Glidewell, O. (1970): *Abstracts of Xth Int. Cancer Congress*, Houston, May 1970, p. 461.
39. Holmes, E. C., Mink, J., Ramming, K. P., Coulson, W. F., and Morton, D. L. (1977): *Lancet*, 2:586–587.
40. Hoover, R., and Fraumeni, J. F. (1973): *Lancet*, 1:55.
41. Horoszewicz, J. S., Leong, S. S., and Carter, W. A. (1979): *Science*, 206:1091–1093.
42. Hreshchyshyn, M. M., Graham, J. B., and Holland, J. F. (1961): *Am. J. Obstet. Gynec.*, 81:688–705.
43. Iles, P. B., et al. (1980): *Lancet*, 1:11–13.
44. Israel, L. (1976): Nonspecific immune stimulation with corynebacteria in lung cancer. In: *Lung Cancer: Natural History, Prognosis, and Therapy*, edited by L. Israel and A. P. Chahinian, pp. 273–280. Academic Press, New York.
45. Jackson, D. V., et al. (1979): *Proc. Am. Soc. Clin. Oncol.*, 20:367.
46. Kersey, J. H., Spector, B. D., and Good, R. (1973): *Int. J. Cancer*, 12:333.
47. Klein, E. (1969): *Cancer Res.*, 29:2351–2362.
48. Krown, S. E., et al. (1982): Phase II trial of human leukocyte interferon (HuLeIF) in non-small cell lung cancer (NSCLC). In: *Immunotherapy of Human Cancer*, edited by W. D. Terry and S. A. Rosenberg, pp. 397–405. Excerpta Medica, New York.
49. Kurvata, T., Fuse, A., Suzuki, N., and Morinaga, N. (1979): *J. Gen. Virol.*, 43:435–439.
50. Lipson, S. D., Chretien, P. B., Makuch, R., Kenady, D. E., and Cohen, M. H. (1979): *Cancer*, 43:863–870.
51. Lowe, J., Iles, P. B., Shore, D. F., Langman, M. J. S., and Baldwin, R. W. (1980): *Lancet*, I:11–13.
52. Ludwig Lung Cancer Study Group (1978): *Cancer Immunol. Immunother.*, 4:69–75.
53. Ludwig Lung Cancer Study Group (1982): Intrapleural cornyebacterium parvum as adjuvant therapy in operable bronchogenic non-small cell carcinonoma. In: *Immunotherapy of Human Cancer*, edited by W. D. Terry and S. A. Rosenberg, pp. 111–114. Excerpta Medica, New York.
54. Ludwig Lung Cancer Study Group (1980): A randomized study with intrapleural corynebacterium parvum in operable non-small cell lung carcinomas. In: *II World Conference on Lung Cancer Abstracts*, edited by Hansen and Dombernowsky. Excerpta Medica, Amsterdam.
55. Mantei, N., Schwarzstein, M., Streuli, M., Panem, S., Nagata, S., and Weissman, C. (1980): *Gene*, 10:1–10.
56. Martini, N., et al. (1977): *J. Thorac. Cardiovasc. Surg.*, 74:499–505.
57. Mathé, G., Amiel, J. L., and Schwarzenberg, L. (1969): *Lancet*, 1:697–699.
58. Mathé, G., Pouillart, P., and Lapeyrague, F. (1969): *Br. J. Cancer*, 23:814–824.
59. Matthay, R. A., Balzer, P. A., Mahler, D. A., Merrill, W. W., Loke, J., Mitchell, M. S., Reynolds, H. Y., Carter, D., and Baue, A. E. (1978): *Chest*, 74:344.
60. Matthews, M. (1974): *Sem. Onc.*, 1:175–182.
61. Maver, C., and McKneally, M. F. (1979): *Cancer Res.*, 39:3276.
62. McCracken, J. D., et al. (1980): *Proc. Am. Soc. Clin. Oncol.* 21:446.
63. McKneally, M. F., Maver, C., and Kausel, H. W. (1976): *Lancet*, I:377–379.
64. McKneally, M. F., et al. (1981): *J. Thorac. Cardiovasc. Surg.*, 81:485–492.
65. McKneally, M. F., Maver, C., and Kausel, H. W. (1978): Regional immunotherapy of lung cancer using postoperative intrapleural BCG. In: *Immunotherapy of Cancer: Present Status of Trials in Man*, edited by W. D. Terry and D. Windhorst, pp. 161–171. Raven Press, New York.
66. Merigan, T. C., Sikora, K., and Breeden, J. H. (1978): *N. Engl. J. Med.*, 299:1449–1453.
67. Miller, A. B., et al. (1979): *Can. Med. Assoc. J.*, 121:45–56.
68. Minasian, H., Lewis, C. T., and Evans, S. J. W. (1978): *Br. Med. J.*, 2:1329–1331.
69. Minks, M. A., West, D. K., Benvin, S., and Baglioni, C. (1979): *J. Biol. Chem.*, 254:10180–10183.
70. Miyazawa, N., et al. (1978): *Igaku-no-ayumi*, 104:181.
71. Miyazawa, N., et al. (1979): *Jpn. J. Clin. Oncol.*, 9:19–26.
72. Morton, D. L., Eilber, F. R., Malmgren, R. A., and Wood, W. C. (1970): *Surgery*, 68:158–164.
73. Nagata, S., Taira, H., Hall, A., Johnsrud, L., Streuli, M., Escodi, J., Boll, W., Cantell, K., and Weissman, C. (1980): *Nature*, 284:316–320.
74. *Natl. Cancer Inst. Monograph No. 44* (1976), 5–148.

75. Osserman, E. F., Sherman, W. H., Alexanian, R., Gutterman, J. U., and Humphrey, R. L. (1980): *Proc. Am. Assoc. Cancer Res.*, 21:161.
76. Penn, I. (1974): *Cancer*, 34:1474.
77. Oldham, R. K. (1976): *Int. J. Cancer*, 18:739–749.
78. Herberman, R. B., et al. (1979): Prospects for immunotherapy of lung cancer with specific immunoadjuvants. In: *Lung Cancer: Progress in Therapeutic Research*, edited by F. M. Muggia and M. Rozencweig, pp. 521–530. Raven Press, New York.
79. Pfreundschuh, M., Shiku, H., Takahashi, T., Ueda, R., Ransohoff, J., Oettgen, H. F., and Old, L. J. (1978): *Proc. Natl. Acad. Sci. USA*, 75:5122–5126.
80. Pines, A., et al. (1976): *Lancet*, 1:380–381.
81. Pouillart, P., Palangie, T., Huguenin, P., Morin, P., Gautier, H., Lededente, A., Baron, A., and Mathé, G. (1977): Attempt at immunotherapy with BCG of patients with bronchus carcinoma: preliminary results. In: *Adjuvant Therapy of Cancer*, edited by S. S. Salmon and S. E. Jones, pp. 225–235. North-Holland, New York.
82. Ram, J. S. (1967): *J. Gerontol.*, 22:92.
83. Ribi, E., Milner, K. C., Granger, D. L., Kelly, M. T., Yamamoto, K., Brehmer, W., Parker, R., Smith, R. F., and Strain, S. M. (1976): *Ann. N. Y. Acad. Sci.*, 277:228–238.
84. Ruckdeschel, J. C., Codish, S. D., Stranahan, A., and McKneally, M. F. (1972): *N. Engl. J. Med.*, 287:1013–1017.
85. Ruckdeschel, J. C., McKneally, M. F., Devore, C., Baxter, D., Sedransk, N., Caradonna, R., and Horton, J. (1980): *Proc. Am. Assoc. Cancer Res.*, 21:374.
86. Samuel, C. E. (1979): *Proc. Natl. Acad. Sci. USA*, 76:600–604.
87. Sarna, G. P., et al. (1978): *Cancer Treat. Rep.*, 62:681–687.
88. Smith, H. C., Bast, R. C., Zbar, B., and Rapp, H. J. (1975): *J. Natl. Cancer Inst.*, 55:1345–1352.
89. Southam, C. M. (1967): *Prog. Exp. Tumor Res.*, 9:1.
90. Stewart, T. H. M., Hollinshead, A. C., Harris, J. E., Belanger, R., Crepeau, A., Hooper, G. D., Sachs, H. J., Klaassen, D. J., Hirte, W., Rapp, E., Crook, A. F., Orizaga, M., Sengar, D. P. S., and Raman, S. (1976): *Ann. N.Y. Acad. Sci.*, 277:436–466.
91. Strander, H., Adamson, U., Aparisi, T., Broström, L. A., Cantell, K., Einhorn, S., Hall, K., Ingimarsson, S., Nilsonne, U., and Söderberg, G. (1979): *Recent Results Cancer Res.*, 68:40–44.
92. Takita, H. (1970): *J. Thorac. Cardiovasc. Surg.*, 59:642–644.
93. Takita, H., Takada, M., Minowada, J., Han, T., and Edgerton, F. (1978): Adjuvant immunotherapy of stage III lung carcinoma. In: *Immunotherapy of Cancer: Present Status of Trials in Man*, edited by W. D. Terry and D. Windhorst, pp. 217–224. Raven Press, New York.
94. Takita, H., Hollinshead, A. C., Edgerton, F., Bhayana, J. N., Moskowitz, R. M., Adler, R. H., Ramundo, M., Han, T., Vincent, R. G., Conway, D., and Takita, L. (1980): Adjuvant immunotherapy of squamous cell lung carcinoma. In: *II World Conference on Lung Cancer Abstracts*, edited by Hansen and Dombernowsky. Excerpta Medica, Amsterdam.
95. Tataryn, D. N., MacFarlane, J. K., Murray, D., and Thomson, D. M. P. (1979): *Cancer*, 43:898–912.
96. Thomson, D. M. P., Ayeni, A. O., MacFarlane, J. K., Tataryn, D. N., Terrin, M., Schraufnagel, D., Wilson, J., and Mulder, D. S. (1981): *Ann. Thor. Surg.*, 31(4):314–321.
97. Wara, D. W., and Ammann, A. J. (1978): *Transplant. Proc.*, 10:203–209.
98. Warren, S., et al. (1977): BCG adjuvant immunotherapy of stage II, III, and IV bronchogenic carcinoma. In: *Neoplasm Immunity: Solid Tumor Therapy*, edited by R. G. Crispen, pp.49–53. Franklin Institute Press, Philadelphia.
99. Wright, P. W., et al. (1977): Immunotherapy of resectable non-small cell cancer of the lung: a prospective comparison of intrapleural BCG + levamisole versus intrapleural BCG versus placebo. In: *Adjuvant Therapy of Cancer*, edited by S. S. Salmon and S. E. Jones, pp. 217–224. North-Holland, New York.
100. Wright, P. W., et al. (1980): Personal communication.
101. Wright, P. W., Hill, L. D., Peterson, A. V., Anderson, R. P., Hammer, S. P., Johnson, L. P., Morgan, E. H., and Pinkham, R. D. (1980): Adjuvant immunotherapy with intrapleural BCG (IP-BCG) and levamisole (L) in patients with resected, non-small cell lung cancer. *Proc. 2nd Conf. on Immunotherapy of Cancer*.

102. Wright, P. W., Hill, L. D., Peterson, A. V., and Bernstein, I. D. (1980): *Proc. Am. Assoc. Cancer Res.*, 21:230.
103. Yamamura, Y., et al. (1979): *Cancer Res.*, 39:3262–3267.
104. Yamamura, Y., Sakatani, M., Ogura, T., and Azuma, I. (1979): *Cancer*, 43:1314–1319.
105. Yeh, M., Hellström, I., Brown, J. P., Warner, G. A., Hansen, J. A., and Hellström, K. E. (1979): *Proc. Natl. Acad. Sci.*, 76:2927–2931.
106. Young, W. (1977): Immunotherapy of resectable bronchogenic carcinoma: A progress report. In: *Neoplasm Immunity: Solid Tumor Therapy*, edited by R. G. Crispen. Franklin Institute Press, Philadelphia.

Thoracic Oncology, edited by N. C. Choi and
H. C. Grillo. Raven Press, New York © 1983.

Role of Chemotherapy in Lung Cancer

Robert W. Carey

Medical Oncology Unit, Massachusetts General Hospital, Boston Massachusetts 02114

Given a reasonably brief average survival of untreated patients, it is a simple matter to judge the relative value of any given modality in a well-defined disease entity.

Thus it was clear that methotrexate induced remission and prolonged survival (1) in acute lymphocytic leukemia of childhood, and similarly, the impact of combined chemotherapy with MOPP (2) (nitrogen mustard, vincristine, procarbazine and prednisone) on response and survival in Hodgkin's disease was immediately evident without the need of the subsequent "dissecting" controlled trial of single components of the MOPP regimen which was carried out in any case.

The situation in lung cancer is more complicated, since except in oat cell carcinoma (3), where 15% 2-year median disease-free survival is now achievable, chemotherapy has not been claimed to offer significant prolongation of survival or "cure" — indeed, it has been difficult to establish the place of chemotherapy in lung cancer management. As clinical management has evolved, a useful generalization is as follows.

For non-small cell tumors (large cell carcinoma, squamous cell carcinoma, and adenocarcinoma), the primary management is surgical, where cure is possible in 40% to 50% of resectable cases (Stage I), and radiotherapeutic, where an overall 8% cure rate is possible in nonresectable but localized disease. The contribution of chemotherapy is minor, and an attempt will be made to assess this more precisely.

For small cell carcinoma chemotherapy is the major effective modality in extensive disease and is of possible principal importance in limited disease. The literature dealing with the results of chemotherapy in lung cancer is difficult to interpret because of the lack of homogeneity of the patient/clinical subset population. Any mix of patients with lung cancer constitutes a heterogeneous population in the following respects: (a) The patients' previous therapeutic experience as related to surgery and previous chemotherapy (Feinstein's work (4) dealing with early symptomatology and attempt to define disease duration more precisely bears upon this issue), (b) variation with respect to disease extent (stage of disease), (c) variation with respect to histology in cell type and grade and hence in growth rate, and biologic behavior, (d) variation in host/tumor response (e.g., performance status and immune factors), (e) variation in prior disease duration.

Each of the above general factors clearly can influence therapy, yet older reports of drug trials in lung cancer are often sadly deficient in reporting elementary considerations such as the extent or stage of disease, the time from diagnosis and/or symptoms to treatment, and performance status. Fortunately, as awareness of the importance of these factors has increased, more recent clinical trials have taken cognizance of these issues allowing a clearer understanding of the impact of treatment. In general, chemotherapeutic treatment has proved to be more effective in patients with excellent performance status and limited extent of disease who have not had prior therapy.

Major improvements in radiologic techniques such as nuclear scans of liver, bone, and brain, computerized axial tomography of chest and brain, and widespread availability of chest tomography have greatly improved the accuracy of clinical staging. A cogent summary of recent staging consideration which elucidates the niceties of TMN Staging is that of Golomb et al (5).

Evaluation of standard response criteria has been helpful in making comparisons possible between various single or combination programs. Thus the standard "objective response" is based upon 50% reduction in the product of longest perpendicular diameters for any given tumor to qualify as a partial regression. Recently Egan et al. (6) have delineated some of the difficulties inherent in attempting to judge responses in bronchogenic carcinoma, e.g., very few tumors readily lend themselves to precise measurements. These authors have shown, however, that in tumors which are "evaluable" (as judged by agreement of two evaluations) the degree of tumor regression can be assessed as well as in more precisely measurable tumors; at least no significant difference was seen in survival rates for patients with measurable as opposed to evaluable regressions.

NON-SMALL CELL TUMORS

The earlier literature on chemotherapeutic agents in this group of malignant pulmonary tumors has been exhaustively researched and tabulated by Selawry and Associates (7–9). Briefly, when older reports are deciphered and allowances made for prior therapy, stage, and duration of disease, it is evident that widely varying "response" rates have been reported for various agents. Those single agents apparently capable of causing responses from 10% to 20% of patients indicate mechlorethamine, cyclophosphamide, methotrexate, procarbazine, CCNU, hydroxyurea, hexamethylmelamine, BCNU, mitomycin, adriamycin, streptonignin, bleomycin, vincristine, and vinblastine. Of these the alkylating agents, nitrogen mustard and cyclophosphamide, and an antibiotic, adriamycin, are probably the most consistently active agents. That responses occur is not really evidence of palliative value since drug toxicity is considerable and remissions are brief with single agents, e.g. of 2 to 3 months duration. Green (10) indicates that in inoperable patients a twofold significant increase in survival was attendant upon mechlorethamine therapy. On the other hand, Edmonson et al. in 1976, using standard responsive criteria, found only 9/109 partial responders, and they saw no improvement in survival of responses (11).

Monochemotherapy after 1974 has been well summarized in the extensive tables of Cohen et al. (12). These newer data are of interest principally in that adriamycin is shown to be active at at least the 20% level in all cell types. Methotrexate is also revealed to be an active agent on a variety of dosage schedules which generally lead to toxicity.

The theoretical rationale for the use of antineoplastic agents in combination has been dealt with extensively by Skipper and associates (13,14), and more recently the basis of cell kinetic data based upon the Gompertzian characteristic of tumor cell growth has been re-examined by Hill (15). Combination chemotherapy has been notably successful in the acute leukemias, Hodgkin's and non-Hodgkin's lymphomas, testis cancer and more recently in ovarian carcinoma. A number of combination programs have been attempted in non-small cell lung cancer. Indeed, several prospective randomized trials comparing monochemotherapy to two or three drug combinations have been carried out.

Only one regimen, cyclophosphamide, adriamycin and CIS-diaminnedichloro, platinum, resulted in a significantly higher response rate than the single agent tested, dihydrogalactitol (16). Several combination regimens have been reported to give a higher response rate than single agents initially; thus the COMB regimen (17) (cyclophosphamide, oncovin, mehtyl-CCNU, and bleomycin) led to 15/33 remission in epidermoid cancer but did not prolong survival even for responders. However in a prospective randomized trial of the COMB regimen reported by Bodey (18) only 1/20 COMB-treated patients and 1/27 cyclophosphamide-treated patients achieved partial remissions. Furthermore, survival among ambulatory patients was better with the single agent than with the combination.

The BACON regimen (Bleomycin/adriamycin, CCNU, vincristine, nitrogen mustard) similarly was initially reported (19) to have a 45% response rate in a single institution, but when subjected to group study only a 21% response rate was found (20). Report on a group study of the MACC regimen (methotrexate, adriamycin, cyclophosphamide, CCNU) originally reported by Chahinian (22) to have a 46% response rate on 27 patients with squamous and adenocarcinoma. In the Eastern Cooperative Oncology Group Study, Vogl et al. (21) found only five partial remissions among 43 evaluable patients and encountered rather severe hematologic and gastrointestinal toxicity. The survival rate was markedly inferior to the median 52-week figure found by Chahinian et al. for adenocarcinoma and the 30-week period found for patients with squamous cell carcinoma. It is hard to account for the differences. Indeed, superficially the characteristics of patients in the Vogl and Chahinian studies seem similar at the outset. One is thus left with possibilities such as overall superiority in supportive care, which may at least be more consistent in a single institution, the problem of case selection and pretreatment duration of disease, and perhaps the investigator's degree of enthusiasm and/or committment— a difficult factor to evaluate that may nonetheless contribute to such disparate clinical results. One regimen which is well tolerated and leads to a reasonable number of remissions is the CAMP regimen (cyclophosphamide, adriamycin, methotrexate, and procarbazine) of Bitran et al. (23). This program was reported to show a response rate of 48% and median survival time of 12.5 months in non-small cell cancer but has not yet been subjected to prospective randomized trial.

The concept of adjuvant chemotherapy, e.g. the use of systemic chemotherapy at or close to the time of surgical or radiotherapeutic "primary" therapy, has had widespread and probably successful application in breast carcinoma, childhood solid tumors, and osteosarcoma. Similarly, a cogent theoretical argument can be made for the adjuvant use of drugs in lung cancer management, since it is not inconceivable that although the available drugs are active at a low and poorly reproducible level in advanced disease, they could be more effective in the "debulked" patient who conceivably might have only micrometastatic disease. The idea is that micrometastases have a higher growth fraction and enhanced susceptibility to the lethal action of anticancer drugs. These available agents have been already tried extensively and reviewed by Legha (24), who analyzed 15 adjuvant trials. Most of these trials took place in the late 1950s. Cytoxan has been the most extensively studied agent (9 of the 15 reported trials). Short-term adjuvant use had little effect. Longer term cyclophosphamide as studied by Brunner (25) suggested that the survival in this controlled study was adversely affected by chemotherapy, although the survival of the control patient at 5 years, which was 61%, is remarkable for a surgically treated group of patients. At least three trials of multiagent chemotherapy have been reported, results of which supported some advantage for chemotherapy. However, Legha et al., in commenting on trials of Kauer (26) and Katsoki (27), conclude that the study design and/or patient selection and/or lack of concurrent controls make evaluation of such data difficult.

Suffice it to say that the record of "adjuvant" chemotherapy in non-small cell lung carcinoma is not a positive one, and recently at least one of the major clinical cooperative groups has been unable to muster sufficient therapeutic optimism to bring to completion planned controlled trials of adjuvant combination chemotherapy.

In general, results of chemotherapy in non-small cell lung cancer are disappointing. Over and over with single agents or with combinations one finds initially hopeful pilot studies the promise of which is not borne out by following trials. It is difficult to maintain a degree of enthusiasm for existing chemotherapeutic agents in the attempt to palliate patients with non-small cell bronchogenic carcinoma. Indeed, our policy is often that of reserving the dubious benefit of such treatment for symptomatic and progressive disease for which radiation is no longer likely to be of benefit. Such patients naturally tend to be more debilitated and perhaps suffer more from the toxicity inherent in such treatment than if they had been treated earlier in their clinical course.

SMALL CELL CARCINOMA

Interest in small cell carcinoma (SCC) has been heightened by the realization that there may be at this time about 15% of patients with limited disease treated wtih modern chemotherapy or combined modality (radiation-chemotherapy) programs free of disease at 2 years, leading Oldham et al. (28) to suggest that the disease may in some cases be "curable." Data published by Greco (29) and Einhorn (30) support this optimistic statement.

Awareness of the unique clinical pathologic feature of oat cell carcinoma followed Azzopardi's delineation of the criteria for diagnosis in 1959 (31). These criteria have been revised: currently the World Health Organization Classification recognizes fusiform, polygonal, lymphocytic-like, and mixed types (32). The significance of subtyping is not clear, although Nixon et al. (33) have felt that the therapeutic outcome may be better for the lymphocyte-like subgroup. This cell type is so named because it is morphologically similar in appearance to the the normal lymphocyte and of about the same size. The cell is believed to have derived from primordial bronchial tissue, hence the high metastatic rate characteristic of epithelial tissue and amine precursor uptake decarboxylation (APUD) — properties which make this disease the endocrinologist's delight. The exact incidence of paraneoplastic syndromes in SCC is not clear, but clinically overt syndromes may occur in up to 5% of cases (34,35) and may precede the diagnosis of small cell carcinoma by a considerable period of time.

The most common syndromes are inappropriate antidiuretic secretion (SIADH), Cushing's Syndrome, and the Eaton-Lambert Syndrome. Indeed North and associates have found determination of plasma neurophysin (a vasopressin pentide) (36) product to represent a tumor marker of oat cell carcinoma correlates well with the overt extent of clinical disease. Gilby et al. (37) reported that water loading leads to demonstration of a defect in water handling in small cell carcinoma patients in the absence of obvious clinical manifestation of SIADH in 40% of 10 patients tested.

The high metastatic rate in SCC has been well established in kinetic studies (38,39). These authors found a higher thymidine labeling index for oat cell cancer than for any other neoplasm. A high growth fraction is no doubt responsible for the following features of small cell carcinoma:

1. Radiologic features: The lesion frequently presents with a very large mediastinal mass and/or hilar adenopathy after the primary tumor is dominated by the mass or absence due to massive nodal metastases; thus the "central" nature of SCC is paramount, and small and/or peripheral tumors, raising the question of resection, are rare.

2. 60% of patients with small cell carcinoma have extra pulmonary spread at the line of diagnosis (40,41), and after staging procedures only 40% appear still localized. Staging studies should include liver scan, bone scan, bone marrow biopsy, CCT of the brain, electrolytes, fasting control level, blood sugar, and neurophysics level. Thus, the higher growth fraction correlates well with the early tendency of this lesion to metastasize.

3. Rapid response to therapy: There is no question in the mind of medical oncologists and radiotherapists that rapid disease regression accompanies either modality or both. These rapidly growing tumors in general are more likely to undergo appreciable cell kill and demonstrate clinical regression than the more slowly growing non-small cell tumors with slower doubling times and less frequent response to treatment.

4. Higher propensity for "obstructive manifestations": Superior vena cava syndrome, bronchial obstruction, and spinal cord compression are common problems; the best "relief" of these symdromes is not certain. Classic radiation therapy has been used with good control of obstructive manifestations. In cases of spinal cord compression, it is perhaps most prudent to use both modalities; indeed since cord compression is often a late manifestation of disease, occurring as a manifestation of relapse after initial chemotherapy, combined modality therapy radiation may be the only practical modality to employ.

THERAPY

The hopeful outlook projected by Greco (29) and Einhorn (30) for possible cure of SCC has brought much recent attention to the entitiy and has lead to several comprehensive reviews (34,41,43,44). Both radiation and chemotherapy may make an important contribution to disease control.

Radiation: The British Medical Research Council's study (45) of radiation as compared to surgery in "operable" localized small cell carcinoma yielded a mean 284-day survival for the radiation treated group as compared with 184 days for the surgical group. This result led to the editorial opinion of Scannell (46) that except for rare peripheral tumors, SCC carcinoma is not a surgical disease. However, recent studies by Cancer and Leukemia Group B and others suggest relapse of SCC in areas given adequate radiotherapy may reach the 50% level, hence leading to the idea, now come full circle, that it would be worth reconsidering surgery's possible contribution in debulking SCC.

As noted, radiation therapy is still an appropriate modality for "obstructive" emergencies although it is not the only way of approaching those problems. It has been difficult to sift out the relative contribution of radiotherapy to programs combining that modality with chemotherapy due to (a) lack of staging data in earlier studies, (b) lack of controlled studies, and (c) change due to improvement in the chemotherapy component of treatment.

Thus Nixon et al. (2) in a nonconcurrent comparison felt the 10-month median survival reported for COPP (cytoxan, oncovin, procarbazine, prednisone) plus radiation was better than a 5-month median survival found for historical radiation controls. The British Medical Research Council study (45) did demonstrate a 22% 5-year survival at 1 year for localized oat cell carcinoma receiving radiation. Recently the contribution of radiotherapy to SCC disease control has had some reappraisal. The early results of Hansen's study (48) comparing a four-drug program with or without radiation etablished a median survival of 14 months for patients not receiving radiation as opposed to 11 months when radiation was given. Similarly, Krauss et al. (49) have early results suggesting that combined therapy with a three-drug program plus radiation is superior to radiation alone. The data of Cohen et al. comparing chemotherapy alone to combination chemotherapy plus radiation therapy suggest the combined modality may ultimately prove to be the superior management. The Cancer and Leukemia Group B is currently piloting a trial which will compare the following.

1. Simultaneous radiotherapy and chemotherapy plus a three-drug program (VP 16, Cytoxan, Vincristine).
2. Sequential chemotherapy and radiation.
3. Chemotherapy alone unless patients fail to respond or relapse, at which point radiation will be given.

The NCI Study (50) and CALGB Study noted above are directed at the 40% of patients with localized disease after staging studies and appropriate central nervous system "sanctuary" therapy. The role of radiation as central nervous system prophylactics in SCC has undergone careful scrutiny. Thus Choi et al. (4) noted only 7% brain metastasis in patients receiving 2800 to 3000 cGy (rad) brain bath. Jackson et al. (51), in a randomized prospective study found 0/14 brain metastases in patients receiving prophylactic radiothetapy to the brain compared to 4/15 in the nontreated control group. Prophylactic brain radiotherapy is now included in virtually all treatment programs of curative intent though some recent data (52) demonstrates that effective chemotherapy alone can result in prolonged survival in the absence of prophylactic brain radiation, as 13% of 72 patients showed no evidence of disease 16 to 18 months from diagnosis.

The status of chemotherapy in SCC has rapidly evolved in the past 10 years. Thus the Veterans Administration Study (58) early on showed cyclophosphamide to increase survival of patients with SCC from a median of 2.7 to 5 months in unstaged patients. A variety of single agents have shown some level of efficacy (Table 1).

A study reported by Edmonsen for the Eastern Cooperative Oncology Group showed CCNU plus cyclophosphamide to be clearly superior to cyclophosphamide alone (53). A similar Cancer and Leukemia Group B study comparing methotrexate plus cyclophosphamide plus vincristine to cyclophosphamide alone failed to demonstrate improvement in remission rate on survival for the combination program in patients with limited disease, although in patients with extensive disease the combination program was associated with a higher response rate. Hansen et al. (55) concluded that vincristine improved results obtained with the combination of CCNU, cyclophosphamide, and methotrexate: Both drugs achieved a 75% response rate,

TABLE 1. *Chemotherapeutic agents active in small cell carcinoma (>20% response)*

Cyclophosphamide
Methotrexate
Vincristine
Procarbazine
CCNU
Adriamycin (Danorubicin)
VP-16 (epipodophyllotoxin)
BCNU
DDEP (Cisdiamminodichtoroplatinum)
Hexamethylmelamine

but patients receiving vincristine in addition had somewhat better survival. The Southwest Oncology Group's combined modality study utilized adriamycin, cyclophosphamide, and vincristine plus radiation and achieved 14% complete regression rate in patients with extensive disease, and 41% in patients with limited disease, the median survival being 26 and 52 weeks respectively. In the Greco study (28) of concomittant radiation and cyclophosphamide, doxorubicin (adriamycin), and vincristine, 29/32 patients with limited disease achieved complete remission and prolonged survival was achieved, suggesting possible cure for a significant fraction. Indeed in the SWOG Study (56) 30% of those achieving complete remission remain in complete remission at 14 months.

The preceding data make clear that some significant progress has been made in managing patients with SCC. However, the 15% or so of patients with limited disease who achieve "cure" constitute only 6% of the total small cell population because it is rare to achieve long-term survival with extensive disease. Thus in fact, only a small fraction of SCC patients achieve prolonged survival and/or cure. It is important to state, however, that the quality of life of patients receiving most combination chemotherapy programs is good, and in fact, attempts to give higher, more myelosuppressive doses of chemotherapy have resulted only in enhanced toxicity and some toxic deaths. Thus one must agree with Sherman (57) that it is important not to overstate the progress in treatment of SCC and to pay close attention to the considerable morbidity and even mortality which can accompany overzealous therapeutic programs. It is particularly important to focus on the patients relapsing from "first line" chemotherapeutic programs because, thus far, attempts to produce palliation in this group with alternative agents have not met with much success, and the toxicity encountered in such relapsed patients is often considerable. Recently Comis et al. (59) reported on use of surgery after cytoreductive chemotherapy in ipselateral stage I–III SCC. 17 of 23 completed resection of disease, and the median survival of the group successfully resected was 20+ months. Lack of local relapse and long survival makes this approach an encouraging alternative to consider in suitable patients with SCC.

Clearly much remains to be done, and, as in the case of non-small cell tumors, additional therapeutic modalities are surely needed.

REFERENCES

1. Farber, S., Diamond, L. K., Mercer, R. D., Sylvester, R. F., Jr., and Wolff, S. A. (1948): Temporary remissions in acute leukemia in children produced by folic acid antagonist 4 aminopteroyl-glutamic acid (Aminopterin). *N. Eng. J. Med.*, 238–287.
2. DeVita, V. T., Serpuck, A., and Carbone, P. P. (1969): Combination chemotherapy of advanced Hodgkin's disease. *Proc. Am. Assoc. Cancer Res. Suppl.*, 10:19.
3. Oldham, R. K., Forbes, J. T., and Niblack, G. D. (1978): Natural killer activity of human thoracic duct lymphocytes. *AACR Abstracts*, 643.
4. Feinstein, A. R., Pritchett, J. A., and Schimpff, C. R. (1969): The epidermology of cancer therapy II, the clinical course data, decisions and temporal demarcations. *Arch. Intern. Med.*, 123:323.
5. Golomb, H. M., and DeMeester, T. R. (1969): Lung Cancer: A combined modality approach to staging and therapy. *CA J. Clinicians*, 29:xx
6. Eagan, R. T., Carr, D. T., Frytak, S., Rubin, J., and Lee, R. E.: VP-16-213 versus polychemotherapy in patients with advanced small cell lung. *Cancer Treat. Rep.*, 60:949–951.

7. Selawry, O. S. (1973): Monochemotherapy of bronchogenic carcinoma with special reference to cell type. *Cancer Chemother. Rep.*, 4:177–188.

8. Selawry, O. S. (1974): The role of chemotherapy in the treatment of lung cancer. *Semin. Oncol.*, L:259–272.

9. Selawry, O. S. (1972): Personal communication of Eastern Cooperative Oncology Group studies of methotrexate in lung cancer. First Int. Workshop Lung Cancer, Airlie, Virginia.

10. Green, R. A., Humphrey, E., Close, H., and Patno, M. E. (1969): Alkylating agents in bronchogenic carcinoma. *Am. J. Med.*, 46:516–525.

11. Edmonson, J. H., Lagakos, S., Stolbach, L., Perlia, C. P., Bennett, J. M., Mansour, E. G., Horton, J., Regelson, W., Cummings, J. F., Israel, L., Brodsky, I., Shnider, B. I., Creech, R., and Carbone, P. P., (1976): Mechlorethamine (NSC-762) plus CCNU (NSC-79037) in the treatment of inoperable squamous and large cell carcinoma of the lung. *Cancer Treat. Rep.*, 60:625–627.

12. Cohen, M. H., and Perevodchikova, N. I. (1979): Single agent chemotherapy of lung cancer. In: *Lung Cancer: Progress in Therapeutic Research*, edited by F. Muggia and M. Rozencweig, pp. 343–376, Raven Press, New York.

13. Skipper, H. E., Schabel, F. M., Jr., and Wilcox, W. S. (1964): Experimental evaluation of potential anticancer agents. XIII. On the criteria and kinetics associated with "curability" of experimental leukemia. *Cancer Chemother. Rep.*, 35:1–113.

14. Skipper, H. E. (1974): Combination therapy: Some concepts and results. *Cancer Chemother. Rep.*, 4:137–145.

15. Hill, B. T. (1978): Cancer chemotherapy: The relevance of certain concepts of cell cycle kinetics. *Biochim. Biophys. Acta*, 516:389–417.

16. Eagan, R. T., Ingle, J. N., Frytak, S., Rubin, J., Kvols, L. K., Carr, D. T., Coles, D. T., and O'Fallon, J. R. (1977): Platinum-based polychemotherapy versus dinhydrogalactitol in advanced non-small cell lung cancer. *Cancer Treat. Rep.*, 61:1339–1345.

17. Livingston, R. B., Einhorn, L. H., Bodey, G. P., Burgess, M. A., Freireich, E. F., and Gottlieb, J. A. (1975): COMB (cyclophosphamide, Oncovin, methyl-CCNU and bleomycin); A four-drug combination in solid tumors. *Cancer*, 36:327–332.

18. Bodey, G. P., Lagakos, S. W., Gutierriez, A. C., Wilson, H. E., and Selawry, O. S. (1977): Therapy of advanced squamous carcinoma of the lung: Cyclophosphamide versus "COMB". *Cancer*, 39:1026–1031.

19. Livingston, R. B., Fee, W. H., Einhorn, L. H., Burgess, M. A., Freireich, E. J., Gottlieb, J. A., and Farber, M. O. (1976): BACON (bleomycin, adriamycin, CCNU, oncovin and nitrogen mustard) in squamous lung cancer. *Cancer*, 37:1237–1242.

20. Livingston, R. B. (1977): Combination chemotherapy of bronchogenic carcinoma I: Non-oat cell. *Cancer Treat. Rev.*, 4:153–165.

21. Vogl, S. E., Mehta, C. R., and Cohen, M. E. (1979): MACC chemotherapy for adenocarcinoma and epidermoid carcinoma of the lung. *Cancer*, 44:864–868.

22. Chahinian, A. P., Arnold, D. J., Cohen, J. M., Purpura, D. P., Jaffrey, I. S., Teirstein, A. S., Kirschner, P. A., and Holland, J. F. (1977): Methotrexate, adriamycin, cyclophosphamide and CCNU (MACC) in bronchogenic carcinoma. *JAMA*, 237:2392–2396.

23. Bitran, J. D., Desser, R. K., DeMeester, T. R., Colman, M., Evans, R., Billings, A., Griem, M., Rubinstein, L., Shapiro, L., and Golomb, H. M. (1976): Cyclophosphamide, adriamycin, methotrexate and procarbazine (CAMP)-effective four-drug combination chemotherapy for metastatic non-oat cell bronchogenic carcinoms. *Cancer Treat. Rep.*, 60:1225–1230.

24. Legha, S. S., Muggia, F. M., and Carter, S. K.(1977): Adjuvant chemotherapy in lung cancer. *Cancer*, 39:1415–1424.

25. Brunner, K. W., Marthaler, T., and Muller, W. (1973): Effects of long term adjuvant chemotherapy with cyclophosphamide (NSC-26271) for radically resected bronchogenic carcinoma. *Cancer Chemother. Rep.*, 4:125–132.

26. Karrer, K., Pridun, N., and Zwintz, E. (1973): Chemotherapy studies in bronchogenic carcinoma by the Austrian Study Group. *Cancer Chemother. Rep*, 4:207–213.

27. Katsuki, H., Shimada, K., Koyama, A. et al. (1975): Long-term intermittent adjuvant chemotherapy for primary, resected lung cancer. *J. Thorac. Cardiovasc. Surg.*, 70:590–599.

28. Oldham, R. K., Greco, F., Richardson, R. L., and Stroup, S. L. (1978): Small cell lung cancer: A potentially curable neoplasm. *Proc. Am. Soc. Clin. Oncol.*, 361.

29. Greco, F. A., Richardson, R. L., Snell, J. O., Stroup, S. L., and Oldham, R. K. (1979): *Am. J. Med.*, 66:625.
30. Einhorn, L. H., Bandy, W. H., Hernback, N., Benk-Tek, J. (1978): Long-term results in combined-modality treatment of small cell carcinoma of the lung. *Semin. Oncol.*, 5:309.
31. Azzopardi, J. G. (1959): Oat cell carcinoma of the bronchus. *J. Pathol. Bact.*, 78:513.
32. Sobin, L. H. (1979): The WHO histological classification of lung tumors. In: *Lung Cancer: Progress in Therapeutic Research*, p. 83, Raven Press, New York.
33. Nixon, D. W. Murphy, G. F., Sewell, C., Cutner, M., Lynn, M. J. (1979): Relationship between survival and histologic type in small cell anaplastic CA of lung. *Cancer*, 44:1045–1049.
34. Ruckdeschel, J. C., Caradonna, R. C., Poladine, W. S., Hillinger, J. M., and Horton, S. (1979): *CA J. Clinicians*, 29–2.
35. Hansen, H. J., Lance, K. P., and Krupey, J. (1971): Demonstration of an ion sensitive antigen site on carcinoembryonic antigen using zirconylphosphate gel. *Clin. Res.*, 19:143.
36. North, W. G. Mauer, L. H., O'Donnell, J. F. (1979): Human neurophysins (HNPs) and small cell carcinoma (SCC). *Clin. Res.*, 27:390A.
37. Gilby, E. D., Rees, L. H., and Bondy, P. K. (1975): Ectopic hormone as markers of response to therapy in cancer. *Excerpta Med.*, p. 202.
38. Muggia, F. M., Krezuski, S. K., and Hansen, H. H. (1974): Cell kinetic studies in patients with small cell carcinoma of the lung: *Cancer*, 34:1683.
39. Strauss, M. J. (1974): The growth characteristics of lung cancer and its application to treatment design. *Semin. Oncol.*, 1:167.
40. Nixon, D., Carey, R. W., Suit, H. D., Aisenberg, A. C. (1975): *Cancer*, 36:867.
41. Choi, C. H., and Carey, R. W. (1976): Small cell anaplastic carcinoma of lung: Reappraisal of current management. *Cancer*, 37:2651–2657.
42. Kane, R. C., Colon, M. H., Broder, L. E., and Bull, M. I. (1976): Superior vena caval obstruction due to small cell anaplastic lung carcinoma. *JAMA*, 235.
43. Bunn, P. A. Cohen, M. H., Ihde, D. C., Fossica, B. E., Matthews, M. J., and Minna, J. D. (1977): Advances in small cell bronchogenic carcinoma. *Cancer Treat. Rep.*, 61:31.
44. Weiss, R. B. (1978): Small cell carcinoma of the lung: Therapeutic management. *Ann. Intern. Med.*, 522.
45. Fox, W., and Scadding, S. G. (1973): Medical Research Council comparative trial of surgery and radiotherapy for primary treatment of small-celled or oat celled carcinoma of the bronchus: Ten year follow-up. *Lancet*, 2:63–65.
46. Scannell, J. G. (1970): The problem of oat cell carcinoma. *N. Engl. J. Med.*, 282:98–99.
47. Mauer, H. (1980): Unpublished data of Cancer and Leukemia Group B.
48. Hansen, H. H., Dambernowsky, P., Hansen, H. S., and Rorth, M. (1979): Chemotherapy versus chemotherapy plus radiotherapy in regional small-cell carcinoma of the lung. *AACR*, Abstr. 1124.
49. Krauss (1979): High dose cyclophosphamide (CTX), doxorubicin (ADR) with vincristine (VCR) HD-CAV in small cell lung carcinoma. C-606, p. 437, ASCO, AACR.
50. Cohen, M. H., Lichter, A. S., Bunn, P. A., Glatstein, E. J., Ihde, B. E., Fossiek, B. E., Matthews, M. J., and Minna, J. D. (1980): Chemotherapy – radiation therapy (CT-RT) versus chemotherapy (CT) in limited small cell lung cancer. *Proc. Am. Soc. Clin. Oncol.*, C-S11.
51. Jackson, D. V., Richards, F., Cooper, R., Ferrec, C., Muss, H. B., White, D. R., and Spurr, C. L. (1977): Prophylactic cranial irradiation in small cell carcinoma of the lung. *JAMA*, 237:2730.
52. Ginsberg, S. J., Comis, R. L., Gottlieb, A. J., King, G. B., Goldberg, J., Zamkoff, K., Elbadaui, A., and Meyer, J. (1979): Long term survivalship in small cell anaplastic lung cancer. *Cancer Treat. Rep.*, 63:8–1347.
53. Edmonson, J. H., Lagakos, S. W., Selawry, O. S., Perlia, C. P., Bennett, J. M., Muggia, F. M., Wampler, G., Brodovsky, H. S., Horton, J., Colsky, J., Mansour, E. G., Creech, R., Stolback, L., Greenspan, E. M., Levitt, M., Israel, L., Ezdinli, E. Z., and Carbone, P. P. (1976): Cyclophosphamide and CCNU in the treatment of inoperable small cell carcinoma and adenocarcinoma of the lung. *Cancer Treat. Rev.*, 60:925.
54. Mauer, H., and Tulloh, M. (1977): Combination chemotherapy and radiation for small cell carcinoma of the lung protocol #7283. CALGB minutes, March 1977.
55. Hansen, H. R., Dombernows, P., Hansen, M., and Hirsch, F. (19xx): Chemotherapy of advanced small cell anaplastic carcinoma.

56. Livingston, R. B., Moore, T. N., Heilbrun, L., Bottomley, R., Le Lanc, D., Rivkin, S. E., and Thiypen, T. (1978): Small-cell carcinoma of the lung: Combined chemotherapy and radiation. *Ann. Intern. Med.*, 88:194.
57. Sherman, C. D. (1979): Feedback: Chemotherapy for small cell lung cancer. *CA*, 296:371.
58. Green, R., Humphrey, E., Close, H., et al. (1969): Alkylating agents in bronchogenic carcinoma. *Am. J. Med.*, 46:516.
59. Comis, R., Meyer, J., Ginsberg, S., Issell, B., Gullo, J., Difino, S.,Tinsley, R., Poiesz, B., and Rudolph, A. (19): The current result of chemotherapy plus adjuvant surgery in limited small cell neoplastic lung cancer (SCALG). *Proc. Amer. Soc. Clin. Onc., 1:147.*

Thoracic Oncology, edited by N. C. Choi and H. C. Grillo. Raven Press, New York © 1983.

Reassessment of the Role of Radiation Therapy Relative to Other Treatments in Small-Cell Carcinoma of the Lung

Noah C. Choi

Department of Radiation Therapy, Harvard Medical School, and Department of Radiation Medicine, Massachusetts General Hospital, Boston, Massachusetts 02114

Ever since the advent in the early 1970s of more effective systemic chemotherapy for small-cell carcinoma of the lung, enthusiasm for this type of treatment has been rapidly growing. There are more than 140 articles listed in the *Cumulated Index Medicus* for 1980 and 1981, including several review articles (1–8), pertaining to the biologic and therapeutic aspects of this tumor. Despite the earlier optimistic view based on the short-term experiences with the current combination chemotherapy, a plateau in the improvement of survival seems to have been reached (1–3,6) and the management of this tumor continues to be a great, challenging problem. It is therefore timely and instructive to draw a few guidelines for the managment of this tumor based on what we have learned during the last decade, but it is also naive to be dogmatic in this field, which is highly susceptible to new developments.

In the 1960s and early 1970s, no patients with extensive stage of small-cell carcinoma of the lung survived longer than 4 to 5 months after the time of diagnosis without treatment (9), and only 7% of patients with the limited stage of the same tumor, when untreated, survived for 12 months (10). In 1973, the Medical Research Council of Great Britain reported that, without effective systemic treatments, only 4% (3 of 73) of patients who received curative radiation therapy were alive at 5 and 10 years, and none of 34 patients who had had complete resection were alive at 5 years (11). With the advent of more effective chemotherapy (12,13), we have witnessed a significant improvement in the median survival time of patients with the limited stage of the tumor, from 5–6 months with radiation therapy alone to 10–14 months with chemotherapy plus radiation therapy (9,14–18) or chemotherapy alone (19–24).

Despite the dramatic improvement in the short-term results achieved by use of the currently effective combination chemotherapy alone or by a combined approach of chemotherapy and regional treatments, such as radiation therapy and/or surgery, the magnitude of improvement of long-term cure by chemotherapy alone remains to be evaluated. This chapter is designed to carefully review the role of radiation therapy and compare it with the role of combination chemotherapy and surgery in the management of patients with small-cell carcinoma of the lung.

233

NEED FOR USE OF TNM STAGING SYSTEM

The current loose staging system, which classifies small-cell carcinoma of the lung into limited versus extensive, based on whether the extent of the tumor can be encompassed in a treatment volume of radiation or not, is no longer adequate for several reasons. Comparison of treatment results for the limited stage of small-cell carcinoma is extremely difficult because of the loose criteria, which vary among different centers. The treatment volume of radiation therapy that is tolerated by patients, of course, varies with the radiation doses on which the control of local and regional tumors by radiation therapy with or without chemotherapy depends. A treatment volume for a stage $T_{1-2}N_2 M_0$ tumor (25) can be given a high dose of radiation of 4,600–5,600 cGy [(time, dose, and fractionation factor (TDF), 76–92)], with a high probability of local and regional tumor control. Conversely, a large treatment volume for a stage $T_3N_2M_0$ SCN (+) tumor[1] can only be given a low-to-moderate dose of radiation of 2,400–4,000 cGy (TDF 40–66), with a high risk of radiation pneumonitis and a low probability of tumor control. There is a rebirth of interest in surgery and innovative radiation therapy for a subset of patients with a limited stage of this tumor—those who had localized and regional tumors had a 30–50% recurrence rate, even with the current most effective chemotherapy alone or with a low-to-moderate dose of radiation, 2,500–4,000 cGy (TDF 46–66). All of us are familiar with the TNM staging system (25) used in the management of patients with non-small-cell carcinoma of the lung. It is hoped that the role of radiation therapy and surgery can be defined more precisely by use of the TNM staging system in the management of patients with small-cell carcinoma of the lung (7,26–28).

ROLE OF RADIATION THERAPY FOR PATIENTS WITH LIMITED STAGE OF SMALL-CELL CARCINOMA OF THE LUNG

According to our current knowledge, a combined approach of local and regional treatments, such as surgery or radiation therapy with chemotherapy, seems to offer the best chance of cure for patients with a limited stage of small-cell carcinoma of the lung (9,28–34). Chemotherapy and radiation therapy are supplementary to the weakness of each method. Analyses of the results in the treatment of this tumor indicate that the most common sites indicating failure of treatment, which vary with the type of treatment, are the primary tumor and involved regional lymph nodes after chemotherapy alone was used (relapse rate of 40–60%) (21,23,35,36), and extrathoracic sites such as the liver, bone, brain and adrenal glands after radiation therapy alone was used (9,11,12,37). The brain, when not electively irradiated, is one of the most frequent sites of metastases (30–40% of patients) after treatment of the lung by both chemotherapy and radiation therapy (9,38–40). When a reasonably tolerable dose of radiation, of the order of 4,600–5,000 cGy

---

[1]SCN (+) = involvement of supraclavicular lymph node.

(TDF 76–82) is used, radiation therapy alone can achieve a control rate of over 80% for local and regional tumors (9). However, because of a high rate of metastases at distant extrathoracic sites (11), only 4% of these patients are cured by radiation therapy alone. The addition of effective chemotherapy to radiation therapy has improved the median survival time of patients with the limited stage of small-cell carcinoma of the lung from 5–6 months to 10–14 months (9,12,15–17,37), and chemotherapy alone has also achieved a median survival time of 10–12 months in a few small series (19,20,23). On the basis of the median survival time of 10–12 months achieved by chemotherapy alone for patients with the limited stage of small-cell carcinoma of the lung, the role of radiation therapy has frequently been questioned without careful evaluation of survival data beyond 1 year and of recurrence rates at the region of the primary tumor and involved regional lymph nodes (Table 1). We should not be content with median survival time alone. Our goal should include not only short-term survival, such as median survival time, but also an ultimate goal of cure. On the basis of a high local and regional recurrence rate of 40–60% after the use of chemotherapy alone and a very dismal survival rate of 12–14% at 2 years, even by combined chemotherapy and radiation therapy (9,32,41), it is premature and risky to use chemotherapy alone for patients with the limited stage of small-cell carcinoma of the lung without the powerful tool of radiation therapy, or surgery for local and regional tumors.

Radiation therapy to the chest has often been delayed, despite incomplete regression of the tumor or slowly progressive recurrence, when chemotherpay alone has been used, until patients become symptomatic from obstructive pneumonia, hemoptysis, or intractable cough. However, such a last-minute recourse is very undesirable because the best form of chemotherapy has already been exhausted and the dose of radiation to control the recurrent tumor is much higher than that required initially to achieve the same goal by a combined use of both treatments (42).

Another unsettled issue in the management of patients with the limited stage of small-cell carcinoma of the lung is how to combine chemotherapy and radiation therapy for the best result. The most reasonable approaches, to take advantage of the strength of each treatment, are either concomitant treatments by starting both at the same time or a sequential approach in which radiation therapy follows after the first two to three cycles of chemotherapy. The use of concomitant treatments seems quite toxic and not suitable for patients in poor general condition, although it may achieve a better control of the local and regional tumor. A sequential approach takes advantage of tumor regression induced by chemotherapy so that the treatment volume to be included in the radiation therapy is usually smaller than that in the concomitant approach. It is also better tolerated by most patients. One drawback of this sequential approach is a potential risk of relapse at extrathoracic sites in the absence of chemotherapy for a period of 5–6 weeks while radiation therapy is given to the chest. One remedy for this potential problem is an addition of one to two cycles of modified chemotherapy in terms of 70–80% of the normal dosage of chemotherapeutic agents without Adriamycin during radiation therapy. Several clinical studies designed to investigate these treatments are under way.

TABLE 1. Chemotherapy plus radiotherapy versus chemotherapy alone in limited stage of small-cell carcinoma of the lung

	Cohen et al. (21)		Oldham et al. (22)		Fox et al. (23)		Hansen et al. (19)		Stevens et al. (20)	
CT program	CTX + MTX + CCNU VCR + ADR + PRC		CTX + ADR + VCR		CTX + ADR + VCR		CTX + CCNU + VCR + MTX		CTX + ADR + VCR + MTX	
RT program	4,500 cGy, 15 F, 3 weeks, to chest 2,000–2,400 cGy, 12 F, to brain		4,000 cGy, 14 F, by split courses, to chest 3,600 cGy, 15 F, by split courses, to brain		4,000 cGy, to chest		4,000 cGy, 10 F, by split courses, to chest		3,500 cGy, by split courses, to chest and brain	
No. of patients	CT + RT (14)	CT (14)	CT + RT (38)	CT (27)	CT + RT (42)	CT (44)	CT + RT (65)	CT (69)	CT + RT (14)	CT (18)
CR	77%	46%	66%	37%	—	—	—	—	71%	50%
NED at 18 months	4 of 8	1 of 9	—	—	—	—	—	—	—	—
Relapse at primary site	4 of 14	10 of 14	—	—	9 of 28	19 of 28	—	—	—	—
MST (months)	—	—	—	—	14.5	15	11	14	13	11.5

Abbreviations used: CT, chemotherapy; RT, radiation therapy; CR, complete remission; NED, no evidence of disease; MST, median survival time; CTX, cyclophosphamide; MTX, methotrexate; CCNU, lomustine; VCR, vincristine; ADR, Adriamycin; PRC, procarbazine; F, fraction. 1 cGy (centigray) = 1 rad.

Patients with severe airway obstruction, superior vena cava obstruction, and obstructive pneumonia distal to the tumor preferably should be given a carefully planned treatment of both radiation therapy and chemotherapy. Symptomatic relief of these medical emergencies can be achieved in 5–10 days by either radiation therapy or intensive chemotherapy. Patients with bronchopneumonia distal to the bronchial obstruction by the tumor preferably should be given first a short course of radiation therapy with a total dose of 2,000–2,600 cGy in 10–13 fractions to relieve the bronchial obstruction, and then the intensive chemotherapy, inasmuch as flare-up of the infection during the period of chemotherapy-induced leukopenia has been a potential problem (43). For the optimum radiation therapy, an additional dose of 2,400–3,000 cGy in 12–15 treatments is necessary to the region of the primary tumor and involved regional nodes after two to three cycles of chemotherapy because there has been a high recurrence rate, of the order of about 50% or greater, in the chest when the dose of radiation therapy used in this combined treatment has been inadequate (9,44).

Elective radiation therapy to the brain should be a part of a comprehensive treatment program aimed at a total cure of patients with the limited stage of small-cell carcinoma of the lung. Patients with the limited stage of small-cell carcinoma have shown a metastatic rate of 30–40% in the brain during the course of their illness, even with a combination of systemic chemotherapy and radiation therapy to the chest (9,38–40,44). The response of gross metastatic tumors in the brain to a moderate dose of radiation therapy of 3,000–4,000 cGy (TDF 62–66) has been rather unsatisfactory, with temporary relief of neurological symptoms for a period of only 3–6 months and a high recurrence rate among survivors for a period of 6–10 months or more (45,46). Because of the high rate of metastases in the brain and the rather unsatisfactory result of radiation therapy for grossly demonstrable metastatic tumors, elective radiation therapy to the brain for potential microscopic metastases has been tried, with dramatic improvement; the rate of metastases in the brain has been reduced from 30–40% without treatment to 10% or less with treatment, using elective irradiation with a radiation dose of 2,500–3,000 cGy (TDF 46–62) (9,16,39,47). Careful evaluation of neurological status before and after elective irradiation to the brain has shown no significant ill effect from this approach (48). Although overall survival of patients with the limited stage of small-cell carcinoma of the lung has not improved by the addition of elective irradiation to the brain, because of uncontrolled tumors elsewhere, it is highly likely that survival of patients who have achieved complete remission will improve with elective irradiation to the brain (49). Another important aspect of elective irradiation to the brain is a potential gain of a better quality of life in terms of a value of ≥70 on the Karnofsky scale (25). There has been a gain of 5–6 months of more active life (≥70 on the Karnofsky scale) when elective irradiation to the brain was compared with therapeutic irradiation for grossly demonstrable metastatic tumors in the brain, according to the series of Rosenman and Choi (46). However, this gain has to be weighed against the expense and inconvenience of elective irradiation to the brain for those who will never develop metastatic tumor in the brain.

ROLE OF RADIATION THERAPY FOR PATIENTS WITH EXTENSIVE STAGE OF SMALL-CELL CARCINOMA OF THE LUNG

The role of radiation therapy for patients with the extensive stage of small-cell carcinoma of the lung should be assessed according to the degree of response to chemotherapy. A routine use of a moderate dose of radiation therapy, 3,000–4,000 cGy (TDF 62–66), to the region of the primary tumor and involved regional lymph nodes in combination with chemotherapy has failed to show any significant improvement of survival because of recurrence elsewhere, although the local and regional recurrence is one of common sites of failure by chemotherapy alone. Approximately 15–20% of these patients achieve a complete remission with current chemotherapy, and their short-term survival is very close to that of those with the limited stage of small-cell carcinoma of the lung (15,16,32). Common sites of recurrence for patients who had achieved a complete remission include the chest and the brain, in addition to the sites of bulky tumors (50,51). This is the group of patients that would benefit from radiation therapy to the chest and elective irradiation to the brain, perhaps with improved survival. For patients whose response to chemotherapy is less than complete remission, the role of radiation therapy is primarily palliation of airway obstruction, superior vena cava obstruction, hemoptysis, and intractable cough caused by a locally progressive tumor, and bone pain and neurological deficit caused by metastatic tumors. With current therapeutic methods, long-term survival of 2 or more years for this group of patients is unusual, and radiation therapy should be used judiciously whenever indicated for a better quality of life.

REASSESSMENT OF RADIATION THERAPY TECHNIQUES

Important variables of radiation therapy that should be taken into consideration in the analysis of the results with this method, with or without other kinds of therapy, include treatment volume, total dose of radiation, radiation dose per each treatment, time interval between treatments, dose rate, and total duration of the treatment. The outcome of radiation therapy depends upon these variables, and every effort should be made to define them as clearly as possible in all published reports, inasmuch as any comparison of results of radiation therapy, either with or without other therapy, is very difficult and could be misleading unless we give careful consideration to these physical factors of radiation therapy.

Definition of Treatment Volume

Careful assessment of the treatment volume is the most important first step toward the successful treatment. I am afraid that a treatment volume that has been chosen on the basis of conventional chest roentgenograms, with or without supplemental tomographic studies, is probably inadequate and has a high risk of geographic miss. Of importance are studies by Emami et al. (52) and Seydel et al. (53) in which data of a computed tomography scan of the chest were judged essential for the planning of radiation therapy in 30–50% of patients with carcinoma of the lung. Gross underestimation of the extent of small-cell carcinoma of the lung by conventional radiographic study without a computed tomographic scan of the chest is clearly demonstrated by a study of Harper et al. (54). In this study, the tumors of 77% (27 of 35) of patients, having been classified as localized T_1 or T_2 on the basis of conventional staging, were subsequently reclassified as extensive T_3 on the basis of computed tomographic scans of the chest. To be successful in controlling the intrathoracic tumors, the treatment volume should include the primary lesion, the ipsilateral hilum, the entire mediastinum including the lymph nodes at the thoracic inlet, and the lower aspect of the mediastinum. A computed tomographic scan of the chest has also been very useful in the evaluation of the subcarinal, lower mediastinal, and retrocrural lymph nodes located along the route of retrograde spread toward the celiac lymph nodes at the upper aspect of the abdomen (Figs. 1 and 2) (55). The study by Harper et al. (54) also demonstrated that the detection rate of involvement of subcarinal lymph nodes was improved from 2% (1 of 50) by the conventional study to 32% (16 of 50) by the addition of the computed tomographic scans of the chest. The optimum treatment volume for the limited stage of small-cell carcinoma of the lung has not yet been clearly established. A small treatment volume is inevitably associated with a high rate of marginal failure, owing to geographic miss, although it is better tolerated by patients (26). However, on the basis of the biological aggressiveness of the tumor and the data of computed tomographic scans of the chest, it seems most logical that the treatment volume should

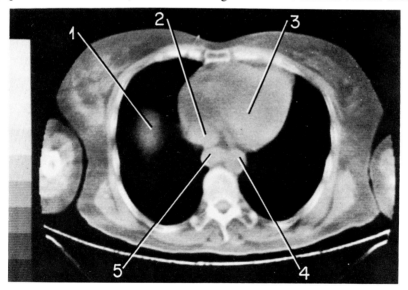

FIG. 1. A computed tomographic scan of the chest at the lower aspect of the mediastinum in patient A, with small-cell carcinoma of the left lower lobe of the lung. A large paraaortic lymph node, which is not demonstrable by conventional radiographic studies, is clearly outlined. 1 = dome of the right diaphragm, 2 = inferior vena cava, 3 = left ventricle, 4 = thoracic descending aorta, 5 = enlarged para-aortic lymph node.

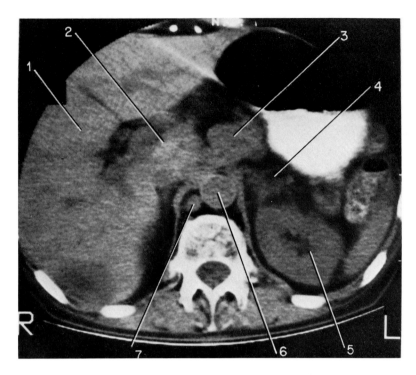

FIG. 2. A computed tomographic scan of the upper aspect of the abdomen at the level of the celiac axis in patient A. Despite a normal scan of the upper aspect of the abdomen initially, gross involvement of the celiac lymph nodes (3), right retrocrural lymph node (7), left adrenal gland (4), and porta hepatis (2) was noted in a repeat study 6 months later. 1 = liver, 5 = left kidney, 6 = abdominal aorta.

include the primary lesion with a 2–2.5-cm margin of radiographically clear pulmonary tissue, the ipsilateral hilum, the entire mediastinum, and both supraclavicular areas (Figs. 3 and 4). The boundary of the treatment volume is outlined on the left by the lateral edge of the aortic arch, on the right by a line drawn 3–4 cm lateral to the right lateral wall of the trachea, inferiorly by the dome of the diaphragm (T_{10-11}), and superiorly by the cricoid cartilage. Both supraclavicular areas are defined laterally by the mid-clavicular lines and inferiorly by a line drawn along the lower border of the first ribs.

Effect of Radiation Dose and Fractionation Schedule on Tumor Response

A reasonable relation between the control rate of local and regional small-cell carcinoma of the lung and radiation doses exists, according to the analysis of the Choi and Carey (9) and of others (Fig. 5) (Table 2) (26,56,57). For patients with the limited stage of small-cell carcinoma, a local control rate of 90% with a minimum follow-up of 4 or more months has been achieved by a radiation dose of 4,500–5,000 cGy (TDF 76–82). However, as median survival time of these patients has

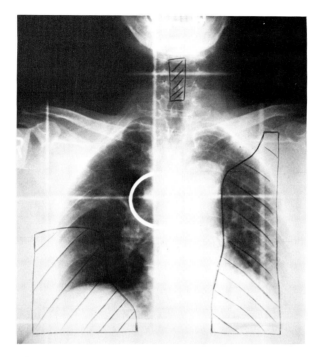

FIG. 3. Patient B has a large small-cell carcinoma of the right mainstem bronchus with partial collapse of the right upper lobe and enlarged right hilum. An anterior simulation film illustrates an initial treatment volume and cerrobend blocks for protection of normal tissues.

improved from 5–6 months to 10–14 months with the advent of more effective chemotherapy, a radiation dose of 5,000–5,400 cGy (TDF 82–89) seems necessary to achieve the same rate of local control for a period longer than 12 months, inasmuch as some local recurrences have been observed up to 3–4 years after the initiation of treatments (29,33,34). One should pay careful attention to the added risk of morbidity associated with increased radiation doses, so that the gain by higher radiation doses can be reflected in improved survival. Of interest is a slight decrease from 32% to 26%, which was less than expected, of the rate of local recurrence in patients with localized tumor when there was the addition of chemotherapy, according to the study of the Medical Research Council (37). The size of the tumor mass, clearly related to the number of clonogenic tumor cells, is an important factor for the control rate of the tumor in relation to the radiation doses. Radiation doses should be graded according to the density of the tumor cells within the treatment volume so that a uniform control–probability of the tumor throughout the treatment volume can be achieved with less likelihood of marginal or central recurrences and less injury to the normal tissue. A carefully designed "shrinking-field technique" is best suited for this situation. It is very desirable to reduce the treatment volume around the primary tumor by using lung blocks that are redesigned according to the degree of tumor regression at the level of a total dose of 2,000–2,400 cGy

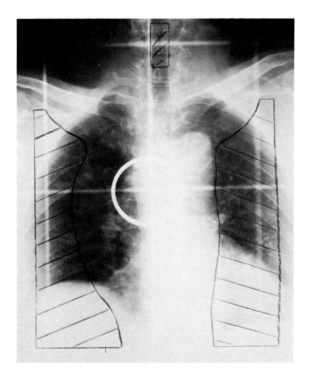

FIG. 4. A repeat anterior simulation film of patient B after a total dose of 2,400 cGy (TDF 73). The treatment volume is reduced around the right hilar mass as the partly collapsed right upper lobe has re-expanded.

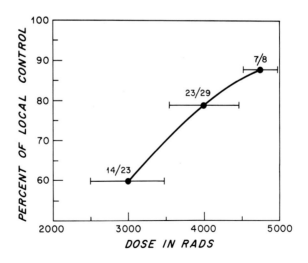

FIG. 5. A dose–response curve for the limited stage of small-cell carcinoma of the lung (9).

TABLE 2. *Relapse rate of local and regional tumors in relation to radiation doses[a]*

Study	Extent of tumor	Treatment methods	Radiation doses (cGy)	TDF	Relapse rate of local and regional tumors
Maurer et al. (16)	LD	CT→RT→CT CTX, MTX, CCNU	3200, 10 F, 2 weeks	68	43% (13 of 30)
MRC Study (37)	LD	RT alone	3000, 15 F, 3 weeks	49	32% (32 of 99)
		RT→CT CTX, MTX, CCNU	3000, 15 F, 3 weeks	49	26% (20 of 76)[b]
Feld et al. (44)	LD	CT→RT→CT CTX, ADR, VCR CCNU, PRC, MTX	2500, 10 F, 2 weeks	46	50% (20 of 40)
Catane et al. (34)	LD + ED	CT + RT, CT→RT CTX, ADR, VCR	2400–4500, 12–45 F, 1–9 weeks	—	37% (19 of 51)
Seydel et al. (58)	LD	RT ± CT CTX, CCNU	4500, 25 F, 5 weeks	70	31% (44 of 141)

[a]Selected series with a minimum of 30 patients.
[b]Local relapse rate is decreased from 32% to 26% by the addition of chemotherapy.
Abbreviations used: LD, limited disease; ED, extensive disease; TDF, time, dose, and fractionation factor. Other abbreviations as in Table 1.

(TDF 33–40) first, and again at a total dose of 3,400–3,600 cGy (TDF 56–59) whenever it is feasible (Fig. 4). With this approach, most patients are able to tolerate the maximum and optimum dose of radiation of 5,400–5,600 cGy (TDF 89–92) to the primary lesion and grossly involved mediastinal lymph nodes without great difficulty. Another important factor to consider in radiation therapy is the dose per treatment. For a specified degree of damage to normal tissue, likelihood of tumor-cell kill is higher when the highly fractionated radiation therapy is used than when fewer, larger doses per treatment are used (59). For this reason, highly fractionated radiation therapy is more desirable for the large treatment volume of this tumor than is a short course of less-fractionated radiation therapy. A fraction size of 180–200 cGy is tolerated better than that of 250–300 cGy, with likelihood of less damage to normal tissue for the same level of probability of tumor control. To remedy the problem of unchecked potential microscopic metastases outside the thorax while patients are treated to the chest for a period of 5–6 weeks with a daily dose of 180–200 cGy, 5 days per week, to a total dose of 5,600 cGy, systemic chemotherapy should be continued with a modified schedule in terms of reduced dose of 70%–80% of the normal dose and an omission of chemotherapeutic agents such as doxorubicin, a potentiator of radiation-induced normal tissue injuries.

Radiation Portal Arrangements

The arrangement of the radiation portals for patients with the limited stage of small-cell carcinoma of the lung is similar to that of curative radiation therapy for non-small-cell carcinoma of the lung. It is dictated by the size and shape of the treatment volume, and total dose and types of radiation. High-energy beams, of the order of 4–25 MeV photon, seem to be the choice, inasmuch as the large penumbra of a Cobalt-60 unit and the scatter radiation of electron or low-energy beams are likely to be more harmful to the already limited pulmonary reserve. Careful selection of radiotherapeutic techniques is essential to be successful in delivering the optimum dose of radiation, 5,00–5,600 cGy (TDF 82–92), to the primary tumor and the areas of grossly involved regional lymph nodes while the remaining pulmonary tissue, the heart, and the spinal cord are spared from excessive and damaging doses of radiation. An arrangement of two parallel, opposing portals (POP) applied anteriorly (AP) and posteriorly (PA) to the chest is a simple, accurate, and commonly used approach for the maximum radiation dose of 4,000–4,400 cGy (TDF 66–73), inasmuch as it reaches the threshold dose for radiation myelitis. To deliver a total dose of 5,000–5,600 cGy (TDF 82–92) to the treatment volume, supplemental portals such as the right posterior oblique (RPO) and the left posterior oblique (LPO) are necessary to keep the spinal cord below the threshold dose of radiation myelitis, 4,000–4,400 cGy (TDF 66–73). The radiotherapeutic technique

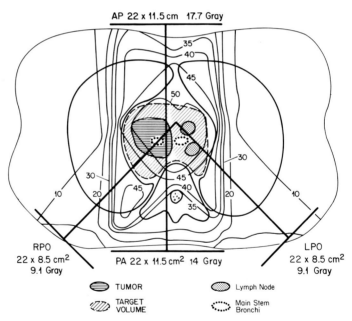

FIG. 6. A composite isodose plan at the level of the central axis designed for a superfractionation schedule of irradiation in which a total dose of 5,000 cGy is delivered by a combination of AP–PA POP for the initial 2,800 cGy and AP–RPO–LPO for the final 2,200 cGy, using a fraction size of 130~150 cGy twice daily for 17~20 treatment days (10 MeV photon). Most of the target volume is encompassed by an isodose line of ≥4,500 cGy, while the cord dose is kept at ≤3,600 cGy. For a conventional schedule of radiation therapy, one can deliver the initial dose up to 3,800–4,000 cGy by AP–PA POP and the final dose of 1,200–1,400 cGy by AP–RPO–LPO.

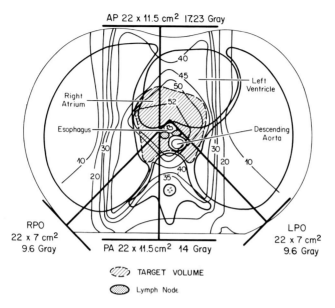

FIG. 7. A composite isodose plan at the level of the lower aspect of the mediastinum, which is the same treatment plan described in Fig. 6. The target volume is well encompassed by an isodose line of ≥4,500 cGy. Radiation doses at the left ventricle and the pulmonary tissue at the path of the oblique beams are kept under their threshold doses for radiation-induced injuries.

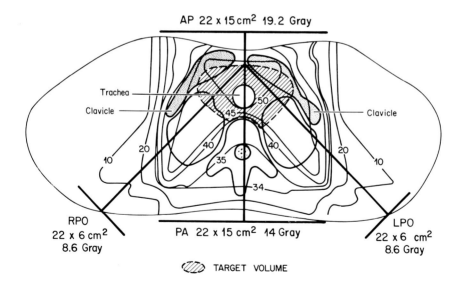

FIG. 8. A composite isodose plan, at the level of the sternal notch, which is the same treatment plan described in Fig. 6. The target volume is well encompassed by an isodose line of >4,500 cGy.

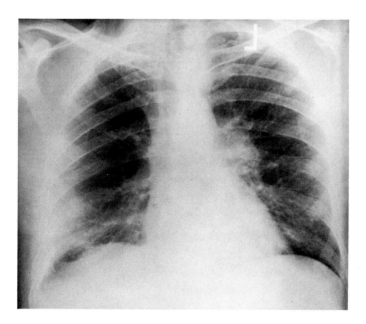

FIG. 9. A PA view of the chest of patient C with small-cell carcinoma of the left lung (stage $T_2N_2M_0$) before a combination of CAV chemotherapy and radiation therapy. The primary tumor is located at the left, upper lobe bronchus, associated with an enlargement of the left hilum.

used by the author consists of a sequential combination of AP–PA POP for the initial 3,800 cGy (TDF 62–64) with a three-field arrangement of AP–RPO–LPO for the final 1,200–1,800 cGy. With this technique, the treatment volume is very well covered by an isodose line of 4,500–5,000 cGy, while the spinal cord, the left ventricle of the heart, and most of the remaining pulmonary tissues are spared from an excessive dose of radiation (Figs. 6–8). Any part of the treatment volume away from the mainstem bronchus and mediastinum, such as a peripherally located tumor, requires supplemental radiation portals of AP–PA oblique opposing fields to secure adequate radiation doses throughout any shape of the treatment volume.

Radiotherapeutic techniques that should be scrutinized include an outright three-field approach, AP–RPO–LPO, and the use of a posterior cord block to reduce the radiation dose to the spinal cord, while other mediastinal structures are given a high dose of radiation of ≥ 5000 cGy by an arrangement of AP–PA POP only. The drawbacks of the outright three-field technique include a relatively high radiation dose, 40–50% of the total dose, to the pulmonary tissue in the path of the oblique beams and the potential risk of a geographic miss along the paravertebral region. The use of the posterior spinal cord block has been associated with an increased incidence of recurrence in the mediastinum. A four-field approach, AP–PA and right and left lateral fields, also has a built-in high risk of geographic miss along the paravertebral region and delivers a significant dose of radiation to a larger

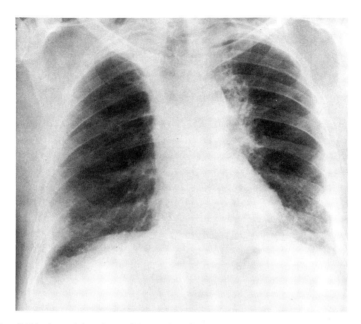

FIG. 10. A PA view of the chest of the patient C, 6.5 years after the initiation of the treatment program. Fibrosis, induced by irradiation, and as a result of repair process of normal tissue injured by the tumor, is present at the left hilar and left paramediastinal regions. The patient is free of recurrence.

volume of pulmonary tissue than does the technique using the sequential combination of AP–PA POP with AP–RPO–LPO.

RESULTS

Survival in Relation to Stages of the Tumor and Treatments

Measurement of tumor-volume doubling time of small-cell carcinoma of the lung has varied greatly from 7 to 160 days, with the mean values ranging from 22 to 77 days (60,61). Tumor-volume doubling time also varies among lesions in the same patient. On the basis of the clinical observations of late recurrences, even 2–3 years after the initiation of the treatment (29,33), and the studies on the tumor-volume doubling time, the likelihood of cure of this tumor should be reserved for patients with disease-free intervals longer than 3–4 years.

Most of long-term survivors who are living over 3 years without evidence of recurrence had been treated by surgery or radiation therapy with or without chemotherapy for early stage of the tumor (Figs. 9–12) (33,62,63). Only a very small number of patients have been reported to be living without evidence of relapse after successful chemotherapy for extensive stage of the tumor. Although median survival time of patients with the limited stage of small-cell carcinoma of the lung has

TABLE 3. *Long-term survival rate for patients with the limited stage of small-cell carcinoma of the lung[a]*

Study	Treatments	MST	2 Years	5 Years
Fox and Scadding (11)	RT	10[b]	10%	4% (3 of 73)
Choi and Carey (9)	RT; RT + CT, S + RT + CT CTX, VCR, PRC	9	10.6% (7 of 66)	3% (2 of 66)
Hansen et al (32)	CT + RT CT only CTX, ADR, VCR, CCNU, VP-16	—	7.2% (12 of 166)	—
Maurer and Pajak (41)	CT→RT→CT CTX, MTX, CCNU	10	12%	—
Catane et al. (34)	CT + RT, CT→RT CTX, ADR, VCR	14	19% (8 of 42)[c]	8–9%[d]

[a]Selected series with a minimum of 42 patients.
[b]Mean survival time in months.
[c]Minimum follow-up period of 30 months.
[d]Projected 5-year survival rate.
Abbreviations as in Table 1.

improved from 5–6 months to 10–14 months by the addition of chemotherapy to radiation therapy, survival rate at 2 years is still 11–14% and projected 5-year survival rate in only 8–9% (Table 3). For patients with the extensive stage of small-cell carcinoma of the lung, long-term survivors (more than 2–3 years) without recurrence of tumor are very rare.

Radiation-Induced Injuries of Intrathoracic Vital Structures

Radiation-induced injuries of the intrathoracic vital structures include radiation pneumonitis, radiation myelitis, radiation carditis, and radiation esophagitis. These serious complications can be prevented or minimized by careful planning of radiation therapy and chemotherapy. Detailed descriptions of these complications and their preventions are described in Chapter 9.

Hematologic Neoplasia Secondary to Anti-Neoplasm Agents

Chemotherapeutic agents, predominantly alkylating agents, and radiation are not only anti-neoplasm but also leukemogenic (64–67). A significant incidence of nonlymphocytic leukemia has been observed in patients who had received alkylating agents alone or in combination with pelvic irradiation for ovarian carcinoma (68). It is significant that there was no appreciable increase of nonlymphocytic leukemia among patients who had received pelvic radiation therapy only for the same type of tumor. According to the studies by Canellos et al. and Coleman et al. (69,70), the incidence of nonlymphocytic leukemia also was markedly increased in patients who had received both MOPP chemotherapy and total nodal irradiation for Hodg-

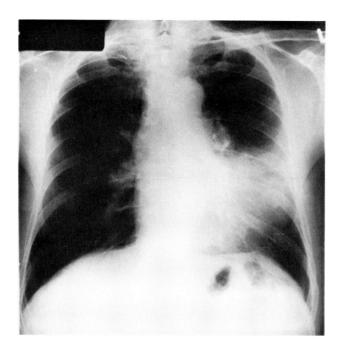

FIG. 11. An anecdotal case of long-term survival by radiation therapy alone. A PA view of the chest of patient D (79 years old) with small-cell carcinoma of the left, upper lobe bronchus, associated with collapse of the left lingular division (stage $T_2N_2M_0$).

kin's disease. No appreciable increase of nonlymphocytic leukemia was observed among patients who had received total nodal irradiation only (320 patients) for Hodgkin's disease in the study by Coleman et al. Acute whole-body irradiation has been associated wtih increased incidence of nonlymphocytic leukemia (66). However, local or regional irradiation does not seem to be associated with any appreciable increase of nonlymphocytic leukemia (71–73). The study by Hutchinson and its update did not show any appreciable increase of leukemia among more than 30,000 long-term survivors who had been treated by intracavitary radiation, external beam radiation, or a combination of both for carcinoma of the cervix (71,73). Potential leukemogenic effects of current chemotherapy programs for patients with small-cell carcinoma of the lung are just appearing among long-term survivors. A report by Bradley et al. (74) is worrisome, inasmuch as one of the eight long-term survivors for over 30 months developed erythroleukemia. The therapeutic program of this patient included cyclophosphamide, methotrexate, lomustine, vincristine, doxorubicin, and procarbazine, and palliative irradiation (2,400 cGy) to the humerus at 18 months. Another patient among the eight long-term survivors has had a persistent pancytopenia with dyserythropoietic features of the bone marrow. There is an urgent need for careful assessment of the relative risk of leukemogenesis by the current chemotherapy program with or without regional radiation therapy. Whatever the mechanism of leukemogenesis by anti-neoplasm agents is, the cumulative dose of

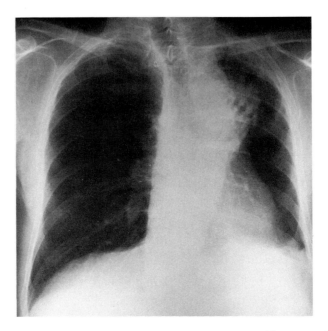

FIG. 12. A PA view of the chest of the patient D (now 84 years old) 5 years after radiation therapy alone without chemotherapy (because of the patient's age). Fibrosis is present at the left hilad and left suprahilar regions. The patient is free of recurrence.

chemotherapeutic agents, the duration of chemotherapy, a combination of chemotherapy and total nodal irradiation, and systemic radiation therapy seem to be significant for induction of leukemia. On the basis of the new information of Bradley et al., the risk factor for nonlymphocytic leukemia, therefore, should be reflected in future therapeutic strategies.

DISCUSSION

Future research in the management of patients with small-cell carcinoma of the lung should be directed to (a) search for new, more effective chemotherapeutic agents, (b) develop specific therapy by using monoclonal antibodies (75) against specific antigens of small-cell carcinoma as vehicles to carry chemotherapeutic agents or radionuclides to the tumor cells for internal specific irradiation (76,77), (c) develop effective immunotherapy, and (d) develop more effective combination therapy of systemic agents with local or regional therapeutic methods.

The role of radiation therapy for patients with the limited stage of small-cell carcinoma has been under investigation by several study groups. As shown in Tables 1 and 3, current chemotherapy alone is good enough to achieve a median survival time of 10–12 months if we are content with short-term results. However, either radiation therapy, surgery, or a combination of both is necessary in addition to chemotherapy for long-term cure of these patients.

Our effort should also be directed at reducing the potential risk of leukemogenesis by the current anti-neoplasm agents. Modern regional radiation therapy alone for malignant tumors does not seem to be associated with increased incidence of leukemia (68,70–73). It may be safer to reduce systemic chemotherapy to a reasonable minimum by using local and regional treatments, such as radiation therapy and surgery to the areas of bulky tumor, as judiciously as possible. Extensive courses of chemotherapy, whole-body irradiation, and hemibody irradiation, with or without chemotherapy, are likely to be associated with increased incidence of nonlymphocytic leukemia among long-term survivors.

Both local and regional recurrences are still major problems for patients with the limited stage of small-cell carcinoma when the treatment program has no radiation therapy at all or inadequate radiation therapy in terms of treatment volume and radiation dose (Table 1 and 2). The optimum radiotherapeutic technique has not yet been clearly established. However, it is quite clear from available data that the treatment volume should be large enough to include the primary tumor, ipsilateral hilum, entire mediastinum, and both supraclavicular areas, and the total radiation dose for grossly involved region should be about 5,000–5,600 cGy (TDF 82–92).

Fractionation schedules of radiation therapy need to be reviewed and redesigned in such a way as to achieve a maximum kill to tumor cells for a given degree of radiation-induced injuries of normal vasculoconnective tissue in the lung (59). Radiation therapy using a fraction size of about 180–200 cGy is preferred to that of 300–400 cGy in terms of the degree of normal tissue injury for the same rate of tumor control. A lack of chemotherapy during a long (6–7 weeks) course of continuous radiation therapy for a total dose of 5,000–5,600 cGy can be remedied by either giving two to three cycles of modified chemotherapy, in terms of 70–80% of the full dose of chemotherapeutic agents during radiation therapy or dividing the 6-week course of radiation therapy into three 2-week courses of radiation therapy and interspersing them with chemotherapy. Superfractionation schedules using fraction sizes of about 120–160 cGy given two to three times daily should be explored on the radiobiological basis of the potential advantage of normal tissue over the rapidly proliferating tumor tissue (78–80).

Elective irradiation to the brain should be part of the comprehensive treatment program for patients with the limited stage of small-cell carcinoma of the lung and also for patients in complete remission after chemotherapy for the extensive stage of the tumor.

Of interest are other therapeutic researches, which include megadose of chemotherapy plus autologous bone marrow transplantation (81), whole or hemibody irradiation as a systemic agent in treatment programs (82–87), use of radio-sensitizer, i.e., misonidazole (88), hyperthermia (89,90), and the use of anticoagulants (91–93).

REFERENCES

1. Weiss, R. B., Minna, J. D., Glatstein, E., Martini, N., Ihde, D. C., and Muggia, F. M. (1980): Commentary: Treatment of small-cell undifferentiated carcinoma of the lung: Update of recent results. *Cancer Treat. Rep.*, 64:539–548.
2. Livingston, R. B. (1981): Small-cell lung carcinoma—Recent advances and current challenges. *Recent Results Cancer Res.*, 76:267–275.

3. Salazar, O. M., and Creech, R. H. (1980): "The state of the art" toward defining the role of radiation therapy in the management of small-cell bronchogenic carcinoma. *Int. J. Rad. Oncol. Biol. Phys.*, 6:1103–1117.
4. Weiss, R. B. (1978): Small-cell carcinoma of the lung: Therapeutic management. *Ann. Intern. Med.*, 88:522–531.
5. Seydel, H. G., Creech, R. H. Mietlowski, W., and Perez, C. (1978): Radiation therapy in small-cell lung cancer. *Semin. Oncol.*, 5:288–298.
6. Cohen, M. H. (1980): Small-cell lung cancer: Restrained optimism. *Int. J. Rad. Oncol. Biol. Phys.*, 6:1119–1120.
7. Meyer, J. A., and Parker, F. B., Jr. (1980): Collective review: Small-cell carcinoma of the lung. *Ann. Thorac. Surg.*, 30:602–610.
8. Greco, F. A., and Oldham, R. K. (1979): Current concepts in cancer. Small-cell lung cancer. *N. Engl. J. Med.*, 301:355–358.
9. Choi, C. H., and Carey, R. W. (1976): Small-cell anaplastic carcinoma of lung. Reappraisal of current management. *Cancer*, 37:2651–2657.
10. Wolf, J., Patno, M. E., Roswit, B., and D'Esopo, N. (1966): Controlled study of survival of patients with clinically inoperable lung cancer treated with radiation therapy. *Am. J. Med.*, 40:360–367.
11. Fox, W., and Scadding, J. G. (1973): Medical Research Council comparative trial of surgery and radiotherapy for primary treatment of small-celled or oat-celled carcinoma of the bronchus. *Lancet*, 2:63–65.
12. Bergsagel, D. E., Jenkin, R. D. T., Pringle, J. F., White, D. M., Fetterly, J. C. M., Klaassen, D. J., and McDermott, R. S. R. (1972): Lung cancer: Clinical trial of radiotherapy alone vs. radiotherapy plus cyclophosphamide. *Cancer*, 30:621–627.
13. Eagan, R. T., Maurer, L. H., Forcier, R. J., and Tulloh, M. (1973): Combination chemotherapy and radiation therapy in small-cell carcinoma of the lung. *Cancer*, 32:371–379.
14. Hornback, N. B., Einhorn, L., Shidnia, H., Joe, B. T., Krause, M., and Furnas, B. (1971): Oat-cell carcinoma of the lung. Early treatment results of combination radiation therapy and chemotherapy. *Cancer*, 37:2658–2664.
15. Livingston, R. B., Moore, T. N., Heilbrun, L., Bottomley, R., Lehane, D., Rivkin, S. E., and Thigpen, T. (1978): Small-cell carcinoma of the lung: Combined chemotherapy and radiation. A Southwest oncology group study. *Ann. Intern. Med.*, 88:194–199.
16. Maurer, L. H., Tulloh, M., Weiss, R. B., Blom, J., Leone, L., Glidewell, O., and Pajak, T. F. (1980): A randomized combined modality trial in small-cell carcinoma of the lung: Comparison of combination chemotherapy-radiation therapy versus cyclophosphamide-radiation therapy: Effects of maintenance chemotherapy and prophylactic whole brain irradiation. *Cancer*, 45:30–39.
17. Greco, F. A., Richardson, R. I., Snell, J. D., Stroup, S. L., and Oldham, R. K. (1979): Small-cell lung cancer — Complete remission and improved survival. *Am. J. Med.*, 66:625–630.
18. Sierocki, J. S., Hilaris, B. S., Hopfan, S., Golbey, R. B., and Wittes, R. E. (1980): Small-cell carcinoma of the lung—Experience with a six-drug regimen. *Cancer*, 45:417–422.
19. Hansen, H. H., Dombernowsky, P., Hansen, H. S., and Rorth, M. (1979): Chemotherapy versus chemotherapy plus radiotherapy in regional small-cell carcinoma of the lung. A randomized trial. *Proc. AACR-ASCO*, 20:277 (Abstr.).
20. Stevens, E., Einhorn, L., and Rohn, R. (1979): Treatment of limited small-cell lung cancer. *Proc. AACR-ASCO*, 20:435 (Abstr.).
21. Cohen, M. H., Lichter, A. S., Bunn, P. A., Jr., Glatstein, E. J., Ihde, D. C., Fossieck, B. E., Jr., Matthews, M. J., and Minna, J. D. (1980): Chemotherapy-radiation therapy versus chemotherapy in limited small-cell lung cancer. *Proc. AACR-ASCO*, 21:448 (Abstr.).
22. Oldham, R. K., Greco, F. A., Einhorn, L., Perez, C., Birch, R., Hester, M., and Krauss, S. (1981): Preliminary results of a randomized trial to evaluate the role of radiotherapy in the combined modality therapy of limited stage small-cell lung cancer. *Proc. AACR-ASCO*, 22:505.
23. Fox, R. M., Tattersall, M. H. N., and Woods, R. L. (1981): Radiation therapy as an adjuvant in small-cell lung cancer treated by combination chemotherapy: A randomized study. *Proc. AACR-ASCO*, 22:502 (Abstr.).
24. Aisner, J., and Wiernik, P. H. (1980): Chemotherapy versus chemoimmunotherapy for small-cell undifferentiated carcinoma of the lung. *Cancer*, 46:2543–2549.
25. American Joint Committee for Cancer Staging and End-Results Reporting (1978): *Staging of Lung Cancer*, pp. 59–64, Chicago.

26. Mira, J. G., and Livingston, R. B. (1980): Evaluation and radiotherapy implications of chest relapse patterns in small-cell lung carcinoma treated with radiotherapy-chemotherapy: Study of 34 cases and review of the literature. *Cancer*, 46:2557–2565.
27. Hoffman, P. C., Golomb, H. M., Bitran, J. D., DeMeester, T. R., Cohen, L., Griem, M. L., Cooksey, J. A., Mintz, U., Gordon, L. I., Desser, R. K., Kinnealley, A. F., and Sovik, C. A. (1980): Small-cell carcinoma of the lung: A five-year experience with combined modality therapy. *Cancer*, 46:2550–2556.
28. Meyer, J. A., Comis, R. L., Ginsberg, S. J., Ikins, P. M., Burke, W. A., King, G. A., Gullo, J. J., DiFino, S. M., Tinsley, R. W., and Parker, F. B., Jr. (1982): Phase II trial of extended indications for resection in small-cell carcinoma of the lung. *J. Thorac. Cardiovasc. Surg.*, 83:12–19.
29. Matthews, M. J., Rozencweig, M., Staquet, M. J., Minna, J. D., and Muggia, F. M. (1980): Long-term survivors with small-cell carcinoma of the lung. *Eur. J. Cancer*, 16:527–531.
30. Holoye, P. Y., Samuels, M. L., Lanzotti, V. J., Smith, T., and Barkley, H. T. (1977): Combination chemotherapy and radiation therapy for small-cell carcinoma. *J.A.M.A.*, 237:1221–1224.
31. Ginsberg, S. J., Comis, R. L., Gottlieb, A. J., King, G. B., Goldberg, J., Zamkoff, K., Elbadawi, A., and Meyer, J. A. (1979): Long-term survivorship in small-cell anaplastic lung carcinoma. *Cancer Treat. Rep.*, 63:1347–1349.
32. Hansen, M., Hansen, H. H., Dombernowsky, P. (1980): Long-term survial in small-cell carcinoma of the lung. *J.A.M.A.*, 244:247–250.
33. Peschel, R. E., Kapp, D. S., Carter, D., and Knowlton, A. (1981): Long-term survivors with small-cell carcinoma of the lung. *Int. J. Rad. Oncol. Biol. Phys.*, 7:1545–1548.
34. Catane, R., Lichter, A., Lee, Y. J., Brereton, H. D., Schwade, J. G., and Glatstein, E. (1981): Small-cell lung cancer: Analysis of treatment factors contributing to prolonged survival. *Cancer*, 48:1936–1943.
35. Byhardt, R. W., Libnoch, J. A., Cox, J. D., Holoye, P. Y., Kun, L., Komaki, R., and Clowry, L. (1981): Local control of intrathoracic disease with chemotherapy and role of prophylactic cranial irradiation in small-cell carcinoma of the lung. *Cancer*, 47:2239–2246.
36. Abeloff, M. D., Ettinger, D. S., Order, S. E., Khouri, N., Mellits, E. D., Dorschel, N. T., and Baumgardner, R. (1981): Intensive induction chemotherapy in 54 patients with small-cell carcinoma of the lung. *Cancer Treat. Rep.*, 65:639–646.
37. Medical Research Council Lung Cancer Working Party (1979): Radiotherapy alone or with chemotherapy in the treatment of small-cell carcinoma of the lung. *Br. J. Cancer*, 40:1–10.
38. Hansen, H. H. (1973): Should initial treatment of small-cell carcinoma include systemic chemotherapy and brain irradiation? *Cancer Chemother. Rep.*, 4:239–241.
39. Jackson, D. V., Richards, F., Cooper, R., Ferree, C., Muss, H., White, D., and Spurr, C. (1977): Prophylactic cranial irradiation in small-cell carcinoma of the lung. A randomized study. *J.A.M.A.*, 237:2730–2733.
40. Komaki, R., Cox, J. D., and Whitson, W. (1981): Risks of brain metastasis from small-cell carcinoma of the lung related to length of survival and prophylactic irradiation. *Cancer Treat. Rep.*, 65:811–814.
41. Maurer, L. H., and Pajak, T. F. (1981): Prognostic factors in small-cell carcinoma of the lung: A cancer and leukemia group B study. *Cancer Treat. Rep.*, 65:767–774.
42. Ihde, D. C., Bilek, F. S., Cohen, M. H., Bunn, P. A., Eddy, J., and Minna, J. D. (1979): Response to thoracic radiotherapy in patients with small-cell carcinoma of the lung after failure of combination chemotherapy. *Radiology*, 132:443–446.
43. Brandman, J., Ruckdeschel, J. C., O'Donnell, M., Horton, J., and Harrington, G. (1980): Unexpected pulmonary complications of intensive therapy for small-cell cancer of the lung. *Proc. AACR-ASCO*, 21:459 (Abstr.).
44. Feld, R., Pringle, J. F., Evans, W. K., Keen, C. W., Quirt, I. C., Curtis, J. E., Baker, M. A., Yeoh, J. L., Deboer, G., and Brown, T. C. (1981): Combined modality treatment of small-cell carcinoma of the lung. *Arch. Intern. Med.*, 141:469–473.
45. Cox, J. D., Komaki, R., Byhardt, R. W., and Kun, L. (1980): Results of whole brain irradiation for metastases from small-cell carcinoma of the lung. *Cancer Treat. Rep.*, 64:957–961.
46. Rosenman, J., and Choi, N. C. (1982): Improved quality of life of patients with small-cell carcinoma of the lung by elective irradiation of the brain. *Int. J. Rad. Oncol. Biol. Phys.*, 8:1041–1043.

47. Moore, T. N., Livingston, R., Heilbrun, L., Eltringham, J., Skinner, O., White, J. H., and Tesh, D. (1978): The effectiveness of prophylactic brain irradiation in small-cell carcinoma of the lung — A Southwest oncology group study. *Cancer*, 41:2149–2153.

48. Catane, R., Schwade, J. G., Yarr, I., Lichter, A. S., Tepper, J. E., Dunnick, N. R., Brody, L., Brereton, H. D., Cohen, M., and Glatstein, E., (1981): Follow-up neurological evaluation in patients with small-cell lung carcinoma treated with prophylactic cranial irradiation and chemotherapy. *Int. J. Rad. Oncol. Biol. Phys.*, 7:105–109.

49. Rosen, S., Bunn, P., Lichter, A., Matthews, M., Ihde, D., Cohen, M., Carney, D., Minna, J., and Glatstein, E. (1981): Prophylactic cranial irradiation in small-cell lung cancer: Benefit restricted to patients in complete response. *Proc. AACR-ASCO*, 22:499 (Abstr.).

50. Vincent, R. G., Wilson, H. E., Lane, W. W., Chen, T. Y., Raza, S., Gutierrez, A. C., and Caracandas, J. E. (1981): Progress in the chemotherapy of small-cell carcinoma of the lung. *Cancer*, 47:229–235.

51. Lininger, T. R., Fleming T. R., and Eagan, R. T. (1981): Evaluation of alternating chemotherapy and sites and extent of disease in extensive small-cell lung cancer. *Cancer*, 48:2147–2153.

52. Emami, B., Melo, A., Carter, B. L., Munzenrider, J. E., and Piro, A. (1978): Value of computed tomography in radiotherapy of lung cancer. *Am. J. Roentgenol.*, 131:63–67.

53. Seydel, H. G., Kutcher, G. J., Steiner, R. M., Mohiuddin, M., and Goldberg, B. (1980): Computed tomography in planning radiation therapy for bronchogenic carcinoma. *Int. J. Rad. Oncol. Biol. Phys.*, 6:601–606.

54. Harper, P. G., Houang, M., Spiro, S. G., Geddes, D., Hodson, M., and Souhami, R. L. (1981): Computerized axial tomography in the pre-treatment assessment of small-cell carcinoma of the bronchus. *Cancer*, 47:1775–1780.

55. Bell, J. W. (1965): Open abdominal biopsy before thoracotomy for lung cancer. *Geriatrics*, 20:715–727.

56. Cox, J. D., Byhardt, R., Komaki, R., Wilson, J. F., Libnoch, J. A., and Hansen, R. (1979): Interaction of thoracic irradiation and chemotherapy on local control and survival in small-cell carcinoma of the lung. *Cancer Treat. Rep.*, 63:1251–1255.

57. McMahon, L. J., Herman, T. S., Manning, M. R., and Dean, J. C. (1979): Patterns of relapse of patients with small-cell carcinoma of the lung treated with doxorubicin-cyclophosphamide chemotherapy and radiation. *Cancer Treat. Rep.*, 63:359–362.

58. Seydel, H. G., Creech, R. H., Pagano, M., Steel, D., and Perez, C. (1980): Sites of relapse following treatment of localized small-cell lung carcinoma. *Proc. AACR-ASCO*, 21:451 (Abstr.).

59. Withers, H. R., and Peters, L. J. (1980): Basic aspects of radiation therapy. In: *Textbook of Radiotherapy*, edited by G. H. Fletcher, pp. 105–180. Lea & Febiger, Philadelphia.

60. Brigham, B. A., Bunn, P. A., Jr., Minna, J. D., Cohen, M. H., Ihde, D. C., and Shackney, S. E. (1978): Growth rates of small-cell bronchogenic carcinoma. *Cancer* 42:2880–2886.

61. Bhaskar, D., Maldonado, A., Ng, A., and Selawry, O. (1977): Volume doubling time of small-cell carcinoma of the lung. *Proc. AACR-ASCO*, 18:335 (Abstr.).

62. Levison, V. (1980): Pre-operative radiotherapy and surgery in the treatment of oat-cell carcinoma of the bronchus. *Clin. Radiol.*, 31:345–348.

63. Wright, P., Schulman, S., Davis, S., Anderson, R., Hammar, S., Hill, L., Li, W., and Thorning, D. (1981): Unexpectedly favorable survival without intensive combination chemotherapy in patients with small-cell lung cancer. *Proc. AACR-ASCO*, 22:493 (Abstr.).

64. Chabner, B. A. (1977): Second neoplasm — A complication of cancer chemotherapy. Editorial. *N. Engl. J. Med.*, 297:213–215.

65. Casciato, D. A., and Scott, J. L. (1979): Acute leukemia following prolonged cytotoxic agent therapy. *Medicine (Balt.)*, 58:32–47.

66. Bizzodero, O. J., Jr., Johnson, K. G., and Ciocco, A. (1966): Radiation-related leukemia in Hiroshima and Nagasaki, 1946–1964. I. Distribution, incidence and appearance time. *N. Engl. J. Med.*, 274:1096–1101.

67. Court-Brown, W. M. C., and Abbatt, J. D. (1955): The incidence of leukemia in ankylosing spondylitis treated with x-ray: A preliminary report. *Lancet*, 1:1283–1285.

68. Reimer, R. R., Hoover, R., Fraumeni, J. F., Jr., and Young, R. C. (1977): Actue leukemia after alkylating-agent therapy of ovarian cancer. *N. Engl. J. Med.*, 297:177–181.

69. Cannellos, G. P., DeVita, V. T., Arseneau, J. C., Whang-Peng, J., and Johnson, R. E. C. (1975): Second malignancies complicating Hodgkin's disease in remission. *Lancet*, 1:947–949.

70. Coleman, C. N., Williams, C. J., Flint, A., Glatstein, E. J., Rosenberg, S. A., and Kaplan, H. S. (1977): Hematologic neoplasia in patients treated for Hodgkin's disease. *N. Engl. J. Med.*, 297:1249–1252.

71. Hutchison, G. B. (1968): Leukemia in patients with cancer of the cervix uteri treated with radiation — A report covering the first 5 years of an international study. *J. Natl. Cancer Inst.*, 40:951–982.

72. Seydel, H. G. (1975): The risk of tumor induction in man following medical irradiation for malignant neoplasm. *Cancer*, 35:1641–1645.

73. Hutchison, G. E. (1976): Late neoplastic changes following medical irradiation. *Cancer*, 37:1102–1107.

74. Bradley, E. C., Schecter, G. P., Matthews, M. J., Whang-Peng, J., Cohen, M. H., Bunn, P. A., Ihde, D. C., and Minna, J. D. (1982): Erythroleukemia and other hematologic complications of intensive therapy in long-term survivors of small-cell lung cancer. *Cancer*, 49:221–223.

75. Kohler, G., and Milstein, C. (1975): Continuous culture of fused cells secreting antibody of predefined specificity. *Nature*, 256:495–497.

76. Goldenberg, D. M., DeLand, F., Kim, E., Bennett, S., Primus, F. J., van Nagell, J. R., Jr., Estes, N., DeSimone, P., and Rayburn, P. (1978): Use of radiolabeled antibodies to carcinoembryonic antigen for the detection and localization of diverse cancers by external photoscanning. *N. Engl. J. Med.*, 298:1384–1388.

77. Order, S. E., Klein, J. L., and Leichner, P. K. (1981): Antiferritin IgG antibody for isotopic cancer therapy. *Oncology*, 38:154–160.

78. Choi, C. H., and Suit, H. D. (1975): Evaluation of rapid radiation treatment schedules utilizing two treatment sessions per day. *Radiology*, 116:703–707.

79. Noron, T., and Onyango, J. (1977): Radiotherapy in Burkett's lymphoma: Conventional vs. superfractionated regime — Early results. *Int. J. Rad. Oncol. Biol. Phys.*, 2:399–406.

80. Suit, H. D. (1977): Superfractionation. [editorial] *Int. J. Rad. Oncol. Biol. Phys.*, 2:591–592.

81. Farha, P., Spitzer, G., Valdivieso, M., Zander, A., Verma, D., Minnhaar, G., Vellekoop, L., Dicke, K., and Bodey, G. (1981): Treatment of small-cell bronchogenic carcinoma with high dose chemotherapy and autologous bone marrow transplantation. *Proc. AACR-ASCO*, 22:496 (Abstr.).

82. Salazar, O. M., Creech, R. H., Rubin, P., Bennett, J. M., Mason, B. A., Young, J. J., Scarantino, C. W., and Catalano, R. B. (1980): Half-body and local chest irradiation as consolidation following response to standard induction chemotherapy for disseminated small-cell lung cancer. *Int. J. Rad. Oncol. Biol. Phys.*, 6:1093–1102.

83. Urtasun, R., Belch, A., Higgins, E., Saunders, W., and MacKinnon, S. (1980): Whole body irradiation of small-cell carcinoma of lung compared to three drug chemotherapy. *Proc. AACR-ASCO*, 21:451 (Abstr.).

84. Rasim, M. M., and The, S. K. (1979): Combined total body irradiation and local radiation therapy in oat-cell carcinoma of the bronchus. *Clin. Radiol.*, 30:161–163.

85. Byhardt, R. W., Cox, J. D., Wilson, J. F., Libnoch, J., and Stein, R. S. (1979): Total body irradiation vs. chemotherapy as a systemic adjuvant for small-cell carcinoma of the lung. *Int. J. Rad. Oncol. Biol. Phys.*, 5:2043–2048.

86. Woods, R. L., Tattersall, M. H. N., and Fox, R. M. (1981): Hemi-body irradiation in "poor prognosis" small-cell lung cancer. *Proc. AACR-ASCO*, 22:502 (Abstr.).

87. Mason, B. A., Richter, M. P., Catalano, R. B., and Creech, R. H. (1981): Upper hemibody and local chest irradiation as consolidation following response to high dose induction chemotherapy for small-cell lung carcinoma—A pilot study. *Proc. AACR-ASCO*, 22:498 (Abstr.).

88. Wasserman, T. H., Phillips, T. L., Johnson, R. J., Gomer, C. J., Lawrence, G. A., Sadee, W., Marques, R. A., Levin, V. A., and Van Raalte, G. (1979): Initial United States clinical and pharmacologic evaluation of misonidazole (RO-07-0582), a hypoxic cell radiosensitizer. *Int. J. Rad. Oncol. Biol. Phys.*, 5:775–786.

89. Manning, M. R., Cetas, T. C., Miller, R. C., Oleson, J. R., Connor, W. G., and Gerner, E. W. (1982): Clinical hyperthermia: Results of a phase I trial employing hyperthermia alone or in combination with external beam or interstitial radiotherapy. *Cancer*, 49:205–216.

90. Parks, L. C., Minaberry, D., Smith, D. P., and Neely, W. A. (1979): Treatment of far-advanced bronchogenic carcinoma by extracorporeally induced systemic hyperthermia. *J. Thorac. Cardiovasc. Surg.*, 78:883–892.

91. Zacharski, L. R., Henderson, W. G., Rickles, F. R., Forman, W. B., Cornell, C. J., Jr., Forcier, J., Edwards, R., Headley, E., Kim, S. H., O'Donnell, J. R., O'Dell, R., Tornyos, K., and

Kwaan, H. C. (1981): Effect of warfarin on survival in small-cell carcinoma of the lung. *J.A.M.A.*, 245:831–835.

92. Stanford, C. F. (1979): Anticoagulants in the treatment of small-cell carcinoma of the bronchus. *Thorax*, 34:113–116.

93. Brown, J. M. (1973): A study of the mechanism by which anticoagulation with warfarin inhibits blood-borne metastases. *Cancer Res.*, 33:1217–1224.

Thoracic Oncology, edited by N. C. Choi and
H. C. Grillo. Raven Press, New York © 1983.

Pathology of Tracheal Neoplasms

Eugene J. Mark

Department of Pathology, Massachusetts General Hospital, Boston, Massachusetts 02114

The trachea cannot be viewed pathologically as a midline bronchus. Surrounded by large vessels, muscles, nerves, thyroid or esophagus, its anatomy, mechanics, physiology and pathology differ from bronchi surrounded by pulmonary parenchyma. C-shaped, imperfect rings of cartilage comprise the anterior and lateral walls of the trachea and a fibromuscular membrane comprises the posterior wall, whereas less regular plates of cartilage comprise the circumference of bronchi. Histologically, the mucosa of the trachea differs from mucosa of bronchi by virtue of greater stratification of nuclei, lesser proportion of goblet cells on the surface, fewer neurosecretory cells, larger mucous glands, thicker basement membrane, and larger fascicles of smooth muscle which are particularly prominent in the posterior wall. Lymphatic drainage of the trachea is segmented by the tracheal rings. The lymph flows in the transverse plane toward the posterior fibromuscular membrane.

Neoplasms of the trachea cover a spectrum of histologic types as wide as those of bronchi but very different in relative frequencies. Adenocarcinomas form a much smaller proportion of cases in the trachea than in the bronchi. Overall, tracheal tumors are approximately 100 times less common than bronchial tumors (24). The ratio of adenoid cystic tumor to carcinoid tumor in the trachea is the reverse of that in the bronchi. Metastasis to the trachea is rare, but direct invasion by carcinoma of the esophagus or thyroid is not uncommon. Sarcomas constitute a higher percentage of neoplasms in the trachea than in the bronchi, and they have a greater variation in histologic type and pattern of growth.

In children, 90% of tracheal tumors are benign (41). In adults, malignant neoplasms of the trachea outnumber benign ones but not to the extent that malignant neoplasms of the bronchus vastly exceed benign ones. The mucous blanket is more complete and flow more laminar and uninterrupted in the trachea than in the bronchi. It has been postulated that this better protection of the tracheal mucosa from carcinogens accounts for the much lower inicidence of carcinoma of the trachea than of the bronchi among smokers (2).

The trachea itself is not uniform in its predispostion to tumors. Malignant tracheal neoplasms arise most frequently from the posterior and distal trachea. Approximately 60% originate from the posterior or postero-lateral wall (5,17). Approximately two-thirds originate from the lower one-third of the trachea including carina (9,33), the portion of the trachea that is unfortunately the most difficult to treat surgically.

The classification of tracheal neoplasms used here is given in Table 1.

TABLE 1. *Tracheal neoplasms*

Epithelial tumors
  Squamous cell carcinoma
  Adenoid cystic tumor
  Adenocarcinoma
  Oat cell carcinoma
  Mucoepidermoid tumor
  Mixed tumor
  Carcinoid tumor

Metastases

Mesenchymal tumors
  Fibroma–fibrosarcoma
  Chondroma–chondrosarcoma
  Leiomyoma–leiomyosarcoma
  Neurofibroma–neurofibrosarcoma
  Lipoma–liposarcoma
  Fibrous histiocytoma
  Granular cell myoblastoma
  Hemangioma
  Intratracheal thyroid

Lymphoma

EPITHELIAL TUMORS

Squamous Cell Carcinoma

Squamous cell carcinoma accounts for approximately 50% of all primary tracheal malignancies (2,14,17,27). It occurs predominantly in male smokers between the ages of 35 and 75 years. Most patients smoke heavily (15). Many develop another primary malignancy, the most common sites for which are the larynx or lung. Tracheal squamous cell carcinoma is usually associated with squamous metaplasia, dysplasia, or carcinoma *in situ* and may be multifocal. The progression of cytologic atypicality leading to malignancy resembles that seen with squamous cell carcinoma of the bronchus (15).

Tracheal squamous cell carcinoma produces an exophytic and usually ulcerated mass obstructing the lumen. At the time of original diagnosis the tumor averages 4 cm in maximal diameter, invasion into tracheal wall has occurred in one-half of cases, extension into mediastinum in one-third, and metastasis to cervical lymph nodes in one-third (15). This early invasion and metastasis contrasts with the behavior of laryngeal squamous cell carcinoma, where the laryngeal cartilages act as a barrier and usually still confine the carcinoma at the time of diagnosis. Metastases in the lymphatic drainage along the recurrent laryngeal nerve may cause paralysis of a vocal cord. At autopsy, metastases from tracheal squamous cell carcinoma are found in mediastinal and cervical lymph nodes, lung, bone, and liver, in order of decreasing frequency, in two-thirds of cases (11,15,33). Tracheo-mediastinal fistula lined by malignant cells occurs in one-fourth of autopsied cases (15).

The histologic spectrum of tracheal squamous cell carcinoma ranges from well-differentiated and verrucous to anaplastic and solid. Well-differentiated carcinoma has large cells, much keratinization, slight nuclear atypicality, and may be difficult to distinguish from squamous papilloma on a superficial biopsy. Poorly differentiated carcinoma has small cells, little or no keratinization, and may reveal its squamous nature only by its continuity with squamous cell carcinoma *in situ* at the surface. Fibrosis, calcification and ossification may occur in the tumor. The degree of histologic differentiation has not been correlated with survival.

Squamous cell carcinoma of the trachea cannot be distinguished histologically from squamous cell carcinoma of the esophagus. Both primary tracheal squamous cell carcinoma and secondarily invasive esophageal squamous cell carcinoma will involve the posterior wall of the trachea more than the anterior or lateral walls. Therefore, invasion of the trachea by an esophageal primary must always be considered when squamous cell carcinoma is first diagnosed by tracheal biopsy.

Adenoid Cystic Tumor

Tracheal adenoid cystic tumor comprises approximately 30% of all primary tracheal malignancies (14,15,17,45). It is proportionately more prevalent in the trachea than in the bronchus. It is slowly growing both before and after it is diagnosed. Patients usually have had symptoms for many months and even for a few years before the correct diagnosis is made (31). Overall, prognosis for adenoid cystic tumor is better than for squamous cell carcinoma. Among those patients whose tumors originally seem to be completely resected, however, a sizeable minority still ultimately succumb, typically after a disease-free interval of 5 to 20 years, followed by local recurrences, followed by metastases (15,31,43,45). At autopsy, tumor will be found invading a lengthy segment of trachea, thyroid, cervical soft tissues or mediastinum. Pericardium, great vessels or pulmonary hila may also be involved. Distant metastases may be present in the lungs, liver, abdominal lymph nodes or bones (15).

Adenoid cystic tumor of the trachea arises usually in the upper third of the trachea, in contradistinction to most other tracheal carcinomas, which arise usually in the lower third. By the time of diagnosis generally the exophytic portion of the tumor measures more than 2 cm in greatest diameter. Extensive, endophytic infiltration often occurs in both horizontal and vertical directions. Horizontally the tumor grows within the tracheal mucosa, thickens the mucosa, and effaces the mucosal folds without producing a distinct mass or ulceration. This endophytic infiltration may extend for a linear distance of as much as 2 cm proximal or distal to the exophytic portion of the tumor and may involve the entire circumference of the trachea (31). Vertically the tumor infiltrates through the fibrous membrane between adjacent cartilage plates or through the posterior fibromuscular membrane into peritracheal adventitial tissue. Respiratory epithelium tends to remain intact over the tumor (31), as is characteristic of slowly growing tumors, although the surface epithelium may exhibit squamous metaplasia. Perineural and intraneural infiltration is characteristic of adenoid cystic tumor (43). Metastasis to regional lymph nodes is uncharacteristic. It is found in only about 10% of cases at time of original resection (31).

The uniform, small, basaloid epithelial cells of adenoid cystic tumor classically arrange themselves in nests or sheets with fenestrations to give a cribriform pattern (Fig. 1). They may align around hyaline cores, which represent basement membrane-like material on ultrastructural examination. They may form true glands and produce mucin. They may form solid nests which undergo central necrosis.

The middle of the tumor generally has the classic histology. Superficial tumor, located immediately beneath the surface epithelium, often consists of non-classic histology with small cellular nests or glands which lack cribriform features. If only such non-classic histology appears on a small superficial tracheal biopsy, the differential diagnosis of adenoid cystic tumor versus adenocarcinoma versus carcinoid may prove difficult. Final diagnosis may have to be postponed until time of excisional surgery.

Frozen section examination of proximal, distal and circumferential resection margins to detect tumor is essential at the time of definitive resection because of the surreptitious manner in which adenoid cystic tumor spreads. Two potential oversights on frozen section diagnosis are noteworthy. First, nests of tumor the size of lobules of normal tracheal mucous glands may partially replace the normal lobules without altering the overall mucosal architecture, thus escaping detection on casual

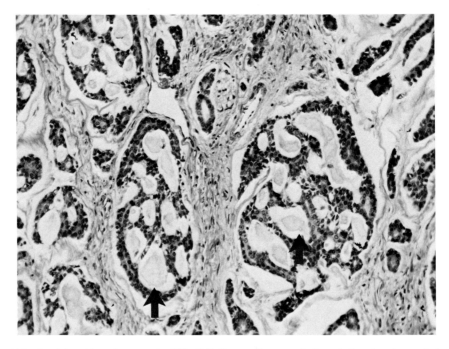

FIG. 1. Adenoid cystic tumor (× 256). Cribriform pattern results from trabeculae, two cells in thickness, separated by hyaline cores *(arrows)* cut in cross and longitudinal section.

examination. Second, perineural infiltration by individual cells may be the only tumor present in the peritracheal adventitia. The tracheal nerves deserve scrutiny.

Cellular pleomorphism may be absent, focal, or extensive and marked (26). Pleomorphism tends to increase in recurrences. If pleomorphism is extensive, histology comes to resemble adenocarcinoma, and tumors with such histology have a bad prognosis. Other histological parameters have not proven to be dependable in prognosis of adenoid cystic tumors in general (26) and have not been analysed for adenoid cystic tumors of the trachea in particular.

Adenocarcinoma

Tracheal adenocarcinoma accounts for approximately 10% of all primary tracheal malignancies (15,28). The proportion would be larger if one included adenocarcinomas arising in main bronchi and extending proximally to involve the carina. Tracheal adenocarcinoma tends to be the most deeply invasive of the tracheal carcinomas at the time of diagnosis. Prognosis is worse than that for tracheal squamous cell carcinoma (15).

Tracheal adenocarcinoma tends to be smaller, firmer and less necrotic than bronchial adenocarcinoma. Histologically, the malignant glands in tracheal adenocarcinoma tend to be more compact and more evenly sized than in bronchial adenocarcinoma. Adenocarcinoma of trachea and of bronchus are histologically and cytologically similar in all other respects. Mucus is found both within the cells and within the lumens of malignant glands. Adenocarcinoma *in situ* associated with the invasive adenocarcinoma rarely can be detected.

Oat Cell Carcinoma

Oat cell carcinoma is one of the most unusual primary tracheal malignancies (33), whereas it is one of the most common primary bronchial malignancies. Primary oat cell carcinoma of the trachea is more common in the upper third than in the middle or lower thirds (35). Oat cell carcinoma involving the carina is statistically more likely to be primary in a bronchus and secondarily invading the trachea rather than primary in the trachea. The natural history of tracheal oat cell carcinoma parallels bronchial oat cell carcinoma.

Mucoepidermoid Tumor

Mucoepidermoid tumors primary in the trachea behave clinically and appear histologically like mucoepidermoid tumors primary in bronchi but are less common (39). Greater degrees of differentiation, as manifested by distinct keratinization and gland formation (Fig. 2), indicate better prognosis. Invasion by broad sheets of cells augurs better than invasion by narrow tongues of cells or single cells. Proximal spread of a bronchial mucoepidermoid tumor into the carina and lower trachea is more common than primary tracheal mucoepidermoid tumor.

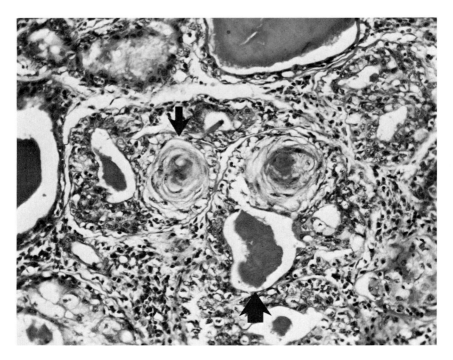

FIG. 2. Mucoepidermoid tumor (×256). Juxtaposed are keratin pearls *(small arrow)* and glands filled with darkly stained mucin *(large arrow)*.

Mixed Tumor

Mixed tumor has as its essential histologic feature joined epithelial and stromal components. The epithelial cells usually form glands and secrete mucus but may also grow as solid sheets. The stroma consists of undifferentiated mesenchyme with variable amounts of hyalinization, myxoid change, cartilage or bone. In the trachea, mixed tumors generally grow as intraluminal polyps which are benign, but in rare instances they may recur after surgery (19). In a series of 18 cases, one tumor recurred 10 years after initial surgery, another patient with tumor died suddenly of respiratory obstruction, and the other 16 patients were cured by excision (25).

Carcinoid Tumor

Tracheal carcinoid tumors are slowly growing polypoid neoplasms which produce hemoptysis, stridor or dyspnea and generally are cured by segmental excision. Most common above the age of 30, they have been reported in children as young as 13 years (42). They arise particularly from the posterior wall of the lower third of the trachea. The uncommonness of tracheal carcinoids compared to bronchial carcinoids presumably reflects the normal distribution of the precursor Kultschitzky cell, which is infrequent in tracheal mucosa but frequent in mucosa of large bronchi. Tracheal carcinoids have the same histology as central bronchial carcinoids, consisting of regular, cuboidal, argyrophilic cells arranged in trabeculae (Fig. 3). Metastasis to regional lymph nodes occurs in approximately 10% of cases and may be anticipated if the cells of the carcinoid have pleomorphism and mitoses. Neither recurrence of tumor nor distant metastases have been reported (3).

METASTASES IN THE TRACHEA

Lymphangitic carcinomatosis within the bronchial mucosa occasionally may extend proximally into the mucosa of the lower trachea. Carcinomas of stomach, breast, and lung, in particular, are prone to extensive lymphangitic spread in the tracheobronchial tree. Malignant melanoma and renal cell carcinoma can produce polypoid metastases in tracheal mucosa. Carcinomas of breast, lung, colon, and uterus have all been reported to form discrete tracheal metastases diagnosed by biopsy.

Esophageal squamous cell carcinoma is the neoplasm which most commonly invades the trachea secondarily. Squamous cell carcinoma arising in a main bronchus or in a medial segmental bronchus of an upper lobe may do so likewise. Histologic distinction from tracheal squamous cell carcinoma will not be possible.

Distinctive involvement of the trachea occurs in carcinoma of the thyroid (6), which invades directly into the trachea either from the primary tumor, from recurrent

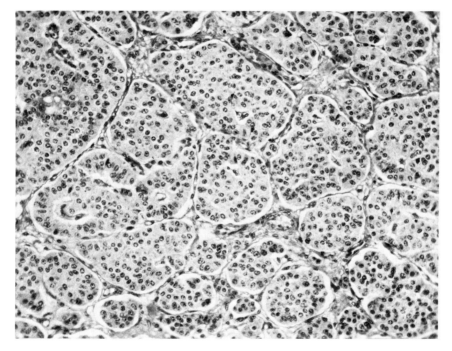

FIG. 3. Carcinoid tumor (×256). Compact islands of monotonous cells are surrounded by delicate fibrous septa. Nuclei are small and oval. Cytoplasm is pale and finely granular.

tumor in cervical soft tissue, or from metastatic tumor in cervical lymph nodes. The primary thyroidal carcinoma need not be clinically obvious. Death due to local disease in cases of thyroidal malignancy is more common with anaplastic than with papillary or follicular carcinomas (34). Anterior or lateral walls of the trachea may be infiltrated by carcinoma of the thyroid, whereas the posterior wall is the site of origin of the primary carcinomas of the trachea. Biopsy of the invasive thyroidal tumor will show, in order of decreasing frequency, anaplastic carcinoma, squamous cell carcinoma, papillary carcinoma, follicular carcinoma, or a combination of these histologic types (Fig. 4).

Hodgkin's disease rarely can extend from a cervical lymph node into and through the wall of the trachea. It may then produce an intratracheal nodule and come to diagnosis on an endoscopic biopsy.

MESENCHYMAL TUMORS

Fibroma–Fibrosarcoma

Fibroma [localized benign fibrous neoplasia (5,15)] outnumbers fibrosarcoma (invasive malignant fibrous neoplasia) (14,27) in the trachea. Both are uncommon because mesenchymal tracheal neoplasms usually exhibit histologic differentiation

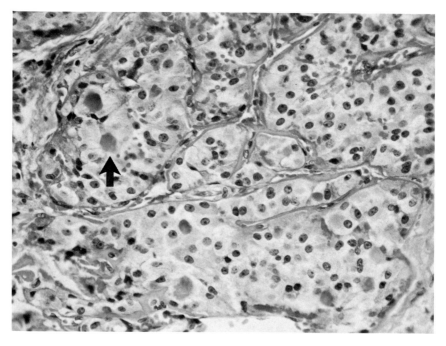

FIG. 4. Recurrent carcinoma of the thyroid invading trachea (×400). Cells with abundant and sharply delineated cytoplasm grow in solid sheets and form a few small follicles *(arrow)* which contain colloid.

more specific than fibrous tissue and then acquire a correspondingly more specific diagnosis, even if the more differentiated tissue (cartilage, smooth muscle, nerve or fat) comprises only a small portion of the tumor. Fibroma may be difficult to distinguish from a fibrous histiocytoma which has minimal inflammation or xanthomatous change. Fibrosarcoma may be difficult to distinguish from a fibrous histiocytoma which invades the tracheal wall.

Chondroma–Chondrosarcoma

Chondroma is the most common of the benign mesenchymal tumors of the trachea (4,13). Chondroma appears grossly as a hard, white, bosselated nodule projecting into the lumen and is composed histologically of chondrocytes without atypicality or mitoses. Extensive ossification may occur. Chondroblastoma, a benign neoplasm composed of smaller and more immature cells, also has arisen in the trachea (14). Chondrosarcoma of the trachea is much less common than chondroma of the trachea. Chondrosarcoma of the larynx may invade distally into the proximal trachea and occurs more frequently than chondrosarcoma of the trachea (18).

Tracheopathia osteoplastica is a pathological entity in which numerous cartilagenous and osseous nodules carpet the tracheal mucosa and may cause tracheal narrowing (44). It is virtually confined to the trachea, never involving the larynx and rarely the bronchi. It occurs primarily in older individuals. A characteristic pattern of calcification may alert the radiologist to the diagnosis, or the endoscopist may unexpectedly encounter tracheopathia osteoplastica either visually or mechanically. It has rarely been implicated as a cause of death. The osseo-cartilagenous nodules form an inner, semicontinuous cylinder contained within an outer, semicontinuous cylinder of normal tracheal cartilages. The inner cylinder is then connected to the outer cylinder by struts of bone, cartilage or fibrous tissue. Tracheopathia osteoplastica is probably a form of ecchondrosis of the internal perichondrium of the tracheal cartilage rings (44).

Leiomyoma–Leiomyosarcoma

Leiomyoma is a benign tumor of smooth muscle. Grossly, it produces a smooth nodule projecting into the lumen of the trachea. Histologically, spindle-shaped cells arrange themselves into characteristic interlacing fascicles. When they occur in the trachea, which is rare, they are found in the lower third (20). Because leiomyomas grow very slowly, some have been successfully treated by endoscopic removal, while others have been resected along with a segment of trachea. Leiomyosarcoma of the trachea is less common than leiomyoma. Histologically, leiomyosarcoma has densely packed cells, pleomorphic nuclei, numerous mitoses, and an infiltrative border. Tracheal leiomyosarcomas invade locally but have not recurred or metastasized after resectional surgery (9,12).

Neurofibroma–Neurofibrosarcoma

Neurofibroma is a benign tumor of Schwann cells. Grossly, it appears as a sessile or pedunculated nodule. Microscopically, richly cellular areas of spindle-shaped cells alternate with poorly cellular areas of myxoid stroma. The proliferating Schwann cells line up in characteristic palisades. The few cases of neurofibroma of the trachea have not been associated with generalized neurofibromatosis (24,38). Tracheal neurofibrosarcoma is very rare. It may permeate diffusely along the tracheal mucosa and through the tracheal wall into the peritracheal adventitia. Histologically, it has atypical nuclei, mitoses, and large areas of myxoid change (Fig. 5). I have seen one case which recurred repeatedly and was extirpated repeatedly. Each recurrence had increased cytologic atypicality.

Lipoma–Liposarcoma

Lipoma of the trachea appears as a yellow, encapsulated nodule of mature fat in the mucosa covered by normal respiratory epithelium. It is rare (4). One case of liposarcoma of the trachea contained pleomorphic nuclei, lipoblasts and mitoses. It did not recur or metastasize (40).

Fibrous Histiocytoma

Fibrous histiocytoma is a histologically benign but locally infiltrative proliferation of fibroblasts and inflammatory cells which may produce an intrabronchial tumor

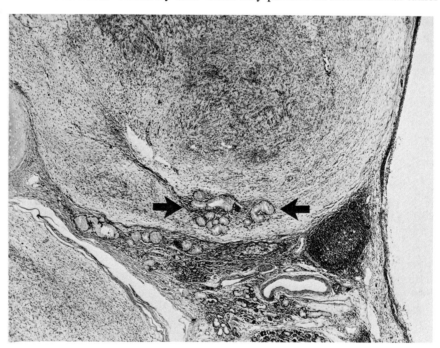

FIG. 5. Neurofibrosarcoma (× 30). Large nodule of fibrillar tumor *(top)* fills the space between cartilage *(left)* and luminal epithelium *(right)* and envelops mucus glands *(arrows)* at its advancing edge.

or, less commonly, an intratracheal polypoid tumor (16,32). When inflammatory cells predominate, the tumor has been termed inflammatory pseudotumor, fibroxanthoma, or plasma cell granuloma (36). The fibroblasts with spindle-shaped nuclei may invade between tracheal cartilages into adventitial tissue and even into thyroid gland (32). The difference between benign and malignant then becomes one of arbitrary definition.

Granular Cell Myoblastoma

Granular cell myoblastoma is a benign neoplasm derived from Schwann cells of peripheral nerves (37). It creates a small and usually solitary nodule in the skin, tongue, gastrointestinal tract or respiratory tract, in order of decreasing frequency. Polygonal cells with uniform nuclei, abundant cytoplasm, and distinct cytoplasmic membranes contain prominent granules which stain positively with the periodic-acid-Schiff technique and ultrastructurally consist of membrane-bound vacuoles containing degenerate cellular organelles. Cells directly beneath the surface epithelium assume a spindle shape.

In the respiratory tract the larynx or bronchi are usually involved. Granular cell myoblastoma is multifocal in approximately 10% of cases, and it is in this group of patients that granular cell myoblastoma usually involves the trachea. The organs involved concurrently with the trachea are bronchus, esophagus or stomach (21,30). Very rarely granular cell myoblastoma presents as a solitary tracheal neoplasm. The neoplastic cells form a mucosal nodule but may also extend for a short distance between the cartilages (21). Malignant and metastasizing granular cell myoblastoma has been reported in some organs but not in the bronchus or trachea.

Hemangioma

Capillary hemangioma is a benign proliferation of blood vessels of small caliber which may cause life threatening tracheal obstruction in infants and children. It may arise in the trachea or extend into it from a hemangioma which is principally in the mediastinum. Within the trachea the hemangioma may diffusely infiltrate the mucosa and inconspicuously narrow the lumen, or it may protrude into the lumen conspicuously as a soft, red, polypoid mass. In children, tracheal hemangiomas consist of closely packed vessels with markedly hyperplastic endothelial cells (10,23). This histology, which in an adult's tumor would raise a suspicion of malignancy, in a child's tumor is innocuous. In adults, hemangiomas of the upper airway are usually in the larynx above the vocal cords, whereas in children they are in the trachea (22).

Tracheal glomus tumor has been reported. Glomus cells surround arteriovenous anastamoses and have functional and morphologic features of smooth muscle cells. Glomus tumor is a highly vascular tumor with proliferating, ectatic, vascular channels surrounded by whorls of glomus cells. In the trachea it is polypoid, circumscribed and benign.

Intratracheal Thyroid

Intratracheal thyroid is an uncommon manifestation of hyperplastic goiter. It typically occurs in middle-aged women who reside in geographic regions where goiter is endemic. Ectopic thyroidal tissue can be discovered in the trachea in approximately one-third of infants. It may or may not be connected to thyroid gland proper (22). Intratracheal thyroid tissue also can be an unusual, incidental microscopic finding in adults. One-fourth of intratracheal goiters occur in patients without clinically obvious external goiters. Upper airway obstruction due to extrinsic pressure by a large thyroid goiter is well recognized, whereas airway obstruction due to intratracheal goiter is less common, less obvious, and less well known, particularly if the thyroid gland has been previously removed by surgery. The hypertrophic thyroid tissue usually appears in the posterolateral wall of the upper third of the trachea as a congested, hemispherical mass covered by smooth, intact mucosa. Histology consists of small and large thyroid follicles, much colloid, and degenerative foci of hemorrhage, inflammation, and fibrosis (7,29).

LYMPHOMA

Lymphocytic lymphoma, Hodgkin's disease, and plasma cell myeloma have all presented primarily as tracheal tumors (1b). Acute leukemia in relapse can produce a localized and obstructing mass in the trachea (1a).

REFERENCES

1. Acquarelli, M. J., Ward, N. O., and Hangos, G. W. (1967): *Ann. Otol. Rhinol. Laryngol.*, 76:843–850.
1a. Barson, A. J., Jones, A. W., and Lodge, K. V. (1968): *J. Clin. Pathol.*, 21:480–485.
1b. Becker, N. H., and Soifer, I. (1971): *Cancer*, 27:712–719.
2. Bennetts, F. E. (1969): *Postgrad. Med. J.*, 45:446–454.
3. Briselli, M., Mark, G. J., and Grillo, H. C. (1978): *Cancer*, 42:2870–2879.
4. Caldarola, V. T., Harrison, E. G., Clagett, O. T., and Schmidt, H. W. (1964): *Ann. Otol. Rhinol. Laryngol.*, 73:1042–1061.
5. Culp, O. S. (1938): *J. Thorac. Surg.*, 7:471–487.
6. Dalby, J. E., and Jones, R. F. M. (1960): *Acta Oto-laryngol.*, 53:12–20.
7. Dowling, E. A., Johnson, I. M., Collier, F. C. D., and Dillard, R. A. (1962): *Ann. Surg.*, 156:258–267.
8. Ellman, P., and Whittaker, H. (1947): *Thorax*, 2:153–162.
9. Eschapasse, H. (1974): *Rev. Fran. Mal. Respir.*, 2:425–446.
10. Flege, J. B., Valencia, G., and Zimmerman, G. (1968): *J. Thorac. Cardiovasc. Surg.*, 56:144–146.
11. Frable, W. J., and Wheelock, M. C. (1962): *Arch. Otolaryngol.*, 76:174–177.
12. Fredrickson, J. M., Jahn, A. F., and Bryce, D. P. (1979): *Ann. Otol.*, 88:463–466.
13. Gilbert, J. G., Mazzarella, L. A., and Feit, L. J. (1953): *Arch. Otolaryngol.*, 58:1–9.
14. Grillo, H. C. (1978): *Ann. Thorac. Surg.*, 26:112–125.
15. Hadju, S. I., Huvos, A. G., Goodner, J. T., Foote, F. W., and Beattie, E. J. (1970): *Cancer*, 25:1448–1456.
16. Hakimi, M., Pai, R. P., Fine, G., and Davila, J. C. (1975): *Chest*, 68:367–368.
17. Houston, H. E., Payne, W. S., Harrison, E. G., and Olsen, A. M. (1969): *Arch. Surg.*, 99:132–140.
18. Huizenga, C., and Balogh, K. (1970): *Cancer*, 26:201–210.
19. Kay, S., and Brooks, J. W. (1970): *Cancer*, 25:1178–1182.

20. Kitamura, S., Maeda, M., Kawashima, U., Masaoka, A., and Manabe, H. (1969): *J. Thorac. Cardiovasc. Surg.*, 57:126–133.
21. Krouse, T. B., and Mobini, J. (1973): *Arch. Pathol.*, 96:95–99.
22. Landing, B. H. (1979): *Am. Rev. Respir. Dis.*, 120:151–185.
23. Littler, E. R. (1963): *J. Thorac. Cardiovasc. Surg.*, 45:552–558.
24. Karlan, M. S., Livingston, P. A., and Baker, D. C. (1973): *Ann. Otol.*, 82:790–799.
25. Ma, C. K., Fine, G., Lewis, J., and Lee, M. W. (1979): *Cancer*, 44:2260–2266.
26. Marsh, W. L., and Allen, M. S., Jr. (1979): *Cancer*, 43:1463–1473.
27. McCafferty, G. J., Parker, L. S., and Suggit, S. C. (1964): *J. Laryngol. Otol.*, 78:441–479.
28. Moersch, H. J., Clagett, O. T., and Ellis, F. H. (1954): *Med. Clin. North. Am.*, 38:1091–1097.
29. Myers, E. N., and Pantangco, I. P., Jr. (1975): *Laryngoscope*, 85:1833–1840.
30. O'Connell, D. J., MacMahon, H., and DeMeester, T. R. (1978): *Thorax*, 33:596–602.
31. Pearson, F. G., Thompson, D. W., Weissberg, D., Simpson, W. J. K., and Kergin, F. G. (1974): *Ann. Thorac. Surg.*, 18:16–29.
32. Sandstrom, R. E., Proppe, K. H., and Trelstad, R. L. (1978): *Am. J. Clin. Pathol.*, 70:429–433.
33. Salm, R. (1964): *Br. J. Dis. Chest.*, 58:61–72.
34. Silverberg, S. G., Hutter, R. V. P., and Foote, F. W. (1970): *Cancer*, 25:792–802.
35. Soorae, A. S., and Gibbons, J. R. P. (1979): *Thorax*, 34:130–131.
36. Spoto, G., Rossi, N. P., and Allsbrook, W. C. (1977): *J. Thorac. Cardiovasc. Surg.*, 73:804–806.
37. Strong, E. W., McDivitt, R. W., and Brasfield, R. D. (1970): *Cancer*, 25:415–422.
38. Thijs-Van Nies, A., Van de Brekel, B., Buytendijk, H. J., and Maesen, F. (1978): *Thorax*, 33:121–123.
39. Trentini, G. P., and Palmieri, B. (1972): *Chest*, 62:336–338.
40. Van den Beukel, J. T. I., Wagenaar, S. J. S. C., and Vanderschueren, R. (1979): *Thorax*, 34:817–818.
41. Weber, A. L., and Grillo, H. C. (1978): *Adv. Oto-Rhino-Laryngol.*, 24:170–176.
42. Weisel, W., and Lepley, D. (1961): *Pediatrics*, 28:394–398.
43. Wilkins, E. W., Darling, R. C., Soutter, L., and Sniffen, R. C. (1963): *J. Thorac. Cardiovasc. Surg.*, 46:279–291.
44. Young, R. H., Sandstrom, R. E., and Mark, G. J. (1980): *J. Thorac. Cardiovasc. Surg.*, 79:537–541.
45. Zunker, H. O., Moore, R. L., Baker, D. C., and Lattes, R. (1969): *Cancer*, 23:699–707.

Thoracic Oncology, edited by N. C. Choi and
H. C. Grillo. Raven Press, New York © 1983.

Tracheal Tumors: Diagnosis and Management

Hermes C. Grillo

*General Thoracic Surgical Unit, Massachusetts General Hospital,
Boston, Massachusetts 02114*

Primary tracheal tumors are among the rarest of the thoracic neoplasms. This very rarity has contributed to the slow accumulation of data about their clinical behavior, to the lag in development of techniques for their surgical management and, particularly, to the limited development of single institutional series (3,6,10,11,12,16).

Between 1962 and 1981 110 patients were seen at the Massachusetts General Hospital with primary tracheal tumors (10). Forty-three had primary squamous cell carcinoma of the trachea. This group excludes extensions of squamous cell carcinoma of larynx, lung, or esophagus. The second most common primary tumor was adenoid cystic carcinoma (formerly cylindroma) seen in 38 patients. Twenty-nine additional patients had tumors of varying diagnoses: chondrosarcoma, carcinosarcoma, carcinoid, spindle cell sarcoma, adenosquamous carcinoma, adenocarcinoma, mucoepidermoid carcinoma, myxoid spindle cell sarcoma, monocytic leukemia, chondroma, chondroblastoma, squamous papilloma, granular cell tumor, hemangioma, and fibroma.

The most common presenting signs and symptoms of primary tracheal tumors are those of upper airway obstruction, cough and hemoptysis (5,20). Shortness of breath, initially on exertion, and, if allowed to progress long enough, even at rest, was common. Varying degrees of wheezing and stridor were also seen. These symptoms were predominant in those patients who did not initially present with hemoptysis, which led earlier to vigorous diagnostic approaches. Several patients presented with unilateral and bilateral recurrent pneumonitis or pneumonia. Delay in diagnosis, especially where hemoptysis did not occur, was common. Patients presenting with wheezing or stridor would often have a chest x-ray which was interpreted as normal since the lung fields were clear. On a number of occasions they were diagnosed as adult onset asthma and so treated. In one extreme case the patient was treated for nine years for asthma and when the diagnosis was finally made of a slowly growing benign tracheal tumor, he was on 50 mg a day of Prednisone.

Symptoms and signs vary with specific types of tumor (15). Hemoptysis occurred in 64% of patients with squamous cell carcinoma and in 28% of those with adenoid cystic carcinoma. While only 39% of those with squamous lesions presented with dyspnea, 69% of those with adenoid cystic carcinoma were short of breath. This variation reflects the rate of progression of the two principal types of primary tracheal cancer. Asthma was a frequent diagnosis especially in patients with slowly growing benign tumors which only infrequently produced hemoptysis.

Simple radiological studies are used to determine the presence of a suspected tracheal neoplasm or to define its extent (20). We have found the use of contrast medium to be unnecessary. Although slightly better definition can be obtained by the instillation of liquid contrast media or the insufflation of powdered tantalum (not approved for general use), careful study using air as the contrast medium gives elegant definition (14). Xerography can provide added detail. Our usual radiological work-up of a patient with a tracheal tumor consists of posteroanterior and lateral chest roentgenograms along with the right and left anterior oblique views. A copper-filtered view of the entire airway from the top of the larynx to the carina gives valuable information, not only about the location of the tumor in relation to other structures and the presence of extramural projection but also, of equal importance, about the amount of grossly normal airway present above and below the tumor. Fluoroscopy is essential to determine functional involvement of the larynx. Spot films taken during the fluoroscopy are also very useful to define specific facets of a tumor's extent. Increasingly, tomography has become unnecessary. In specific instances, however, both anteroposterior and lateral tomograms are useful. For any tumor which does or is likely to extend beyond the tracheal wall a barium swallow may give added information about such extension. Full lung tomograms are useful, particularly in lesions such as adenoid cystic carcinoma, to establish the presence of pulmonary metastases, all too common with this disease. Radiologic definition should usually precede endoscopy since it serves as a road map for the broncho-scopist. This does not preclude use of bronchoscopy as an initial scanning mode where a tumor is suspected on the basis of such symptoms as persistent cough or recurrent localized pneumonitis.

On a few occasions pulmonary function studies, particularly flow volume loops, have led to the suspicion of an upper airway tumor in a patient previously considered to have an asthmatic wheeze (19). Generally, function studies contribute little of practical interest to the management of patients with primary tracheal tumors. The obstruction usually requires relief and most patients are able to tolerate procedures required for this relief.

Sooner or later bronchoscopy is necessary. With a radiologically well defined tumor which appears to be potentially resectable for cure, bronchoscopy may be deferred until the surgeon is prepared to go ahead with resection. Biopsy will generally be done at this time and frozen section diagnosis obtained. Surgical treatment of tracheal tumors should not be undertaken without excellent frozen section diagnosis facilities, not alone for initial diagnosis but for determination of margins and nodal involvement. In the case of some extensively infiltrating tumors, biopsies taken proximally and distally to the visible extent of tumor may demonstrate infiltration far beyond this point, declaring the lesion to be surgically irremovable.

With lesions of questionable resectability, bronchoscopy is done as an initial, separate procedure.

Patients may present initially with life endangering obstruction. Partial endoscopic removal of tumor obstructing the lumen of the airway may occasionally be needed to obtain time for the initiation of palliative irradiation treatment or, more rarely, for further study of a patient's medical status. In my own practice such emergency provision of airway has been possible with conventional instruments through a rigid bronchoscope. The laser has also been utilized for this purpose (13). Obviously, laser removal of that portion of a tumor which obstructs the lumen is not curative.

We are still in a period of determining what is the best method of treatment of the various primary tumors of the trachea. At the present time, however, direct surgical resection with primary reconstruction appears to offer the most prompt relief of symptoms, the most prolonged palliation, and in many cases the probability of cure. Resection and primary reconstruction of the trachea and carina have only been utilized to any degree since 1962 when the techniques of anatomic mobilization were first applied to extend the possibilities of these procedures. Of the 110 patients seen in this 19 year period, 41 were not subjected to resection. Some had lesions which were clearly too extensive for surgical removal, some had multiple distant metastases, and others had lesions which appeared to be best treated conservatively. The latter included juvenile papillomas, extensive squamous papillomas with atypism, and a hemangioma presenting in the trachea with evidence of extensive congenital vascular malformation involving the mediastinum widely. Patients with squamous cell carcinoma who did not undergo resection generally had lesions which were clearly either too extensive along the length of the trachea or had extended too deeply into mediastinal structures to be considered for surgical resection. Several patients with adenoid cystic carcinoma also had invasion of the mediastinum or mucosal or submucosal extension over too long a length to permit primary resection. In several cases adenoid cystic carcinoma was centered at the carina but invasion was demonstrated by biopsy as far down as the right and left upper lobe takeoffs on both sides.

Sixty-two of the 110 patients underwent some type of surgical resection either with primary reconstruction, or in some cases, with the hope or attempt at reconstruction at a second stage. Seven more underwent laryngo-tracheal resection, usually for adenoid cystic carcinoma involving the larynx as well as a large part of the trachea. During the same period 33 patients with secondary tumors involving the trachea were treated by attempts at surgical extirpation. This group principally included carcinoma of the thyroid although there were some patients with other primary tumors, such as esophageal carcinoma or carcinoid tumors of bronchi recurrent in the stump of the main bronchus. Table 1 summarizes the distribution of these patients, primary and secondary, and their methods of treatment. Resection and primary reconstruction was possible in 19 patients with squamous carcinoma, 16 with adenoid cystic carcinoma, and 19 with other types of primary tumors. Where squamous cell carcinoma involved the carina resection was often not possible.

TABLE 1. *Management of tracheal tumors at Massachusetts General Hospital (1962–1981)*

Treatment	Primary tumors			Secondary tumors	Total
	Squamous cell	Adenoid cystic	Other		
Resection and anastomosis	19	16	19	19	73
Resection for staged reconstruction	2	5	1	4	12
Laryngo-tracheal reconstruction	1	5	1	10	17
Exploration	2	2	1	1	6
Irradiation, tracheostomy, or no treatment	19	10	7	—	36
Total	43	38	29	34	144

Lateral resection was only possible in two patients with small secondary tumors of thyroid involving the tracheal wall.

The techniques of tracheal resection and reconstruction have been well described in other publications (4,7,9). Tumors of the upper trachea were approached generally through an anterior exposure, with the potential provided for extending the exposure into the right hemi-thorax if necessary (8). This contrasts with the approach to benign inflammatory lesions of the trachea. In most cases of primary malignant tumors it is wise for the surgeon to consider the possibility of such an extension in nearly every case. Tumors in the lower half of the trachea, on the other hand, and those of the carina, are approached through a transthoracic incision. After an initial experience utilizing a trap-door type of approach, which involved a partial median-sternotomy with extension into the right hemi-thorax, I chose posterolateral thoracotomy as the preferred route of approach. The neck, however, is prepared so that laryngeal release, if necessary, may be accomplished with ease. There is great variability in the approach which must be used for specific problems. On occasion the approach has been through the left side where a special problem presented which was likely to require a left pneumonectomy and only limited approach to the carina. At times the effort was made to preserve the anterior chest wall skin in situations which might have ended up requiring a mediastinal tracheostomy either as a definitive or as part of a staged approach. Median sternotomy does not provide a truly adequate approach to the carina where significant dissection is necessary.

An extensive *en bloc* approach is not really possible if reconstruction is to be done. Other mediastinal structures prevent such an approach even as they do in surgery of the esophagus. Fortunately, many of these lesions do not extend widely into the mediastinum. In contrast to the surgery of inflammatory disease where the dissection is kept close to the trachea itself, as a way of avoiding injury to the recurrent nerves which may be involved in scar, in the case of tumor the surgeon deliberately identifies the nerves at some distance from the tumor and then attempts to encompass as much of the peritracheal tissue in the region of the tumor as is possible. The blood supply, however, of the residual trachea must be carefully preserved.

The multiple techniques for obtaining sufficient length for reconstruction have been detailed (7). These include mobilization of the hilum of the right lung, including intrapericardial release, elevation of the right main bronchus to the trachea, and flexion of the neck to devolve the trachea into the mediastinum as far as possible. Laryngeal release has been a useful adjunct also. In extreme situations other techniques have also been additionally used. The effort is made, however, to attempt to plan the extent of the resection as much as possible before actually embarking upon irrevocable steps.

Carinal reconstruction is accomplished in a variety of ways depending on the individual problem (9). It is difficult in most cases to plan precisely what will be the safest and easiest method in a given situation until the tumor itself has been removed. While it is attractive experimentally and theoretically to think of reapproximating the right and left main bronchi and then suturing the trachea to form a new carina, usually this is disadvantageous. The left main bronchus is tethered in position by the level of the aortic arch. If the right bronchus is then sewed to the left, the carinal point is fixed and it is necessary for the trachea to be advanced distally to reach the new carina. Where a greater extent of trachea has been removed, it is much simpler to anastomose the trachea either to the elevated right main bronchus or to the left main bronchus. If the length of trachea which has been removed has been extensive, usually it is necessary to anastomose the trachea to the right main bronchus, which can be elevated. In that case, the left main bronchus is sutured into the bronchus intermedius using the technique first described by Barclay, McSwan, and Welsh (1). In other situations, the right or left main bronchi may be more simply anastomosed to an opening made in the lateral margin of the lower trachea following the primary anastomosis between the end of the trachea and the appropriate main bronchus. The length of trachea which can be removed and anastomosis yet accomplished primarily varies enormously with the age, anatomic build of the patient, and extensibility of the tissues.

In 73 patients with both primary and secondary tumors who underwent surgical resection with direct reconstruction there were five hospital deaths related to the surgical procedure. In one case the cause of failure was surgery done in the face of very high-dose irradiation given years before. This has been avoided in subsequent cases. Three of the other four patients had undergone carinal reconstruction. These operations were done for extensive malignant lesions, one of which required a concomitant pneumonectomy. In general, where the lesions were so extensive that staged reconstructions were undertaken with the hope of later reconstruction, the disease proved to be incurable. On the basis of this experience it was concluded that patients with such extensive disease would better receive palliative irradiation than undergo this type of extended surgery—whether with later reconstruction or with a prosthesis placed at the time of the resection.

The number of patients treated by attempts at curative resection is small and, therefore, makes it difficult to predict what will be the eventual outcome. In 1978

(6) a group of 36 resected patients were studied. There were five patients of the group with squamous cell carcinoma alive and without known disease, over periods ranging from 10 months to 13½ years after operation. Three of those had been followed for more than 2 years. One additional patient had developed recurrent disease 1½ years after resection and one had further squamous carcinomas of both oro-pharynx and respiratory tree. Another had died 2 years later from myocardial infarction or pulmonary embolism without known recurrence. An additional patient had gone nearly 3 years after resection but with the use of irradiation when positive lymph nodes appeared subsequently. There were six with adenoid cystic carcinoma known to be living without disease. The heterogenous group of patients with benign tumors of the trachea or with tumors of low-grade malignancy did best on the whole. It is worth noting that respectable palliation was obtained in some of the patients who had resections for secondary tumors, particularly in those with low-grade thyroid carcinoma. Current survival figures are listed in Table 2.

While this series is a small one, it does compare closely with the cumulative results tabulated by Eschapasse (3) in 1974. He collected a series of 152 patients with primary tracheal tumors treated by 12 French and two Russian groups. Thirty-two cylindrical resections had been accomplished with primary anastomosis and a further 18 reconstructions. The largest number of these cases were reported from the work of Perelman (17). The longterm results were similar to the series just reported in that the best results were seen with benign tumors and carcinoid tumors. Those with adenoid cystic carcinoma demonstrated prolonged survival but late recurrences. Squamous cell carcinoma produced the poorest results. Pearson and his associates (16) reported a series of 14 patients with adenoid cystic carcinoma treated by circumferential resection and two with lateral resection. Five underwent primary anastomosis, six were treated by prosthetic replacement and three by laryngotracheiectomy. There were eight alive and free of tumor 2 to 18 years later. Houston and coworkers (12) reported a small series of patients treated by primary resection. Most of the other reports in the literature are of single cases or very small numbers of cases treated surgically or by other means (11). Pearson and his group applied radiotherapy in medium dosage preoperatively. We have generally used irradiation for adenoid cystic carcinoma either as primary treatment in extensive lesions or postoperatively in those lesions demonstrated to have either tumor close

TABLE 2. *Results of primary resection and reconstruction (1962–1981)*

	Squamous cell	Adenoid cystic	Other primary	Secondary	Totals
Total resected	19	16	19	19	73
Operative survivors	17	15	18	18	68
Alive without disease	12	12	15	12	51
Alive with disease	1	0	2	0	3
Dead with disease	3	3	1	6	13
Dead—Other disease	1	0	0	0	1

to the margins, at the margins of resection or in lymph nodes. Most adenoid cystic carcinoma is responsive to irradiation despite earlier feelings to the contrary. Patients receiving primary radiotherapy have remained apparently tumor-free for as long as 5 years or more. In time, recurrence is usually the rule. Whereas squamous cell carcinoma has also responded to irradiation, recurrence has been much more prompt, parallel with the experience in squamous carcinoma of the lung.

At the present time, on the basis of the results just described, I continue to use surgical resection in squamous cell carcinoma and adenoid cystic carcinoma primary in the trachea as the procedure of choice, provided I feel that primary repair can be done after the tumor has been encompassed. Irradiation hasthen been added in accord with the indications described above. Irradiation is used primarily in "curative" doses if the lesion is deemed to be beyond the scope of resection. Although I have not seen such a circumstance yet, I agree with the suggestion of Eschapasse (3) that, given the long course of most patients with adenoid cystic carcinoma, even palliative resection would be indicated for a tumor of limited extent despite the presence of pulmonary metastases. Primary radiotherapy has been proposed for all tracheal tumors (18), but the data do not seem to support this election. Surgical resection seems clearly to be the treatment of choice for most other primary tumors of the trachea whether benign in character or of low-grade malignancy.

REFERENCES

1. Barclay, R. S. McSwan, N., and Welsh, T. M. (1957): Tracheal reconstruction without the use of grafts. *Thorax*, 12:177.
2. Briselli, M., Mark, E. J., and Grillo, H. C. (1978): Tracheal carcinoids. *Cancer*, 42:2870.
3. Eschapasse, H., (1974): Les tumeurs tracheales primitives: Traitement chirurgical. *Rev. Fr. Malad. Resp.*, 2:425.
4. Grillo, H. C. (1970): Surgery of the trachea. *Current Prob. Surg.*, July.
5. Grillo, H. C. (1977): Tracheal tumors. In: *Rhoads Textbook of Surgery*, 5th ed., edited by J. Hardy, pp.1364–1371. Lippincott, Philadelphia.
6. Grillo, H. C. (1978): Tracheal tumors: Surgical management. *Ann. Thor. Surg.*, 26:112.
7. Grillo, H. C. (1981): Surgery of the trachea. In: *Operative Surgery and Management*, edited by G. Keen, pp. 651–660. John Wright, Ltd., Bristol, England.
8. Grillo, H. C. (1981): Tumors of the cervical trachea. In: *Cancer of the Head and Neck*, edited by J. Y. Suen and E. N. Myers, pp. 500–523. Churchill Livingstone, New York.
9. Grillo, H. C. (1982): Carinal resection. *Ann. Thorac. Surg.*, 34:356.
10. Grillo, H. C. (1982) Management of tracheal tumors. *Am. J. Surg.*, 143:697.
11. Hajdu, S. I., Huvos, A. G., Goodner, J. T., Foote, F. W., Jr., and Beattie, E. J., Jr. (1970): Carcinoma of the trachea: Clinicopathologic study of 41 cases. *Cancer*, 25:1448.
12. Houston, H. G., Payne, W. S., and Harrison, E. G., Jr. (1969): Primary cancers of the trachea. *Arch. Surg.*, 99:132.
13. Laforet, E. G., Berger, R. I., and Vaughan, C. W. (1976): Carcinoma obstructing the trachea. Treatment by laser resection. *N. Engl. J. Med.*, 294:941.
14. Momose, K. R., and MacMillan, A. S., Jr. (1978): Roentgenologic investigations of the larynx and trachea. *Radiol. Clin. N.A.*, 16:321.
15. Morgan, R. J., and Grillo, H. C. (1982): Clinical presentation of primary tracheal tumors—a frequently misdiagnosed entity. (*Submitted for publication.*)
16. Pearson, F. G., Thompson, D. W., Weissberg, D., Simpson, W., Jr., and Kergin, F. G. (1974): Adenoid cystic carcinoma of the trachea. Experience with 16 patients managed by tracheal resection. *Ann. Thorac. Surg.*, 18:16.
17. Perelman, M. I., and Koroleva, N. (1980): Surgery of the trachea. *World J. Surg.*, 4:583.

18. Rostom, A. Y., and Morgan, R. L. (1978): Results of treating primary tumors of the trachea by irradiation. *Thorax*, 33:387.
19. Strieder, D. J. (1975): Case records of the Massachusetts General Hospital: Case 42, 1975. *N. Engl. J. Med.*, 293:866.
20. Weber, A. L., and Grillo, H. C. (1978): Tracheal tumors: A radiological clinical and pathological evaluation of 84 cases. *Radiol. Clin. N.A.*, 16:227.
21. Weber, A. L., Shortsleeve, M., Goodman, M., Montgomery, W. W., and Grillo, H. C. (1978): Cartilaginous tumors of the larynx and trachea. *Radiol. Clin. N.A.*, 16:261.

Thoracic Oncology, edited by N. C. Choi and
H. C. Grillo. Raven Press, New York © 1983.

Carcinoma of the Esophagus: A Current Perspective

Mark R. Katlic and Hermes C. Grillo

*General Thoracic Surgical Unit and the Surgical Services, Massachusetts General
Hospital, and the Department of Surgery, Harvard Medical School,
Boston, Massachusetts 02114*

A paper published over a decade ago was entitled "Carcinoma of the Esophagus:
A Disaster" (44); indeed, few diagnoses embody more morbid or mortal prospects.
In esophageal cancer one is faced with malignancy in an advanced state, often with
a cachectic patient who is unable to swallow. A century after Czerny's first esophageal resection the surgeon can offer such a patient palliation and increased survival
but a very limited possibility of cure. Carcinoma of the esophagus remains a disaster,
but perhaps less so than ever before.

INCIDENCE

In the United States, esophageal carcinoma represents 1.1% of all cancers in
both sexes, excluding skin tumors; the average age-adjusted incidence rate for
esophageal cancer is 3.4 cases per 100,000 (30). Silverberg and Holleb (72) estimated in 1975 that approximately 7,400 cases occurred annually in the United States
and that there were approximately 6,300 deaths annually due to esophageal carcinoma.

It is more often a disease of the elderly, with the majority of cases occurring in
the sixth and seventh decades of life. In a series of 142 resected cases from the
Massachusetts General Hospital, 1962–1970, the average age was 63 years (range,
41–84 years), and was equal in males and females. Esophageal cancer is virtually
unknown in childhood; Pickett and Briggs (64) in 1967 reported only three cases
in a 5-year survey of cancer of the gastrointestinal tract in childhood. Males are
affected more often than females by a ratio, in the United States, of 3 to 1.
Esophageal cancer accounts for a higher percentage of all cancers among blacks
(3.1%) than among whites (0.9%), and is particularly important among black males:
the average age-adjusted incidence rate for black males is 16.7 per 100,000, 3.6
times that of white males (17). The incidence may be rising in black males, although
reasons for this are unclear.

Geographical variations in the occurrence of esophageal cancer are great (20).
Within the United States, males living in industrial areas, such as the northeast or
Chicago, have a greater chance of developing esophageal cancer, irrespective of

their smoking or drinking habits. There is increased incidence for females in certain states such as North Carolina, Georgia, and Texas, as well as in the northeastern states. Within the western hemisphere there is lower incidence in Canada and increased occurrence in Puerto Rico and Jamaica. In some areas of Europe, namely Normandy and Brittany, the incidence is markedly increased for males; the male-to-female ratio in these regions approaches 23 to 1. Esophageal cancer is virtually unknown in western Africa; however, in other areas of the continent hyperendemic areas, such as South Africa among the Bantu, alternate with areas of low frequency. Parts of Iran show striking variations in incidence of esophageal carcinoma, variations that appear to parallel those of climate and landscape; there seems to be increased incidence, for example, in areas of arid climate and alkaline soil irrespective of alcohol or tobacco use (47). In Ceylon, esophageal cancer is the most common gastrointestinal tumor, and this may be related to the chewing of betel gum.

Some of the most interesting epidemiologic data has come from the Lin Xian valley of China. In this 20-square-mile area, one in four people dies of esophageal cancer, yet 30 miles away the incidence falls by one-half (15).

ETIOLOGY

Proposed etiologic factors in esophageal cancer have been nicely summarized by Haas and Schottenfeld (30). Alcohol can clearly be related to esophageal cancer in the United States and Europe. Virtually all recent series of esophageal cancer patients show a heavy preponderance of drinkers. At the Massachusetts General Hospital, heavy drinkers comprise 65% of patients with esophageal cancer. Wynder and Bross (90) showed that in two New York City hospitals, average daily alcohol intake of male esophageal cancer patients was greater than that of male control patients with cancers at other locations. Binge drinkers and those drinking excessively made up 34% of the esophageal cancer group and only 13% of the control group. These relationships pertained irrespective of smoking habits. Although the exact mechanism whereby alcohol leads to esophageal cancer is unclear, it seems not to be related to nitrosamine compounds (12), but may be related in some way to the introduction of maize products as a major ingredient in alcoholic drinks (13). Prohibition of alcohol may be related to the low incidence of esophageal cancer seen in certain religious groups in the United States. On the other hand, those areas of Iran which see high rates of esophageal cancer are inhabited by Islamic peoples for whom alcohol is disallowed.

Tobacco use has been strongly associated with esophageal cancer, particularly smoking cigarettes. Wynder and Bross (90) found that more esophageal cancer patients than controls smoked more than 21 cigarettes per day, or smoked cigars or pipes; smokers in the esophageal cancer group also smoked to a shorter butt length than did controls. It has been estimated that the risk of esophageal cancer in smokers is 2 to 6 times that of nonsmokers, with increased risk proportional to the amount smoked. Cigar and pipe smokers also are felt to have risks 2 to 4 times that of controls (90). At the Massachusetts General Hospital, 77% of esophageal cancer patients used tobacco, 64% using cigarettes. A synergism between alcohol and tobacco has been proposed but not proven. At the Massachusetts General Hospital, 59% of patients used both alcohol and tobacco. In 1978, Norton et al. (57) reported a 10-fold increase in the incidence of esophageal carcinoma in patients with previous head and neck carcinomas, and suggested performing screening barium swallows in this high-risk group of head and neck carcinoma patients. It is likely, however, that this association reflects the excessive use of alcohol and tobacco by these patients.

Other esophageal abnormalities, particularly those predisposing to mucosal irritation, have been associated with esophageal carcinoma. Kirivanta, in 1952 (41), found nine esophageal cancers in 381 individuals with esophageal corrosions, 90% of which were due to lye ingestion. He estimated that the risk of developing esophageal cancer in this group was, therefore, a 100-fold greater than for others in the same age group. There may, however, be increased resection rate and chance of long survival in these patients (36). The latency period between lye ingestion and cancer ranged from 24 to 44 years. Others (40) have reported esophageal cancer developing as early as 12 years after lye stricture.

Achalasia has been associated with esophageal cancer. Just-Viera and Haight, in 1969 (39), studied 160 cases collected from English literature of esophageal cancer in patients with achalasia. They estimated that in those patients with prior achalasia there was a three- to ten-fold increase in risk of developing esophageal cancer compared to the normal population; the esophageal cancer in their patients developed an average of 17 years after the onset of initial symptoms of achalasia. Wychulis et al. (89) at the Mayo Clinic found seven cases of esophageal cancer in 1,318 patients treated for achalasia, an incidence rate of 41 cases per 100,000 per year. Achalasia symptoms had been present an average of 28 years prior to development of esophageal cancer.

Plummer-Vinson syndrome has long been felt to be associated with esophageal cancer, though recent widespread recognition and treatment of this disorder have made few cases available for study. In some rural areas of Sweden, for example, iron deficiency anemia and vitamin B deficiencies are endemic, and in these areas there is both an increased incidence of Plummer-Vinson syndrome and carcinoma of the upper third of the esophagus. In these areas, there are more upper-one-third lesions in females than in males, in keeping with the syndrome (91). In 142 patients undergoing resection for esophageal carcinoma at the Massachusetts General Hospital, one patient had a prior history of Plummer-Vinson syndrome, one caustic stricture, and two achalasia.

In areas of the world where tobacco and alcohol use are common, dietary and soil factors may play a special role. In the Lin Xian region of China, for example, soil has been found to be low in molybdenum, prohibiting plants from concentrating vitamin C and thereby leading to a diet low in vitamin C. At the same time, the diet here is high in nitrates, as well as in amines from moldy bread products. The lack of vitamin C further interferes with the body's defense against these high nitrates, and nitrosamine compounds may therefore accumulate (8). As noted above, in areas of Iran such as the Caspian littoral, the dietary effects of local soil characteristics, e.g., alkalinity, may be significant. Molds that produce carcinogens such as aflatoxin may be limited to particular geographic areas and may be responsible for the high incidence of carcinoma here.

The one hereditary disorder associated with esophageal cancer is tylosis, an autosomal dominant trait characterized by hyperkeratosis of the palms and soles. Two English families with this form of tylosis have been followed; it is estimated that 95% of the members of these families with tylosis will have died of esophageal cancer before age 65, while no cases of esophageal cancer have been found in those family members without tylosis (33).

PATHOLOGY

Histology

Nearly all esophageal carcinomas are squamous cell carcinomas. In a review of 1,918 patients with cancer of the esophagus seen at Memorial Hospital, 1926–1968 (83), only 3.4% were not squamous cell and a proportion of these were atypical squamous cell. Raphael et al. in 1966 (68) reviewed 1,312 patients seen at the Mayo Clinic, 1946–1963, and also the literature on primary adenocarcinoma of the esophagus. Their conclusion was that only 0.6% of these patients had primary adenocarcinoma. It seems reasonable to conclude that while a rare primary adenocarcinoma of the esophagus may arise in an esophageal gland or an area of Barrett's esophagus, most adenocarcinomas near the gastroesophageal junction are of gastric origin, and that esophageal carcinoma is a squamous cell cancer.

Site

For purposes of classification, staging, and reporting of cancer, the esophagus may be divided into three anatomic areas: the upper, the middle, and the lower thirds. The American Joint Committee for Cancer Staging and End Results Reporting (4) defines these regions as follows: (a) The cervical esophagus extends from the pharyngoesophageal junction, the cricopharyngeal sphincter, down to the level of the thoracic inlet, approximately 18 cm from the upper incisor teeth. (b) The middle third extends from the thoracic inlet to a point 10 cm above the gastroesophageal junction, a point usually at the level of the border of the eighth thoracic vertebra and approximately 31 cm from the upper incisor teeth. (c) The lower third extends from a point 10 cm above the gastroesophageal junction to the cardiac orifice of the stomach, a point approximately 40 cm from the upper incisor teeth. Postlethwait (65), in a collected series of 14,181 cases of squamous cell carcinoma of the esophagus, found 15% in the upper one-third, 52% in the mid–one–third, and 33% in the lower one-third of the esophagus. Of 142 recently resected cases from the Massachusetts General Hospital, 20% were in the upper one-third, 49% in the mid–one-third, and 31% in the lower one-third.

Gross and Microscopic Appearance

In the Lin Xian valley of China, an area hyperendemic for esophageal cancer, screening for this lesion is carried out yearly by scraping for cytology with an endoesophageal balloon catheter. Evidence from this ongoing study (8) has shown that 50% of all people screened switch from normal mucosa to hyperplasia and back again. Twelve percent of individuals went on to severe hyperplasia, a condition that appears to be a precursor to esophageal carcinoma. Of these patients with severe hyperplasia, one-third regressed to normal mucosa, one-third remained with severe hyperplasia, and one-third evolved into frank carcinoma. The earliest gross appearance of carcinoma of the esophagus, therefore, may be an area of hyperplastic mucosa, though this has rarely been found in this country. Esophageal carcinoma is generally seen as an infiltrative, fungating, or ulcerative lesion, or occasionally a polypoid one. The most common gross presentation is as a combination of these forms with a fungating, ulcerated intraluminal appearance with infiltration of the esophageal wall, causing concentric luminal narrowing by means of fibrous growth and contraction. Undermining of the edges may occur, with pale, friable tumor tissue extending beneath normal-appearing mucosa. In other cases, necrotic friable tissue may cover the ulcer bed. Extensive submucosal spread of tumor may occur 4 cm or more from the gross margin of the tumor (10). Microscopically, the lesion is that of squamous cell carcinoma, though of variable differentiation. Some are well-differentiated with evidence of keratin formation, flat squamous cells, and intracellular bridging, but the majority are less well-differentiated.

Metastasis

Local spread of esophageal cancer is favored by many features including extensive lymphatics and lack of serosal covering. All structures of the neck, mediastinum, and thorax may potentially be involved by local spread of an esophageal cancer. There is frequent spread to the tracheobronchial tree, more often the trachea or left mainstem bronchus; extension may also involve the pericardium, diaphragm, aorta, or great vessels. The recurrent laryngeal nerves may become involved. Metastases to lymph nodes are frequent and, while generally near the primary lesion, may also occur in more distant groups of nodes. Submucosal lymphatics travel several centimeters longitudinally before joining lymphatics in the adventitia, which then also run longitudinally before draining to a node group. McCort's classic study in 1952 (50) identified eight groups of lymph nodes to which esophageal cancer might spread. Upper one-third lesions were drained by internal jugular, paratracheal, and, in some cases, perihilar lymph nodes; mid–one-third lesions were drained by nodes around the esophagus and near the carina; lower one-third and gastroesophageal junction nodes were drained, in addition to nodes near the cardia, by left gastric and celiac nodes. Postlethwait (65), in a collected series of 2,440 autopsy cases, found 564 cases with lymph node metastases. The most frequent sites of nodal metastases were mediastinal (484 cases), abdominal (236 cases), paratracheal and paraesophageal (220 cases), and cervical and supraclavicular (136 cases). The most frequent sites of distant metastases in that series were liver, lung, bone, and kidney. The brain appears to be a rare site for metastasis from esophageal carcinoma.

STAGING

Carcinoma of the esophagus is staged on the basis of the TNM system. The various categories of T, N, and M are grouped into appropriate combinations to categorize three stages of the disease. Classification may then be carried out clinically, at the time of surgical exploration, and postsurgically when pathologic information is available. Simply speaking, Stage I represents a tumor limited to the esophagus and involving 5 cm or less of esophageal length and which produces no obstruction. A Stage II lesion involves more than 5 cm of esophageal length or produces obstruction; if it is a cervical lesion, it may also involve palpable, moveable, regional nodes. A Stage III lesion is any esophageal cancer at any level with distant metastases, extra esophageal spread, or fixed lymph node metastases; any intrathoracic esophageal cancer with any positive regional lymph node is Stage III.

Stage I carcinoma is rare in the United States. Postlethwait and Musser (66), in a series of 1,000 autopsy specimens of the esophagus, found only three cases of carcinoma *in situ*. With cytologic screening, however, it appears that a great many more Stage I lesions might be detected. At the Lin Xian county hospital in China, 1,156 esophageal cancers were resected over the 10-year period, 1964–1974; 81 cases were carcinoma *in situ* and 89 additional cases were early carcinomas limited to mucosa and submucosa only. Mass survey has been carried out in people over 30 years of age in recent years (14). During this survey, 70.6% of detected cancers were in an early stage. In comparison, only 6.6% of cases diagnosed at the county hospital itself were early cancers. In striking contrast to the Chinese screening program, and due to the characteristics of the esophagus noted above, symptoms in esophageal cancer occur late and nearly all patients are Stage II or Stage III at diagnosis. In the 142 resected Massachusetts General Hospital cases noted above, one-third were Stage II and two-thirds were Stage III.

DIAGNOSIS

Symptoms

Symptoms that actually cause the patient to seek medical attention may be termed iatrotropic symptoms. With esophageal carcinoma the iatrotropic symptom is nearly always dysphagia or difficulty swallowing. Various forms of pain including odynophagia or painful swallowing comprise the remainder of iatrotropic symptoms. In the 1961 series of Parker et al. (62), 58% of patients sought medical attention because of dysphagia, 13% for substernal distress, 6% for odynophagia, and 5% for pharyngeal pain. In 142 patients from the Massachusetts General Hospital, 85% sought attention for dysphagia. Weight loss alone almost never brings the patient to medical attention. In addition to dysphagia, though, weight loss is frequently elicited as a symptom during history taking. Average weight loss is 15 to 25 pounds, but may range from several pounds to over half the patient's body weight. Other symptoms include fatigue, substernal pain, hoarseness, anorexia, back pain, or epigastric pain. Average duration of symptoms is 3 to 4 months. Parker et al. (62) found, however, that duration of symptoms related poorly to the size or location of the lesion, to ultimate survival, or to complications; he described three patients with tracheoesophageal fistulae who had had symptoms for less than 3 weeks.

Examination

Physical findings are rare in the patient with esophageal carcinoma. Weight loss may be evident, as may be dehydration or poor dentition. Fever is occasionally found, the result of concomitant pneumonia or fistula. Although Ong et al. (59) found palpable cervical adenopathy in 20% of 152 patients in 1977, such adenopathy has been only an occasional finding in our experience.

Laboratory Data

Laboratory evaluation is rarely helpful. The hematocrit may often be falsely elevated secondary to dehydration. Liver function tests are nearly always normal and, although 26 patients have been described in the literature with ectopic hyperparathyroidism associated with esophageal malignancy (25), hypercalcemia remains rare. The one Massachusetts General Hospital patient with esophageal carcinoma and hypercalcemia was found to have a concomitant parathyroid adenoma.

Radiology

Chest radiographs are generally unremarkable in these patients. Chronic obstructive pulmonary disease is frequent but evidence of metastatic nodules or signs characteristic of esophageal cancer are unusual. Liver and bone scans have not been helpful in our experience. Barium swallow is the mainstay of radiologic diagnosis and is diagnostic in over 80% of patients. Many physicians, particularly the Japanese (37), feel that the barium swallow may be used to predict resectability of a given tumor. Akiyama (2) evaluates abnormalities of "esophageal axis," including proximal tortuosity (representative of prestenotic dilatation and elongation), angulation of the long axis of the esophagus or axis deviation (representing fixation or traction), or increased distance of the esophagus from the spine (suggesting a bulky tumor). Narrowing, obstruction, or shift of the azygos vein on azygogram have been used by Mori et al. (53) to predict resectability of an esophageal tumor. They found that the azygogram gave the best information in terms of predicting resectability, followed by esophageal axis; neither tumor length nor radiologic type of tumor were helpful. Finally, Dafner et al. (19) found that thoraco-abdominal computed tomography correctly predicted extra-esophageal spread of carcinoma in 23 of 24 patients; there was one false positive result in a patient who had severe cachexia. Computed tomography correctly predicted absence of mediastinal extension in four of six patients; one of the false negative results occurred in a patient who had had earlier radiotherapy. Hepatic metastases were correctly predicted by computed tomography in two of three patients, the false negative occurring in a patient whose liver was replaced by tumor.

Endoscopy

Esophagoscopy is carried out in nearly all patients in whom a diagnosis of esophageal carcinoma is entertained, and is positive in nearly all patients with carcinoma. Bruni and Nelson (9) found an overall accuracy of histologic diagnosis of 96% using fiberoptic endoscopy with directed biopsy and brush cytology. At the Massachusetts General Hospital, of 134 ultimately proven at resection to have squamous cell carcinoma of the esophagus, 96% had positive biopsy at esophagoscopy. In a patient suspected of having esophageal carcinoma but with a negative biopsy, a second or third esophagoscopy should be performed. Parker et al. (62) found one esophagoscopy to be needed in 77% of patients, two in 6%, and three in 3%. Bronchoscopy should be performed at the time of the esophagoscopy in order to identify tracheo-bronchial invasion or tracheo-esophageal fistula; bronchial involvement in some series of upper one-third cancers exceeds 60% of patients (46). Mediastinoscopy has been used by some (54) to assess operability of appropriate lesions.

HISTORY OF SURGICAL TREATMENT

In 1946, Ivor Lewis (45) said, "There are few things in surgery to match the courage and enterprise with which the great surgeons of the last century attacked this problem." Although there are hints that a veterinarian in 1833 removed a tumor from a ram's esophagus, Billroth (7) is credited with having performed the first documented esophageal resection, in a large yellow dog. He resected 1½ inches of cervical esophagus, allowed the ends to heal by primary intention, and 2 months later found a healed esophagus amenable to dilatation. Seven years later, his pupil Czerny (18) performed the first esophageal resection in a human, resecting a 6-cm portion of the cervical esophagus of a 51-year-old woman and leaving the distal end open, through which the patient took nourishment. In 1884, another pupil, Mikulicz (51), resected a portion of cervical esophagus and later carried out plastic reconstruction.

In the early 1900s, successful resections via the abdominal route were added to these successful cervical resections. However, no one had performed a successful transthoracic resection of the esophagus. Sauerbruch (69) had previously said that growths in the middle one-third of the esophagus were not removable (he had performed five unsuccessfully) due to inaccessability under the aortic arch, danger of injury to the "pneumogastric" or vagus nerves, and uncertainty of closure of the upper stump. Notwithstanding this warning, Torek (82) in 1913 resected a mid-esophageal carcinoma in a 67-year-old woman via left thoracotomy; he performed gastrostomy and cervical esophagostomy. Although pathology revealed that this lesion had grown through the esophageal wall, his patient was able to eat bread, cereal, potatoes, and eggs through an external tube (Fig. 1) and died of pneumonia 13 years later.

Palliative procedures were also being undertaken at this time. As early as 1840, esophageal intubation with a decalcified animal tusk had been used once or twice. It was not until 1924 that Souttar (73) demonstrated consistent results using a spiral silver intraluminal esophageal tube. Although Adams and Phemister (1) in 1938 are credited with having performed the first thoracic esophagectomy with primary esophagogastrostomy, several of these operations had been performed previously. Ohsawa (58) had previously performed thoracic esophagectomy with esophago-gastrostomy on eight patients and esophagojejunostomy in two patients. Although he reported 50% operative mortality, his report was still looked upon with incredulity until his results were reproduced later. In 1937, Samuel Marshall (49) of the Lahey Clinic performed thoracic esophagectomy and esophagogastrostomy on a 46-year-old man, a case he later reported in June 1938. Still, Adams and Phemister (1) are generally credited with having performed the first thoracic esophagectomy with esophagogastrostomy. In looking back to this time, Lewis (45) has said, "It seems likely that 1938 will come to be looked upon as the turning point in the surgery of the esophagus—a year which marked the end of 40 years wandering after elaborate and ingenious devices and a return to simple, straightforward and meticulous sur-gery." The year 1938 also marks the first Massachusetts General Hospital esopha-gectomy with skin tube reconstruction (11). By 1945, however, Sweet had essentially abandoned the Torek operation and was routinely performing primary esophago-gastrostomy for reconstruction after resection of mid-thoracic carcinoma. The first supra-aortic anastomosis was performed by Sweet in 1944 (79). During this time,

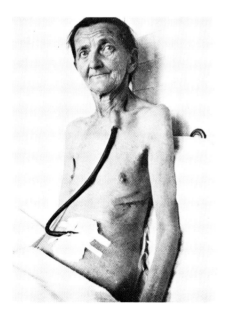

FIG. 1. Torek's first transthoracic eso-phagectomy patient. (From Torek, ref. 81, with permission.)

Wookey (86) had also described his skin tube esophageal reconstruction, and Lewis (45) his right-sided approach to mid-esophageal lesions. In 1954, Sweet (77) was able to report a series of 450 patients (1939–1952) of which 303 had undergone esophageal resection. Surgical therapy of esophageal carcinoma had become established.

RESECTIONS

Operability and Resectability

Most surgeons agree that palliation of symptoms is a worthy goal, and some assert it is the only realistic goal in treating the patient with carcinoma of the esophagus. A given surgeon's operability and resectability rates will reflect his particular treatment philosophy, e.g., the surgeon who feels that resection offers the best palliation, irrespective of potential for cure, will report higher resectability rates. Operability generally reflects the percentage of patients in whom operation may be performed with a reasonable chance for resection without excessive morbidity or mortality. Of 448 cases of squamous cell carcinoma seen recently at the Massachusetts General Hospital, 200 (about 45%) were felt to be operable. This is consistent with collected reports from the literature (65). Of those 200 patients, 58 were found unresectable at operation and 142 underwent resection. Thus, 70% of those operated were resected, or about 30% of all patients underwent resection. These figures have remained stable throughout the history of esophageal resections at the Massachusetts General Hospital (77,78,79). Much higher resectability rates may be achieved if the goal of surgical treatment is strictly palliative. Belsey and Hiebert (6) in the last 5 years of their study (reported in 1974), resected 97% of mid-thoracic esophageal carcinomas. Based on an aggressive surgical approach to the management of patients with carcinoma of the esophagus or cardia, Ellis and Gibb (23) in 1979 reported resectability of 82.3%. A later report of Ellis (22) found 88% of patients were resectable. Particularly noteworthy is the Chinese Lin Xian experience. This series, which included a number of very early carcinomas detected by frequent population screening, showed a resectability rate in 1,228 cases of 94.1%. Rates from other Chinese hospitals not involved in screening for early cancers range from 60% to 80%.

Causes of inoperability generally relate to the poor condition or age of the patient, or to advanced disease of other systems. Preoperative evidence of local invasion or distant metastases are other causes. Nonresectability usually relates to the degree of local invasion, for example, fistula into the trachea or bronchi, or invasion of diaphragm or pericardium. Not infrequently, metastases to liver or abdominal lymph nodes cause a patient to be judged inappropriate for resection.

Selection of Operation

Carcinoma of the lower one-third of the esophagus, and in particular that of the esophagogastric junction including adenocarcinoma, is most often treated surgically by resection of a generous portion of the esophagus through a left thoraco-abdominal incision (Fig. 2), with advancement of the mobilized stomach, pedicled on the right gastro-epiploic and right gastric arteries, into the thorax. The resection includes oblique division of the stomach to include the left gastric and celiac lymph nodes, which preferably are dissected to the origin of the left gastric artery. The spleen is left in place unless there is visible involvement of nodes on the greater curvature, in which case, more often than not, the lesion is beyond the bounds of resection. While the procedure may be done through a left thoracotomy, it is our preference to use the thoraco-abdominal approach to allow easier access to the pylorus, where either pyloromyotomy or pyloroplasty is routinely done. This is added because of the necessary vagotomy. While many patients have functioned well in the past without division of the pylorus, there are just enough complications related to failure of emptying so that we feel this is a worthwhile addition. With a minimum margin of at least 5 cm of esophagus, recurrence at the suture line has not been a major problem, and total thoracic esophagectomy has not been deemed necessary in all cases. It must be remembered that it is possible to free the normal esophagus quite easily beneath the aortic arch from the left side if more length is necessary, pulling the esophagus over the aortic arch to allow a high intrathoracic anastomosis. If necessary, a rib above the incision may be "shingled" by removal of a small proximal segment, or a second incision may be made through the bed of the fourth rib higher in the chest but through the same thoracic incision. These additions are not often needed. The anastomosis we prefer is a classical one described by Sweet and Churchill (11,81). This is an end-to-side anastomosis of the esophagus to a circular

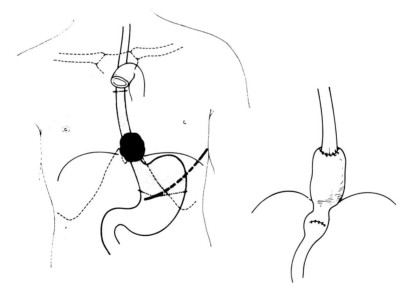

FIG. 2. Thoraco-abdominal esophagogastrectomy and esophagogastrostomy. (From Grillo, ref. 28, with permission.)

resection of a button of gastric wall placed judiciously away from the gastric turn-in. A two-layer, 4-0 silk anastomosis is still utilized. The incidence of leakage in such anastomoses, carefully performed, is negligible.

The selection of approach to lesions of the mid-esophagus and higher intra-thoracic esophagus is less uniform. At the present time, our most commonly used approach is essentially that described by Lewis (45). The stomach is initially mo-bilized through a midline laparotomy (Fig. 3, left). Esophagectomy is performed through a right thoracotomy and the mobilized stomach advanced high into the apex of the chest or to the base of the neck. The anastomosis is performed either intra-thoracically or through a third incision in the base of the neck. The same technique of anastomosis is used. A useful variant for exposure in this operation is that described by Lawrence (43). A right fifth interspace thoracotomy is performed, which transects the costal margin and continues subcostally on the left (Fig. 3, right). This provides much better access for mobilization of the stomach. The physiological impact postoperatively is greater than the two incisions described by Lewis, so that we have confined the use of this incision to the younger patient with good pulmonary function.

For a period of approximately 5 years, in an effort to improve the results of resection of middle third esophageal lesions, patients who were deemed to be operative candidates had an initial substernal total esophageal bypass performed through cervical and abdominal incisions. Usually, the left colon, pedicled on the left colic artery (Fig. 4A), was advanced substernally and an anastomosis done in the neck, turning in the distal cervical esophagus. The patient was then subjected to 4,500 rads of irradiation. If there was no evidence of metastatic disease, the patient was subjected to radical block excision of the esophagus through a right thoracotomy 4 weeks later. This excision included the entire esophagus from the cervical turn-in to the esophagogastric junction and all of the nodal tissue from the

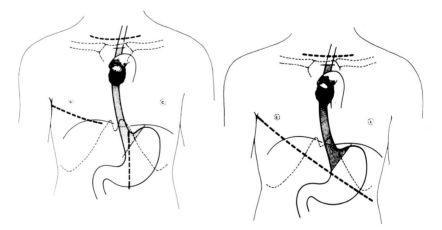

FIG. 3. **Left:** Ivor Lewis esophagogastrectomy. **Right:** Lawrence modification. (From Grillo, ref. 28, with permission.)

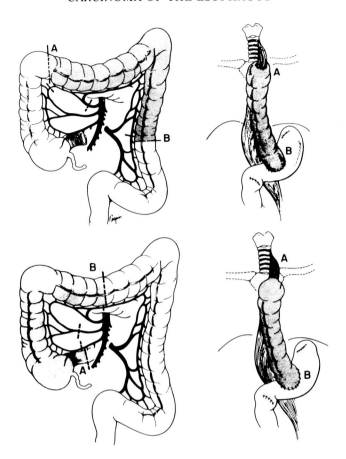

FIG. 4. **A:** Left colon esophageal bypass. **B:** Right colon esophageal bypass. (From Grillo, ref. 28, with permission.)

prevertebral fascia to the subcarinal pericardium anteriorly. No improvement in results was obtained by this procedure.

On occasion, however, colonic replacement is still used. The left colon is preferred because greater length may more easily be obtained and the left colic blood supply is more dependable in its arcades, even across the splenic flexure, than is the right side. Preoperative angiography allows one to predict the adequacy of the blood supply in advance (84). After the age of 70, the blood supply becomes more tenuous because of atherosclerotic changes.

Although short segment colon replacements, jejunal replacements, and reverse gastric tubes have been used for various benign diseases, they have been used much less often in our hands for malignant disease. Similarly, antethoracic placement of colon replacements or antethoracic cutaneous or synthetic tubes have found little use. Free jejunal (34) or ileal grafts (32) with microvascular anastomoses have been used only in very special circumstances.

The management of cervical esophageal cancer presents a special spectrum of problems. In a small number of apparently confined cases of postcricoidal carcinoma of the esophagus, without evidence of extensive lymph node or distant metastases, we have given 4,500 rads of preoperative therapy, restudied them, and, in the persisting absence of demonstrable metastases, have done radical excision. The excision is done through a transverse cervical incision, often with either an upper sternal division or, if necessary, excision of a plaque of upper sternum and medial ends of clavicles, and excision of the first and second costal cartilages. The lower pharynx, the esophagus to the carina, and the larynx and trachea as far as necessary are excised *en bloc*. Through an abdominal incision, the left colon is mobilized and is anastomosed to the pharynx above and to the stomach below. An end-tracheal stoma is brought out either at the base of the neck above the sternal notch or, if the cancer is more extensive, as a mediastinal tracheostomy after resection of the bony plate, as described. We prefer this to closing off the lower end of the esophagus or to blunt total esophagectomy and advancement of the stomach substernally to the neck. In these patients, recurrence has usually been in lymph nodes of the neck rather than more distally, so that there seems to be little brief for total esophagectomy.

In a small number of cancers confined to the thoracic inlet, we have used a similar approach of preoperative irradiation with subsequent excision, preserving the larynx and the cricopharyngeus. A segment of trachea may be resected if it is involved by the tumor. The right colon is used preferentially (Fig. 4B). Anastomosis behind the cricoid cartilage of a segment of left colon to the cricopharyngeus is difficult. A small segment of ileum, which is left attached to the right colon, may be more easily anastomosed to the cricopharyngeus, using two layers of fine silk. The majority of cervical and postcricoidal carcinomas are still treated by irradiation. Operations for removal of cervical esophageal carcinomas are of great magnitude; patients must be selected carefully for potential for cure and for physiological ability to withstand such a surgical assault (71).

In all surgery for cancer of the esophagus, the procedure must be done with meticulous care and with special attention to anastomotic precision. In the advancement of the colon, great attention must be paid to maintaining perfect viability of the tissues. If there is any question of viability at the conclusion of an advancement, it is unlikely that healing will be successful. With increasingly precise attention to anastomotic details the leak rate for esophagogastric anastomosis should be close to nil. It is somewhat more difficult to maintain a similar record in esophagocolonic anastomosis but, with increasing experience, the rate of difficulties with such anastomoses has also declined markedly (84). Cologastric anastomoses are rarely the site of leakage. On occasions, stenosis of such anastomoses may occur.

Since many patients with cancer of the esophagus are older and have chronic obstructive pulmonary disease, often related to a long cigarette-smoking history, pulmonary function may be borderline. Such patients may have difficulty weaning from respirators postoperatively. The physiological impact of the operations appears to increase serially from those done in the lower third through a left thoraco-abdominal incision, to those done in the mid-esophagus through an abdominal and right thoracic incision, to those done through a right thoraco-abdominal incision. If there is any virtue to esophagectomy done by the "blunt" modifications of the Gray-Turner technique (60,75) it would be to minimize postoperative ventilatory problems.

Complications

In 1947 and 1948, Sweet (76,80) reported complications in 18% to 20% of his patients. Around the world today, complication rates range from 15% (23) to 40% (55). Complications frequently relate to anastomotic problems, e.g., leak or stricture, or to pulmonary problems. Traumatic injury to the spleen may occur.

Perioperative Death

Perioperative deaths occur in 10% to 20% of patients after resections for esophageal carcinoma (2,16,28,29,35,70) but may be as high as 40% (59). Mortality rates as low as 2% to 5%, however, have been reported (22,23,55,88). Causes of death often relate to sepsis, e.g., secondary to anastomotic leak, or to cardiopulmonary causes. An additional dramatic cause of death is rupture of innominate artery, subclavian or carotid artery, or aorta. Ong et al. (59) reported this complication in 10 of 108 patients, resulting in six deaths. Of 142 patients at the Massachusetts General Hospital, five deaths were caused by great vessel rupture; four of these were in patients who had undergone extensive cervical resections with mediastinal tracheostomy, obviously a special problem. In 1982 there were no deaths after esophagectomy at this hospital.

Late Death

Respiratory failure and pneumonia, particularly aspiration pneumonia, are frequent causes of late death. Cardiac deaths are not unusual in this group of patients, and rupture of a great vessel may occur months to years postoperatively as the result of recurrence or mediastinal sepsis.

Survival

In a group of 123 survivors of resection for esophageal carcinoma at the Massachusetts General Hospital, 31% survived 2 years and 12% survived 5 years (Fig. 5). These figures are consistent with those of collected series in the literature (16,24,28), although some report 5-year survival figures as high as 25% to 34% (2,3). Of special interest are the recent reports from China (14,87,88); their overall 5-year survival after resections is 25%, and in their most recent series approaches 30% to 40%. The 44% 5-year survival of 250 resections in the Lin Xian province attests to the favorable nature of the early lesions detected there.

Staging is predictive of survival even in more advanced lesions. As early as 1952, Sweet (78) indicated that the survival of patients with uninvolved lymph

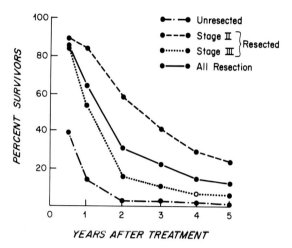

FIG. 5. Survival in 448 cases of squamous cell carcinoma of the esophagus at the Massachusetts General Hospital.

nodes was triple that of those with involved nodes. More recent experience from the Massachusetts General Hospital (Fig. 5) mirrors Sweet's early data; 2-year survival for Stage II patients was 58%, for Stage III patients, 16%; 5-year survival for Stage II patients was 24%, compared to 6% for Stage III patients. The effect of early stage is particularly evident once again in the Lin Xian experience (88). Of 163 resections of "very early carcinoma," 5-year survival so far is 90.3%; there has been one late recurrence 9 years postoperatively.

PALLIATIVE OPERATIONS

Three general types of palliative procedures are (a) bypass operation without resection (e.g., colon interposition, esophagogastrostomy, reverse gastric tube, jejunal interposition); (b) intraluminal esophageal tubes; and (c) feeding tubes (e.g., gastrostomy or jejunostomy). Although these operations are generally less stressful than resections with reconstruction, they still have associated morbidity and mortality that equal or exceed those of resections (85).

Colon Bypass

Since the mid-1950s (48), right or left colon, placed intrathoracically, have been recognized as suitable substitutes for the esophagus (Fig. 4). The chief advantage of the colon as a surrogate esophagus is its length. Disadvantages include the variable blood supply, high bacterial content, and need for additional bowel anastomoses. Many surgeons feel that colon interposition is associated with increased morbidity and mortality, compared to other esophageal bypass or reconstructive procedures. Schuchmann et al. (70) found an operative mortality rate of 33% for resection plus colon interposition, compared to 19% for resection plus esophagogastrostomy. Overall, the operation appears to carry with it an operative mortality of 20% to

25% (16,26,67), though Wilkins (84) in 1980 reported only nine deaths in 100 cases. It remains the most common form of bypass procedure at the Massachusetts General Hospital.

Intraluminal Esophageal Tubes

An ingenious variety of these tubes exists, the most common now being synthetic latex or polyethylene tubes. These are designed either to be pulled through the lesion via gastrostomy or pushed through perorally (5). In concept, esophageal intubation is attractive, providing palliation with a minor endoscopic procedure. Complications such as tube dislodgement or obstruction, wound infection, bleeding, or aspiration occur in 25% of patients, however, and mortality ranges from 10% to 43% (31,38,63). Recently, we have preferred the peroral route, placing a silicone rubber tube as described by Montgomery (52). Results have been very satisfactory and morbidity is low.

Gastrostomy

Gastrostomy alone is felt by most to be poor palliation for esophageal carcinoma. The patient's nutritional needs may be met but he remains unable to swallow. In addition, even this minor procedure is not benign. In 61 patients with esophageal carcinoma treated at the Massachusetts General Hospital since 1962 with gastrostomy tube alone, seven patients (11%) had complications, the majority being wound infections, and 11 patients (18%) died postoperatively, nearly half of pneumonia.

Survival after Palliative Operation

Review of 126 esophageal carcinoma patients who had survived palliative surgery showed that only 3% lived 2 years, only 1% lived 5 years. In the same time period, 123 patients who had survived resection had a 2-year survival of 31% and a 5-year survival of 12%. Even the most advanced, i.e., Stage III, carcinomas had greater survival when resected, compared to the unresected group (16% 2-year survival, 6% 5-year survival) (Fig. 5).

ADJUNCTIVE TREATMENT

Adjunctive Radiotherapy

The value of preoperative or postoperative radiotherapy remains unproven. One of the strongest proponents of preoperative radiotherapy is Nakayama (56), who feels that it extends resectability, decreases lymph node metastases associated with surgical manipulation, and increases survival. His patients receive a dose of 2,000 to 2,500 rads given over 4 to 5 days. The 5-year survival rate in this group of patients was 37.5%, compared to 19.1% in patients treated by resection only. Parker and Gregorie (61) also advocate preoperative radiotherapy. They gave 4,500 rads preoperatively and found increased 2-year survival to 12%, based on historical controls. Drucker et al. (21) found no difference in survival when 4,000 to 6,000 rads were given postoperatively, regardless of the stage of the lesion. At the Massachusetts General Hospital, 43 patients who underwent resection only were compared to 80 patients who had received 4,000 to 6,000 rads either preoperatively or postoperatively; there was no difference in survival (Fig. 6).

Between 1965 and 1970, 87 patients with squamous cell carcinoma of the mid-esophagus were studied by Drs. H. C. Grillo, G. L. Nardi, C. C. Wang and E. W. Wilkins, Jr., *(unpublished)* at the Massachusetts General Hospital. Five of these patients had such advanced disease that no treatment was given; they died within 6 months. Four patients had single-stage esophagectomies, three were treated with irradiation alone, and 35 with irradiation and various adjunctive measures such as inlying intraluminal tube or gastrostomy. Forty patients were entered into a study protocol, which consisted first of substernal colon bypass to establish the patient's swallowing, then 4,500 rads delivered to the tumor and mediastinum, and, finally, if there was no evidence of distant metastasis or irresectability, block excision of the entire intrathoracic esophagus and adjacent mediastinal tissue including subcarinal lymph nodes. In this early phase of this type of surgery, there were four postoperative deaths in these 40 patients. Another five developed obvious metastatic disease following completion of the bypass and during irradiation. Thirty-one of the original 40 completed the surgical bypass and irradiation phases. During the period of waiting prior to block excision, 15 developed evidence of deterioration such as tracheo-esophageal fistula, appearance of metastatic disease, or general debilitation. All of them died of their disease, although several lived for nearly a year. Only 16 patients arrived at the point of radical esophagectomy. There was one postoperative death. Of the others, four were dead in less than 6 months and seven died in periods between 6 months to 3½ years. Three additional patients died of their disease, but the length of survival could not be precisely determined. Only

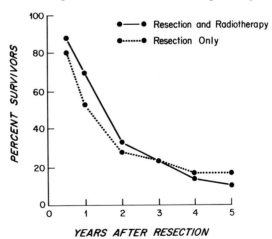

FIG. 6. Effect of adjunctive radiotherapy on survival in 123 cases of squamous cell carcinoma of the esophagus at the Massachusetts General Hospital.

one patient was living disease-free to die of other causes 6 years following completion of the three stages. Thus, only one of the 16 pateints who underwent the entire treatment survived over 5 years without disease. Four had prolonged survival between 1 and 3½ years, but did die of their disease.

Adjunctive Chemotherapy

An aggressive search continues for effective chemotherapeutic agents. However, at the present time, none has shown clear efficacy. Bleomycin has received considerable attention. In a prospective randomized study (42), 16 patients treated with bleomycin and adriamycin showed a response rate of 19%; 15 patients treated with these drugs plus radiation showed a response rate of 60%. Side effects, though, were much more severe in the latter group. Steiger et al. (74) have reported 68% 1-year survival in a series of patients treated with 5-fluorouracil and mitamycin C or *cis*-platinum in addition to radiotherapy and surgery. Long-term survival is not yet known. In China, an anti-pyretic herbal medicine called "kang-I-e-san" or, literally, "anti-tumor B-3" is being tested (8). Patients discovered to have severe esophageal hyperplasia on the basis of screening cytologies were randomized. In the untreated group, 30% of severe hyperplasia cases regressed to normal mucosa and 7% went on to frank carcinoma; of those treated with "kang-I-e-san," 75% regressed to normal and only 1.5% went on to carcinoma. In the United States, hypoxic cell radiation sensitizers such as misonidazole are being studied in squamous cell carcinoma of the esophagus (J. G. Schwade, personal communication). Multiple trials of preoperative and postoperative multi-drug chemotherapeutic regimens are in progress, modelled on protocols used in treatment of squamous carcinoma of head and neck.

Adjunctive Immunotherapy

Postoperative immunotherapy with *bacilli Calmette-Guerin* (BCG) and beta streptococcal preparations have been attempted. Akiyama (2) found slightly favorable effects of one such streptococcal compound in cases with markedly positive lymph node metastases, but felt it too early to report definitively.

OUTLOOK

The prospects of a patient with esophageal carcinoma remain grim, though perhaps less so than ever before. Improvements in perioperative mortality and morbidity have already occurred and are likely to continue. It is also possible that some combination of adjunctive radiotherapy, chemotherapy, or immunotherapy will result—if not in a breakthough, at least in an incremental improvement in survival. The most exciting recent development, the Lin Xian screening program in China, unfortunately is applicable to few areas around the world. For the present, we can offer cure to some, increased survival to many, and palliation to most patients.

REFERENCES

1. Adams, W. E., and Phemister, D. B. (1938): Carcinoma of the lower thoracic esophagus: Report of a successful resection and esophagogastrostomy. *J. Thorac. Surg.*, 7:621–632.
2. Akiyama, H. (1980): Surgery for carcinoma of the esophagus. *Current Problems In Surgery*, 17:1–120.
3. Akiyama, H., Tsurumaru, M., Kawomura, T., and Ono, Y. (1981): Principles of surgical treatment for carcinoma of the esophagus. *Ann. Surg.*, 194:438–446.
4. The American Joint Committee for Cancer Staging and End Results Reporting (1973): *Clinical Staging System for Carcinoma of the Esophagus.*
5. Angorn, I. B. (1981): Intubation in the treatment of carcinoma of the esophagus. *World J. Surg.*, 5:535–541.
6. Belsey, R., and Hiebert, C. A. (1974): An exclusive right thoracic approach for cancer of the middle third of the esophagus. *Ann. Thorac. Surg.*, 18:1–15.
7. Billroth, T. (1872): Resection of the esophagus. *Arch. Klin. Chir.*, 13:65–69.
8. The British Broadcasting Corporation (WGBH Educational Foundation) (1980): *The Cancer Detectives of Lin Xian.* WGBH transcripts ("Nova").
9. Bruni, H. C., and Nelson, R. S. (1975): Carcinoma of the esophagus and cardia: Diagnostic evaluation in 113 cases. *J. Thorac. Cardiovasc. Surg.*, 70:367–370.
10. Burgess, H. M., Baggenstoss, A. H., Moersch, H. J., and Clagett, O. T. (1951): Carcinoma of the esophagus: Clinicopathologic study. *Surg. Clin. North Am.*, 31:965.
11. Churchill, E. D., and Sweet, R. H. (1942): Transthoracic resection of tumors of the stomach and esophagus. *Ann. Surg.*, 115:897–920.
12. Collis, C. H., Cook, P. J., Forman, J. K., and Palframan, J. F. (1971): A search for nitrosamine in East African spirit samples from areas of varying esophageal cancer frequency. *Gut*, 12:1015–1018.
13. Cook, P. (1971): Carcinoma of the esophagus in Africa: A summary and evaluation of the evidence for the frequency of occurrence, and a preliminary indication of the possible association with the consumption of alcoholic drinks made from maize. *Br. J. Cancer*, 25:853–880.
14. Guojun, H., Lingfang, S., Dawei, Z., Zhangcai, L., Guoqing, W., Shuxian, L., and Fubao, C. (1981): Diagnosis and treatment of early esophageal carcinoma. *Chinese Med. J.*, 94:229–232.
15. Coordinating Group for Research on the Etiology of Esophageal Cancer of North China (1974): Epidemiology and etiology of esophageal cancer in North China. *Chinese Med. J.*, 54:671.
16. Cukingnan, R. A., and Carey, J. S. (1978): Carcinoma of the esophagus. *Ann. Thorac. Surg.*, 26:274–286.
17. Cutler, S. J., and Young, J. L., Jr. (1975): Third national cancer survey: Incidence data. *Nat. Cancer Inst. Monograph*, 44.
18. Czerny, J. (1877): Neue operationen. *Zentralbl Chir.*, 4:433.
19. Daffner, R. H., Halber, M. D., Postlethwait, R. W., Korobkin, M., and Thompson, W. M. (1979): Computed tomography of the esophagus. II. Carcinoma. *Am. J. Roentgenol.*, 133:1051.
20. Doll, R. (1969): The geographical distribution of cancer. *Br. J. Cancer*, 23:1–8.
21. Drucker, M. H., Mansour, K. A., Hatcher, C. R., and Symbas, P. N. (1979): Esophageal carcinoma: An aggressive approach. *Ann. Thorac. Surg.*, 28:133–137.
22. Ellis, F. H., Jr. (1980): Esophagogastrectomy for carcinoma: Technical considerations based on anatomic location of lesion. *Surg. Clin. North Am.*, 60:265.
23. Ellis, F. H., Jr., and Gibb, S. P. (1979): Esophagogastrectomy for carcinoma: Current hospital mortality and morbidity rates. *Ann. Surg.*, 190:699–705.
24. Giuli, R., and Gignoux, M. (1980): Treatment of carcinoma of the esophagus. Retrospective study of 2400 patients. *Ann. Surg.*, 192:44–52.
25. Grajower, M., and Barzell, U. S. (1976): Ectopic hyperparathyroidism (pseudophyerparathyroidism) in esophageal malignancy: Report of a case and a review of the literature. *Am. J. Med.*, 61:134–135.
26. Gregorie, H. B. (1972): Esophagocoloplasty. *Ann. Surg.*, 175:741.
27. Griffith, J. L., and Davis, J. T. (1980): A 20-year experience with surgical management of carcinoma of the esophagus and gastric cardia. *J. Thorac. Cardiovasc. Surg.*, 79:447–452.
28. Grillo, H. C. (1982): The thorax. In: *Surgery: Essentials of Clinical Practice*, edited by G. L. Nardi and G. D. Zuidema. Little, Brown, Boston.

29. Gunnlaugsson, G. H., Wychulis, A. R., Roland, C., and Ellis, F. H., Jr. (1970): Analysis of the records of 1657 patients with carcinoma of the esophagus and cardia of the stomach. *Surg. Gynecol. Obstet.*, 130:997–1005.

30. Haas, J. F., and Schottenfeld, D. (1978): Epidemiology of esophageal cancer. In: *Gastrointestinal Tract Cancer*, edited by M. Lipkin and R. A. Good, pp. 145–172. Plenum, New York.

31. Hankins, J. R., Cole, F. N., Attar, S., Satterfield, J. R., and McLaughlin, J. S. (1979): Palliation of esophageal carcinoma with intraluminal tubes: Experience with 30 patients. *Ann. Thorac. Surg.*, 28:224–229.

32. Harashina, T., Kakegawa, T., Imai, T., and Suguro, Y. (1981): Secondary reconstruction of the esophagus with free revascularized ileal transfer. *Br. J. Plast. Surg.*, 34:17–22.

33. Harper, P. S., Harper, R. M. J., and Howel-Evans, A. W. (1970): Carcinoma of the oesophagus with tylosis. *Quart. J. Med.*, 39:317–333.

34. Hester, T. R., McConnel, F. M. S., Nakai, F., Jurkiewicz, M. J., and Brown, R. G. (1980): Reconstruction of cervical esophagus, hypolarynx, and oral cavity using free jejunal transfer. *Am. J. Surg.*, 140:487–491.

35. Hoffman, T. H., Kelley, J. R., Grover, F. L. and Trinkle, J. K. (1981): Carcinoma of the esophagus: An aggressive one-stage palliative approach. *J. Thorac. Cardiovasc. Surg.*, 81:44–49.

36. Hopkins, R. A., and Postlethwait, R. W. (1981): Caustic burns and carcinoma of the esophagus. *Ann. Surg.*, 194:146–148.

37. Japanese Society for Esophageal Diseases (1976): Guidelines for the clinical and pathologic studies on carcinoma of the esophagus. *Japan. J. Surg.*, 6:69.

38. Jirardet, R. E., Ransdell, H. T., and Wheat, M., Jr. (1974): Palliative intubation in the management of esophageal carcinoma. *Ann. Thorac. Surg.*, 18:417–430.

39. Just-Viera, J. O., and Haight, C. (1969): Achalasia and carcinoma of the esophagus. *Surg. Gynecol. Obstet.*, 128:1081–1095.

40. Kinnmann, J., Shinn, H. I., and Wetteland, P. (1968): Carcinoma of the oesophagus after lye corosion. *Acta. Chir. Scand.*, 134:489–493.

41. Kirivanta, U. K. (1952): Corosion carcinoma of the esophagus. *Acta Otolaryngol.*, 42:89–95.

42. Kolaric, K., Maricic, Z., Roth, A., and Kujmovic, I. (1980): Combination of bleomycin and adriamycin with and without radiation in the treatment of inoperative esophageal cancer: A randomized study. *Cancer*, 45:2265.

43. Lawrence, G. H. (1957): Right thoracoabdominal approach to esophageal resection. *Surg. Gynecol. Obstet.*, 105:641–644.

44. Leon, W., Strug, L. H., and Brickman, I. D. (1971): Carcinoma of the esophagus: A disaster. *Ann. Thorac. Surg.*, 11:583–592.

45. Lewis, I. (1946): The surgical treatment of carcinoma of the esophagus with special reference to a new operation for growth of the middle third. *Br. J. Surg.*, 34:18–31.

46. Lira, E. (1979): Tratamiento quirurgico del covier esofago. Experiencia de 1012 cases. *Adv. Med. Oncol. Res. Ed.*, 9:359–367.

47. Mahboubi, E., Kmet, J., Cook, P. J., Day, N. E., Ghadirian, P., and Salmasizadeh, S. (1973): Oesophageal cancer studies in the Caspian littoral of Iran: The Caspian cancer registry. *Br. J. Cancer*, 28:197–214.

48. Mahoney, E. B., and Sherman, C. D., Jr. (1954): Total esophagoplasty using intrathoracic right colon. *Surgery*, 35:937.

49. Marshall, S. F. (1938): Carcinoma of the esophagus: Successful resection of lower end of esophagus with re-establishment of esophageal gastric continuity. *Surg. Clin. North Am.*, June: 643–648.

50. McCort, J. J. (1952): Radiographic identification of lymph node metastases from carcinoma of the esophagus. *Radiology*, 59:694.

51. Mikulicz, J. (1886): A case of resection of carcinoma of the esophagus. *Prag. Med. Wschr.*, 9:92–95.

52. Montgomery, W. W. (1978): Salivary bypass tube. *Ann. Oto. Rhinol. Laryngol.*, 87:159.

53. Mori, S., Kasai, M., Watanabe, T., and Shibuya, I. (1979): Preoperative assessment of resectability for carcinoma of the thoracic esophagus: Part 1. Esophagogram and azyogogram. *Ann. Surg.*, 190:100–105.

54. Murray, G. J., Wilcox, B. R., and Stark, B. J. K. (1977): The assessment of operability of esophageal carcinoma. *Ann. Thorac. Surg.*, 23:393.

55. Nakayama, K. (1974): Surgical treatment of esophageal malignancy. In: *Gastroenterology*, edited by H. L. Bockus, pp. 307–318. W. B. Saunders, Philadelphia.

56. Nakayama, K., and Kinoshita, Y. (1974): Carcinoma of the esophagus: Surgical treatment combined with preoperative concentrated irradiation. *J.A.M.A.*, 227:178–181.
57. Norton, G. A., Postlethwait, R. W., and Thompson, W. M. (1980): Esophageal carcinoma: A survey of populations at risk. *South. Med. J.*, 73:25–27.
58. Ohsawa, T. (1933): The surgery of the esophagus. *Arch. Japan. Chir.*, 10:605.
59. Ong, G. B., Lam, K. H., Wong, J., and Lim, T. K. (1978): Factors influencing morbidity and mortality in esophageal carcinoma. *J. Thorac. Cardiovasc. Surg.*, 76:745–754.
60. Orringer, M. B., and Sloan, H. (1978): Esophagectomy without thoracotomy. *J. Thorac. Cardiovasc. Surg.* 76:643–654.
61. Parker, E. F., and Gregorie, H. B. (1976): Carcinoma of the esophagus. Long term results. *J.A.M.A.*, 235:1018–1020.
62. Parker, E. F., Gregorie, H. B., and Hughes, J. C. (1961): Carcinoma of the esophagus. *Ann. Surg.*, 153:957–970.
63. Payne, W. S. (1979): Palliation of esophageal carcinoma. Editorial. *Ann. Thorac. Surg.*, 28:208–209.
64. Pickett, L. K., and Briggs, H. C. (1967): Cancer of the gastrointestinal tract in childhood. *Pediatr. Clin. North Am.*, 14:223–234.
65. Postlethwait, R. W. (1979): *Surgery of the Esophagus*, pp. 341–414. Appleton-Century-Crofts, New York.
66. Postlethwait, R. W., and Musser, A. W. (1974): Changes in the esophagus in one thousand autopsy specimens. *J. Thorac. Cardiovasc. Surg.*, 68:953–956.
67. Postlethwait, R. W., Sealy, W. C., Dillon, M. L., and Young, W. G. (1971): Colon interposition for esophageal substitution. *Ann. Thorac. Surg.*, 12:89.
68. Raphael, H. A., Ellis, F. H., Jr., and Dockerty, M. B. (1966): Primary adenocarcinoma of the esophagus: 18-year review and review of the literature. *Ann. Surg.*, 164:785–796.
69. Sauerbruch, F. (1905): Die Anastomose zwischen Magen und Speiserohre und die Resecktion des Brustabschnittes der Speiserohre. *Zentralbl. Chir.*, 32:81.
70. Schuchmann, J. F., Haydorn, W. H., and Hall, R. V., et al. (1980): Treatment of esophageal carcinoma: A retrospective review. *J. Thorac. Cardiovasc. Surg.*, 79:67–73.
71. Silver, C. E. (1981): Surgical treatment of hypopharyngeal and cervical esophageal cancer. *World J. Surg.*, 5:499–507.
72. Silverberg, E., and Holleb, A. I. (1975): Major trends in cancer: 25-year survey. *Cancer*, 25:2–20.
73. Souttar, H. C. (1924): A method of intubating the esophagus for malignant stricture. *Br. Med. J.*, 1:782.
74. Steiger, Z., Franklin, R., and Wilson, R. F., et al. (1981): Eradication and palliation of squamous cell carcinoma of the esophagus with chemotherapy, radiotherapy, and surgical therapy. *J. Thorac. Cardiovasc. Surg.*, 82:713–719.
75. Steiger, Z., and Wilson, R. F. (1981): Comparison of the results of esophagectomy with and without a thoracotomy. *Surg. Gynecol. Obstet.*, 153:653–656.
76. Sweet, R. H. (1947): Carcinoma of the esophagus and cardiac end of the stomach: Immediate and late results of treatment by resection and primary esophagogastric anastomosis. *J.A.M.A.*, 135:485–490.
77. Sweet, R. H. (1954): Late results of surgical treatment of carcinoma of the esophagus. *J.A.M.A.*, 155:422–425.
78. Sweet, R. H. (1952): The results of radical surgical extirpation in the treatment of carcinoma of the esophagus and cardia with five-year survival statistics. *Surg. Gynecol. Obstet.*, 94:46–52.
79. Sweet, R. H. (1945): Surgical management of carcinoma of the mid-thoracic esophagus: Preliminary report. *N. Engl. J. Med.*, 233:1–7.
80. Sweet, R. H. (1948): The treatment of carcinoma of the esophagus and cardiac end of the stomach by surgical extirpation : 203 cases of resection. *Surgery*, 23:952–975.
81. Sweet, R. H. (1943): Total gastrectomy by the transthoracic approach. *Ann. Surg.*, 118:816–837.
82. Torek, F. (1913): The first successful case of resection of the thoracic portion of the esophagus for carcinoma. *Surg. Gynecol. Obstet.*, 16:614–617.
83. Turnbull, A. D., Rosen, P., Goodner, J. T., and Beattie, E. J. (1973): Primary malignant tumors of the esophagus other than typical epidermoid carcinoma. *Ann. Thorac. Surg.*, 15:463–473.
84. Wilkins, E. W., Jr. (1980): Long-segment colon substitution for the esophagus. *Ann. Surg.*, 192:722–725.

85. Wong, J., Lam, K. H., Wei, W. I., and Ong, G. B. (1981): Results of the Kirschner Operation. *World J. Surg.*, 5:547–552.
86. Wookey, H. (1942): The surgical treatment of carcinoma of the pharynx and upper esophagus. *Surg. Gynecol. Obstet*, 75:499–506.
87. Wu, Y., Chen, P., Fong, J., and Lin, S. (1980): Surgical treatment of esophageal carcinoma. *Am. J. Surg.*, 139:805–809.
88. Wu, Y., and Kuo-Chun, H. (1979): Chinese experience in the surgical treatment of carcinoma of the esophagus. *Ann. Surg.*, 190:361–365.
89. Wychulis, A. R., Woolam, G. L., Anderson, H. A., and Ellis, F. H., Jr. (1971): Achalasia and carcinoma of the esophagus. *J. A. M. A.*, 215:1638–1641.
90. Wynder, E. L., and Bross, I. J. (1961): A study of etiologic factors in carcinoma of the esophagus. *Cancer*, 14:389–413.
91. Wynder, E. L., Hultberg, S., Jacobson, E., and Bross, E. J. (1957): Environmental factors in cancer of the upper alimentary tract: Swedish study with special reference to Plummer-Vinson syndrome. *Cancer*, 10:470–487.
92. Wynder, E. L., and Mabuchi, K. (1973): Etiologic and environmental factors. *J.A.M.A.*, 226:1546–1548.

Thoracic Oncology, edited by N. C. Choi and H. C. Grillo. Raven Press, New York © 1983.

Radiation Therapy for Carcinoma of the Esophagus

James G. Pearson

Division of Radiation Oncology, University of Alberta; and Cross Cancer Institute, Edmonton, Alberta, Canada T6G 1Z2

Esophageal carcinoma usually is diagnosed so late that the tumor has spread beyond hope of cure by loco-regional treatment. Management frequently is complicated by starvation, cardiovascular disease, emphysema, and the effects of overuse of alcohol and tobacco. In North America, only 5% of these patients survive 5 years after diagnosis. Good palliation is not easy to accomplish. Nevertheless, during the last 40 years there have been important improvements in diagnosis and in radiation and surgical treatment; there have been isolated reports of an overall 5-year survival rate of 10% and occasionally more, and further improvement is expected.

ATTEMPTED CURE BY RADIATION THERAPY

Indications

Curative radiation therapy for carcinoma of the esophagus is indicated if (a) histology shows squamous or undifferentiated carcinoma, (b) there are no detectable distant metastases, (c) the demonstrable length of the primary tumor and any detectable lymph node metastases extends over no more than 9 cm (less for a frail patient), (d) there is no invasion of trachea, bronchi, thyroid, stomach, or vertebrae (the commonly present bulging of the posterior tracheal wall without demonstrable invasion is not a contraindication), and (e) the patient's general condition is good enough to tolerate a course of radiation therapy. Emaciation does not rule out an attempt at cure if the tumor is localized and small.

The greater the number of unfavorable factors (e.g., advanced age, emaciation, advanced circulatory, respiratory, or metabolic disease), the smaller must be the tumor for cure to be attempted. Werner et al. (58,60) have described the indications for treatment.

Diagnosis of Tumor Extent

In order to plan the site, size, and shape of the volume of tissue to be irradiated, it is highly desirable to have complete information about the true extent of the tumor. Unfortunately, such complete information is impossible, because metastases of less than 10^8 cells (0.5 cm) are rarely detected during the course of pretreatment evaluation. The radiation therapist, even more than the surgeon, works in blind ignorance of the true distribution of malignant cells throughout the body. Normally the history and physical examination are followed by a complete noninvasive investigation that includes esophagogastric barium studies, chest and mediastinal radiography, computerized tomography of the neck, chest, and upper abdomen, radionuclide imaging, hematology, and a biochemical profile. These investigations are followed by esophagoscopy, brushings, washings, and biopsies. Bronchoscopy is necessary unless the tumor is remote from the trachea. More invasive investigations such as mediastinoscopy, laparotomy, and thoracotomy are not usual preliminaries to irradiation (4,27,50). The target volume chosen for irradiation without the evidence from these more aggressive investigations usually will cover all the tumor if it is indeed curable. A tumor that can be encompassed only by a much larger volume usually will not be controlled by the lower radiation dose that must be prescribed for a larger volume, and such an extensive tumor usually will be accompanied by distant metastases, making cure by any means impossible.

In North America the type of patient most frequently seen with esophageal cancer is a user of tobacco or alcohol or both who has already suffered some functional impairment of the respiratory, cardiovascular, and digestive systems. The tumor is usually a rather undifferentiated squamous carcinoma, and in the average patient accepted for radical radiation therapy the demonstrable length of tumor is 6 cm or more.

Technique

Corrections of starvation, dehydration, anemia, and infection are commenced, and without delay radiation therapy is started. If it is decided to give a moderately high radical dose, then it is reasonable to prescribe, for example, 20 equal fractions, one fraction per day, five times a week, to a total dose ranging between 4,800 and 5,300 rads throughout a 15-cm-long by 6.5-cm-diameter cylindrical volume. Rider and Mendoza (48) and Beatty et al. (5) have reported experience with a wide range of doses and have concluded that a close range around 5,000 rads in 20 fractions in 4 weeks is probably optimal. There are other combinations of dose, number of fractions, and overall time that may be chosen to give the same biological effect. A 4-, 6-, or 8-MeV linear accelerator usually is used, but higher photon energies can be used with advantage, as reported by Beatty et al. (5) and as suggested by the dose distributions illustrated in Fig. 1. If unusually low tolerance is expected, a reduction in volume rather than in dose is indicated. Only for the larger, very undifferentiated carcinomas is a dose of 200 to 500 rads less given to a volume rarely exceeding an 18-cm by 7.5-cm cylinder. Rarely is the volume less than a 12-cm by 6-cm cylinder, even for the small tumors. The irradiated volumes vary over a smaller range than the estimated tumor volumes. A patient with a small

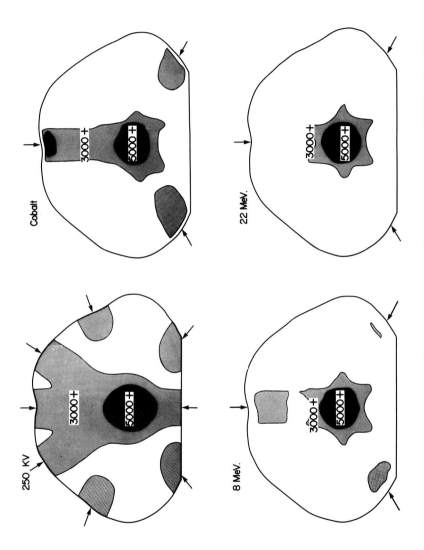

FIG. 1. Four dose distributions for the mid-tumor cross section of the same patient using 250-kV, ^{60}Co, 8-MeV, and 22-MeV photons. The higher the energy, the better the localization of the absorbed radiation in the target volume. (From Pearson, ref. 43, with permission.)

tumor is given the benefit of a slightly wider margin around the tumor and, if the patient is not too frail, an extra 250 rads of dose. For a patient with a slightly larger tumor, the margin allowed is less, and the risk of geographic miss is greater, so the standard dose is given. Even when given the same dose, a larger tumor is more likely to recur locally. Because most of the larger tumors are associated with occult distant spread, a higher treatment morbidity is not inflicted on all for the sake of

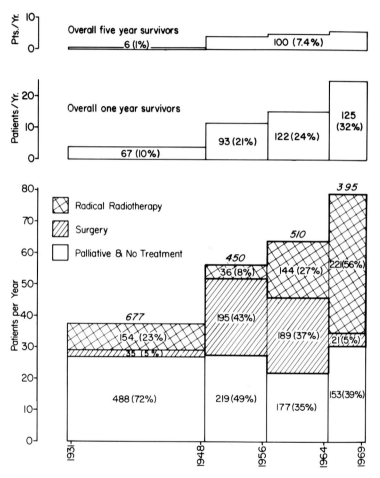

FIG. 2. Distribution of 2,032 patients with squamous carcinoma of the esophagus seen in hospitals in the Edinburgh area during four periods of 18, 8, 8, and 5 years between 1931 and 1969. The vertical scale shows the absolute numbers of patients per year. The trend toward more patients per year represents the increasing proportion referred rather than increasing incidence. The percentages are out of the total number of patients that were seen in each period. From 1949 to 1969 the trend toward wider use of radiation therapy for initial treatment was associated with an increasing 1-year survival rate, a maintained overall 5-year survival rate, and increasing absolute numbers of 1- and 5-year survivors in the community. (Reproduced by permission from Pearson, J. G.: Management of cancer of the oesophagus. In: *Topical Reviews in Radiotherapy and Oncology*, edited by T. J. Deeley. John Wright & Sons, London, 1979.)

the rare additional cure that would be at the expense of optimum palliation for the majority.

The above regimen is attended by a local failure rate of 50%. The achievement of a lower failure rate awaits earlier diagnosis, improved definition of the extent of the tumor, and an improved therapeutic ratio. An improved therapeutic ratio may be achieved by improved fractionation, hypoxic cell sensitizers, hyperbaric oxygen, irradiation by neutrons, pions, or heavy ions, or superadditive combinations with hyperthermia or cytotoxic drugs—or whatever other improvements lie in the future.

For radical irradiation of esophageal cancer, anteroposterior opposed ports should not be used. Even that "moderate radical dose" which locally eradicates only 50% of these large esophageal cancers is too great a threat to the functional integrity of the spinal cord. There have been numerous published reports of paraplegia resulting from the treatment of esophageal cancer using techniques that irradiate the spinal cord to the same dose as the esophagus, and radiation pneumonitis has been a frequently reported complication. Not one of the 401 patients radically irradiated in Edinburgh from 1949 to 1969 (Fig. 2) was treated with an anteroposterior opposed pair. Over 180 of these patients lived more than a year, but only one developed partial, transient transverse myelitis, and only one (who had scleroderma) suffered significantly from radiation pneumonitis.

In the Edinburgh series referred to above and reported by Pearson (41,43), from 1956 to 1969 radical irradiation of the thoracic esophagus was usually done using three symmetrically arranged ports at 120 degrees to one another, the anterior port applied with the patient supine and the two posterolateral ports applied with the patient prone. Orthogonal planning films were prepared separately for the supine and prone positions, and the two plans were integrated using the center of the target volume placed at the isocenter as the common reference point. In every case the planning was three-dimensional in that the relationship of the spinal cord to the target volume was determined 1 cm within the rostral and caudal ends of the target volume as well as in the central transverse plane. In the central plane a more detailed calculation was performed. The long axis of the target volume usually lay at an angle to the horizontal (coronal) plane, and sometimes at an angle to the sagittal plane, so as best to fit the volume suspect of invasion by tumor without encroaching on the spinal cord at any level.

Most centers now use a linear accelerator that can swing below the couch; the patient remains supine throughout treatment,and either an anterior and two poster-olateral ports or a vertically upward posterior and two anterolateral ports may be used. Supine is the most relaxed, precisely reproducible treatment position, and for this reason is preferable. With a modern machine the oblique ports can be shaped by lead blocks bolted to a shadow tray so that the treated volume is sausage-shaped, to fit the curve of the spine, thus affording greater security to the spinal cord without loss of tumor coverage (12). Lewinsky et al. (24) and Prager (45) have studied the attractions of the prone position to increase the separation between the esophagus and the spinal cord; however, given precise treatment planning and execution, the greater stability and reproducibility of the supine position may outweigh the advantage of increasing the separation of esophagus and spinal cord.

The shape of the lung can be reconstructed in the main-plane plan from the orthogonal planning films and anatomic knowledge, and the decreased absorption in the lung can be calculated separately for each port, but a computerized tomographic (CT) cut angled to coincide with the main plane of the plan, and further cuts parallel to this, all prepared with the patient precisely in the treatment position, facilitate the localization and measurement of lung, bone, and other tissues of various densities that are important to precise dosimetry. It is hoped that in the future the calibration of CT numbers to indicate electron density and atomic number distribution will lead to more precise computerized treatment planning.

For the more complexly varying tissue depths and lung thicknesses between the neck and the upper thorax, a volume angled to fit snugly in front of the spinal cord, if necessary from cricoid to main carina, is irradiated using two anterolateral ports, again with the patient supine. Two planning films are prepared with a diagnostic beam perpendicular to the intended treatment beam, barium in the esophagus, and the appropriate body surface contour outlined by malleable wire. Then contours are prepared, the lung shape is drawn in, and planning is done in the main plane and in planes 1 cm within either end of the target volume. Compensation for varying tissue thicknesses and inhomogeneity may be achieved rather crudely by introducing wedge filtration for an appropriate number of fractions across the long axis and then across the short axis of each field. Deeley (8) solved this problem with a combination of a stepped port in the long axis and wedge filtration across the short axis of each of the anterolateral ports. In the early 1950s in Liverpool a standard brass block wedged diagonally across each rectangular anterolateral port was used to make this correction (14). Now these needs are more elegantly and precisely met using computerized tomographic cuts at the appropriate levels, prepared with the patient in the treatment position, simulator fluoroscopy and planning films with barium, and a perspex shell and compensators, still with the patient supine (21,53).

Occasionally, for a small tumor at the upper end of the esophagus in a long-necked patient, two laterally opposed ports treat a satisfactory volume in front of the spinal cord and include such lymph nodes on either side of the neck as are in line with the esophagus.

For the lower neck, cures can be achieved with the patient supine, head and neck flexed to the left, steadied in a head clamp, and a horizontal right "superolateral" beam, with its long axis angled to fit the spine, directed somewhat caudally into the thorax (and usually perpendicular to the midsagittal plane of the skull), using an appropriate couch angle, all angles being recorded, and reproduced for each daily treatment. Then a similar setup is used with the head and neck flexed to the right and a left superolateral beam. Both right and left superolateral ports are treated each day. Plans are prepared at each of the three levels on either side and integrated using reference points along the axis of the esophagus. An inescapable complexity results from the changing relationships of the surrounding normal tissues as the head and neck are moved from left to right lateral flexion, but reasonably accurate dosimetry can be achieved along the changing curvature of the axis of the esophagus and spinal cord.

Most radically treated patients start radiation therapy while still able to swallow liquids or soft solids. Many can be treated as outpatients. Each benefits from skilled dietary advice and supervision. Usually a creamy soft or liquid diet is necessary, and for those patients unable to swallow sufficient liquid, intravenous supplements are used. If patient and medical delays have been so disastrous that a diagnosis is not made until dysphagia is complete, total intravenous alimentation is instituted. Intravenous hydration and feeding is preferred to either intubation or enterostomy. As Marcial (26) reported, intravenous management usually successfully tides the patient over until the tumor shrinks. Delay in commencing irradiation is avoided. For the patient who can still swallow liquids and whose tumor is soon to regress, intubation contributes nothing but an unnecessary hazard. The presence of a tube through the tumor adds to the fibrosis that attends healing as the tumor regresses. Without intubation, the stricture at the site of healing may be less severe or may be avoided (41).

Usually the tumor starts to shrink and swallowing improves toward the end of the second week of treatment, and the patient then improves rapidly. The symptoms of irradiation esophagitis also commence during the second week of treatment and are a great burden to the few patients whose dysphagia was insignificant at the start of treatment, but they cause little additional suffering to the more typical patient who starts treatment with severe dysphagia. Irradiation esophagitis reaches a maximum during the fourth and final week of a 4-week course, continues unabated for the first week after treatment, and takes another 2 weeks (sometimes longer) to settle down. An antacid mucilage with a mild mucosal analgesic may give comfort. Strong mucosal anesthetics are to be avoided because of the danger of aspiration into the lungs of retained esophageal contents. The main supportive measure is a copious, very bland, nutritionally rich liquid diet flavored and timed to the patient's taste.

There is considerable variation in the rate of shrinkage of the tumor following radiation therapy. The average tumor is halved in bulk by the end of the treatment, and 2 months later mucosal healing is complete. Healing may occur with minimal fibrosis and complete relief of dysphagia (Fig. 3), or the tumor may be replaced by a fibrous stricture. If this residual stricture seriously impairs nutrition, gentle bouginage should be attempted. Of the 48 5-year survivors in the Edinburgh series, half never required bouginage, a quarter needed one dilatation, and the remaining quarter needed repeated bouginage, in some cases for over a year. Bouginage is hazardous; it must not be started until 2 months or more after irradiation, and it must be very gentle. Several such patients, cancer-free at autopsy, have died as a consequence of rupture of the esophagus by a bougie.

If the philosophy of the treatment team is to administer moderate radical-dose radiation therapy such as 20 fractions of 250 rads in 4 weeks (or 28 fractions of 200 rads in 5.5 weeks) to a 15-cm by 7-cm cylindrical volume, half of the 5-cm-long tumors will be locally eradicated (more than half of the smaller tumors and

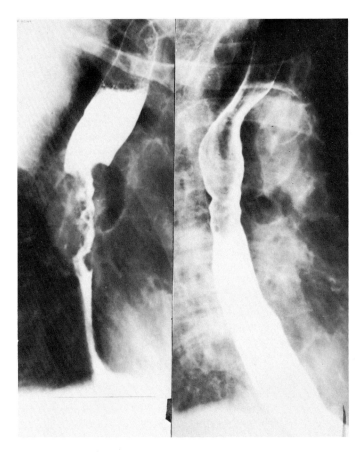

FIG. 3. Squamous carcinoma of the esophagus at the level of the left main bronchus in an 80-year-old woman, irradiated in October 1960, and restored to clinical normality. Re-X-rayed in October 1965, when treated for a new cancer of the breast. In 1970, the patient, then aged 90, was well and free from any evidence of either malignancy. (From Pearson and Le Roux, ref. 44, with permission.)

less than half of the larger tumors), and for the majority of patients so treated who are not cured because of local failure or occult spread beyond the target volume, such a moderate radical dose and volume achieve good palliation, with quite moderate radiation morbidity. There are some patients embarked on radical irradiation in whom previously occult remote lymphatic or distant metastases become manifest before completion of irradiation. For these, radical treatment is converted to palliation by aborting the course at about 80% of the radical dose or by reducing the treated volume or both. In this way some treatment morbidity is saved while useful (although less long-lasting) relief from dysphagia is achieved, and the patient may die from distant metastases, but euphagic. There is justification for delaying the full investigation for distant metastases until three-quarters through the course of irradiation, just before the patient is finally committed to the full radical dose.

When local failure occurs, the recurrence usually can be detected between 6 and 12 months, but occasionally as much as 30 months after irradiation (44). A potentially operable patient must be followed closely with a view to salvage by surgical resection should a local recurrence develop. Such surgery is technically more difficult than esophageal resection in an unirradiated patient, but is occasionally very successful (41). The majority of the patients who suffer local failure of radiation therapy are not suitable for surgery, some because distant metastases have appeared since irradiation, and some because of various criteria of inoperability that were present before the initial decision to irradiate. As dysphagia worsens, a strictly liquid but rich diet is advised. When nutrition is no longer adequate with this regimen, the esophageal lumen can be kept open a little longer and occasionally many months longer by means of intubation.

Results

The most important benefit is restoration of months or years of enjoyable life that otherwise would be lost. Of the 228 patients radically irradiated in Edinburgh from 1949 to 1967, 41% survived 1 year, and 17% survived 5 years (Fig. 4). For those whose cancer is not eradicated, the main concern is the quality of their remaining life. Most live more than 6 months. If local recurrence occurs, the outlook is indeed gloomy, but even these patients usually have had restoration of normal or improved swallowing for a period of months up to a year or two. Elkon et al. (10) also has recorded this feature. For radiation failure, surgical salvage is occasionally possible but always difficult. Intubation is the next resort but it is not without mortality and its benefits are short-lived. Enterostomy is avoided once it is recognized that cure is not possible. Of those dying within 5 years from causes other than local recurrence, half die from distant metastases, and half die from causes other than cancer. After the first 3 years, most of the deaths are due to causes other than cancer (40).

Forty-eight of the 288 patients irradiated for cure in Edinburgh between 1949 and 1967 (Fig. 4) lived more than 5 years, and each had a dormal voice and a normal stomach and had regained normal or excessive weight. Those under retirement age were working, and nearly all were taking a normal diet.

Using these techniques, the worst complication is local recurrence of the esophageal cancer. Otherwise, the morbidity is low. Treatment mortality is less than 1%. Radiation esophagitis occurs in all patients. Less than 1% suffer symptoms from lung or skin reactions. A faint paramediastinal lung opacity may be detected on chest X-rays in nearly all cases. Radiation osteitis of the spine occurs after 3 years in 10% of the long-term survivors (especially if there is already senile osteoporosis), but the symptoms are minimal (22,44). Radiation myelitis does not occur with good radiation therapy technique unless there is some unusual extra hazard, such as the need to attempt cure in a patient who has had previous radiation therapy but refuses alternative surgical treatment. Esophagotracheal fistula is not a complication of the techniques described earlier, but Rider and Mendoza (48) have reported that it

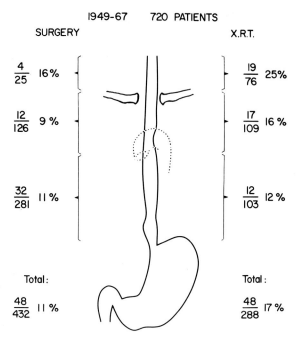

FIG. 4. The 5-year survival fractions and percentages are shown for 720 patients treated radically for squamous esophageal cancer in Edinburgh from 1949 to 1967; 432 patients were treated by surgery and 288 by radiation therapy. Ninety-six survived 5 years. The site differences in the 5-year survivals are partly attributable to age and sex factors, but, in part independent of age and sex, survival by site varies with treatment. Radiation therapy is most successful toward the upper end and surgery toward the lower end (the number of cervical esophageal tumors resected was too small for significant comparison). The difference between radiation therapy and surgical 5-year survivals is significant ($p < 0.05$) for the upper and middle esophagus, and overall, but not for the lower third. (From Pearson, ref. 43, with permission.)

becomes a problem when higher radiation doses are used in an attempt to reduce the incidence of local recurrence of the cancer. Beatty et al. (5) now favor more moderate doses for radical irradiation. A patient with detectable tumor invasion through to the tracheal mucosa is not irradiated for cure but is treated with lower-dose palliative irradiation. High-dose irradiation of such a patient might well cause a fistula. A patient with an established esophagotracheal fistula is rarely irradiated. In such a case, even moderate-dose irradiation would be expected to enlarge the fistula as the tumor shrinks. Esophagotracheal fistula commonly results from the advance of untreated or recurrent esophageal cancer. In a report of 111 patients with esophagorespiratory fistula, Martini et al. (29) found no evidence that radiation therapy was a significant cause. In fact, they reported one unusual patient whose fistula was healed by irradiation.

Following curative irradiation, half of the long-term survivors require dilatation of a stricture. This is not a radiation stricture. When a tumor that has destroyed the whole thickness of the esophageal wall around its whole circumference is eradicated by radiation therapy, healing occurs by fibrosis and causes a stricture.

If the cancer destroys both muscle layers around only half the circumference, healing following radiocure will produce a fibrous scar that will merely kink the esophageal wall, may be asymptomatic, and will not require bouginage (Fig. 5). If the cancer infiltrates without destroying the muscle, radiocure leaves a normally functioning stricture-free esophagus that is also radiographically normal (Fig. 3).

Prognostic Factors

If patients with squamous esophageal cancer are treated by irradiation for cure, 40% or more or much less may survive a year, and 20% or more or much less may survive 5 years. The most important measurable prognostic factors that influence the length and quality of survival following radiation therapy for cure are (a) tumor

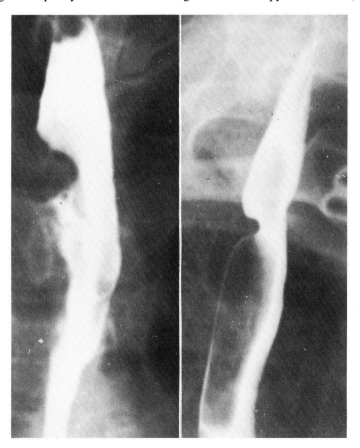

FIG. 5. A 7-cm squamous carcinoma at the level of the suprasternal notch, presenting mainly on the posterolateral wall of the esophagus, treated by megavoltage irradiation in October 1963, leaving a kink in the esophageal wall where the large malignant ulcer has been replaced by a fibrous scar. In 1968, swallowing was normal for all food except large pieces of meat. (From Pearson and Le Roux, ref. 44, with permission.)

extent, (b) sex, (c) age and general condition, (d) site (level), (e) histology, (f) treatment technique, and (g) the community where the patient lives. Other patient factors are important but are less measurable or thus far unrecognized. Certainly the unpredictability of the radiation response suggests that there is much worthwhile research still to be done.

Tumor Extent

Given current diagnostic methods, there is always conjecture about the true extent of the cancer. In most sites, a metastasis of 100 million cells (0.5 cm in diameter) goes undetected. Nevertheless, the extent of demonstrable tumor remains the best guide to prognosis.

The UICC TNM classification (55) is the standard classification most representative of various interests and is now increasingly being adopted. Of the many other classifications, the clinical and pathological classification of the Japanese Society of Esophageal Diseases (18) is especially detailed.

In the esophagus, as in other sites, early cancer is highly curable. In Linhsien County Hospital, Honan, China, 58 (86%) of 69 patients with "stage 0" esophageal cancer are alive 5 years after surgical treatment, and 133 (52%) of 255 stage I and stage II patients survived 5 years (1). There is no published account of the radiation therapy for such early esophageal cancer, but in 701 patients with carcinoma of the esophagus and cardia treated by radiation therapy or surgery, Appelqvist (3) reported 5-year survival rates among patients with tumors less than 4 cm, 4 to 8 cm, and more than 8 cm of 21%, 9%, and 1%, respectively. In the Edinburgh series, of those treated radically by irradiation from 1949 to 1969 the shorter the radiographically demonstrable length of the tumor, the better the prognosis, but only 1 patient had a tumor not demonstrably more than 2 cm long. For patients in whom loco-regional eradication of an esophageal cancer more than 8 cm long is achieved, death usually occurs later from distant metastases.

As Appelqvist (3) reported, although a patient's untreated cancer always increases in extent with time, the length of the history by itself is not a useful guide to prognosis. Some slow-growing tumors with a long history are still at an early stage when treated, and some aggressive, rapidly growing tumors present at a late stage with a short history.

Lymph node invasion often indicates incurable disease, but when confined to nodes lying close to the primary tumor, long survival is still possible following loco-regional treatment by irradiation or surgery (17).

Sex

Female patients have a better prognosis than males, whether they are young or old, whether they are treated by irradiation or surgery, and whether their tumors are in the upper or lower half of the esophagus (39,42). The better prognosis for females has been observed by many (3,5,22,30–32,54,57,63).

Age and General Condition

Advanced age, cardiovascular and respiratory disease, smoking, heavy alcohol consumption, and prolonged starvation militate against successful irradiation. However, it must not be overlooked that a patient may be in very poor condition solely because of starvation caused by a relatively small, metastasis-free, radiocurable esophageal cancer.

Site (Level)

In a center where both radiation therapy and surgery are available and collaboration between the disciplines is close, prognosis may not vary greatly with the site of the tumor in the esophagus (3). However, many primarily surgical series show a worse prognosis for tumors in the upper thorax linked with the early invasion of trachea, bronchi, and aorta that occurs at that level. Such invasion may not prevent successful irradiation to the same degree as it limits surgery (Figs. 4 and 6).

Histology

Patients with well-differentiated squamous carcinoma have the best prognosis following irradiation. Adenocarcinoma is worse because it is commonly associated with a large primary tumor and a higher incidence of distant mestastases (3,7,11,17,23,30). Resection, if possible, is superior to irradiation for adenocarcinoma because adenocarcinoma is marginally less radiosensitive than squamous carcinoma and because irradiation below the diaphragm is complicated by reduced tolerance of the normal tissues.

Undifferentiated carcinoma has the worst prognosis (3,23). The local response of undifferentiated carcinoma to radiation therapy is excellent, with rapid relief of

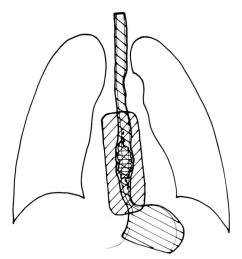

FIG. 6. Comparison of the shorter, wider volume of tissue that can be radically irradiated around an esophageal cancer and the larger but overly narrow volume removed by total esophagectomy. (Reproduced by permission of the editor of *Gann*, Monograph No. 9, 1970.)

symptoms and eradication of tumor within the irradiated volume, but the patient usually dies from distant metastases within a few months. As Vaeth (56) has indicated, it would be helpful to institute a uniform and widely applied system of histological grading of esophageal carcinoma. The Japanese Society of Esophageal Diseases (18) made recommendations for an integrated system of staging and histological grading.

Younghusband and Aluwihare (63) reported a series of 77 patients treated by esophagectomy among whom those with histological evidence of an immune response in the tumor and lymph nodes had a reduced incidence of tumor extension beyond the esophagus, fewer lymph node metastases, and longer survival. These findings are likely to be as relevant to irradiation as to surgical treatment.

Treatment Technique

Untreated esophageal cancer usually kills the patient within a year of the onset of symptoms; the mean survival is 7.5 months (37,52). Yet even the short life remaining to a very old patient or one with extensive cancer may be further shortened by radiation therapy to too high a dose or too great a volume. It is essential to match the aggressiveness of the investigation and treatment to the fortitude of the patient. Radiation therapy applied with skill and wide experience of the disease will shorten the lives of few, improve the quality of remaining life for many, and restore to a few the expectation of a life normal in both length and quality.

The Patient's Community

In affluent communities in which large resources are devoted to alcohol, tobacco, education, and medical facilities, patients with esophageal cancer usually present with late disease. Between 2% and 9% are alive 5 years later.

In some less affluent communities (even in some of the communities in Africa in which esophageal cancer is epidemic and the esophagus is the commonest site of cancer), late presentation, too late for it to be possible to modify the course of the disease, is so common that 5-year survival is unknown (46).

In another less affluent community (Linhsien County of Honan in China) where the disease is epidemic and radiation therapy is primitive, education of the populace and the medical profession, together with a screening campaign, has resulted in early diagnosis, high operability and a high resection rate, low operative mortality, and 507 (43%) of 1,308 patients alive 5 years later (1,61). Modern radiation therapy is not yet available in Linhsien County, and no other community has yet reported a sizable number of patients with esophageal cancer diagnosed early; therefore the contribution that irradiation might make to the management of such early esophageal cancer still remains to be demonstrated.

RADIATION THERAPY FOR PALLIATION

To palliate is to improve the quality of the patient's remaining life.

Quality of Life when Attempted Cure Fails

In addition to offering as good a chance of cure as is available for most of the patients as they present with squamous or undifferentiated carcinoma of the esophagus, radiation therapy has the additional merit of low treatment morbidity and good palliation, with relief of dysphagia for a few months, or even a year or two, should the attempt at cure fail (10).

Palliative Irradiation

When cure is seen to be impossible, there is rarely occasion for a major procedure that itself induces symptoms. To prolong a life of suffering is not good palliation. In the Edinburgh series, 35% of the patients were demonstrably incurable, and for another 10% the chance of cure was remote (Fig. 2).

Those with very advanced disease received excellent nursing and anxiety- and pain-relieving medication, but no direct attack on the tumor. Of the 35% judged incurable, about half received palliative irradiation of the primary tumor: 4,500 to 4,800 rads in 20 fractions in 4 weeks to a restricted volume, allowing a smaller margin around the detectable tumor than is used for radical treatment, or appropriately lower doses given over 1 or 2 weeks. Significantly smaller doses than these risk the mere prolongation of an unsatisfactory existence characterized by persistent distressing dysphagia. The results of palliative irradiation in Edinburgh were similar to those of other authors, who have observed that 75% of patients experience worthwhile relief of dysphagia and that some remain euphagic until they die from distant metastases (10,20,22,26). If a patient is going to die of cancer within a year (as do 95% of those not suitable for radical treatment) and there is dysphagia requiring relief, palliative irradiation usually is the preferred initial treatment (59). It is less of a burden to the patient than intubation or a bypass operation. If relief of dysphagia following irradiation is inadequate, or if after a few months of improved swallowing a local recurrence develops, palliative intubation is carried out. Beatty et al. (5) recommend a more aggressive approach to effect surgical relief of persistent or recurrent dysphagia after irradiation. Sedation is the final resort.

For a patient with painful metastases remote from the primary tumor, satisfactory short-term palliation frequently results from simple single-fraction or five-fraction radiation treatment.

COMPARISON OF RADIATION THERAPY AND SURGERY

Localized Treatment

Radiation therapy, like surgery, can eradicate only the primary tumor, nearby infiltration, and local lymph node metastases, but there are differences from surgery in details that can be critical for some patients. The surgeon may resect the whole esophagus but leave tumor behind on the trachea, aorta, pericardium or in lymph nodes. The radiation therapist will irradiate a larger volume circumferentially around the esophagus than the surgeon can resect, but the length of esophagus irradiated will be less than the surgeon removes in a total esophagectomy (Fig. 6). An esophagogastrectomy performed below the aortic arch may well remove a smaller margin of esophagus above the tumor than would be irradiated.

Local Irradiation Failure versus Operative Mortality

Radiation therapy frequently fails because the tumor recurs at the primary site. Such failures are less common in favorable patients with smaller tumors, which are also associated with less occult distant spread. The treatment mortality for moderate-dose radical irradiation is much less than the operative mortality for radical surgery. These disastrous features of the two methods of treatment tend to have similar effects on long-term survival, but operative death kills a patient about 6 months earlier than a local recurrence following radiation therapy (Fig. 7).

Squamous Carcinoma versus Adenocarcinoma

Surgery is preferable to irradiation for the initial treatment of adenocarcinoma. If surgery is impossible, irradiation may palliate.

Level of the Tumor

It has been observed by many radiation therapists that irradiation tends to be rather more effective in the upper two-thirds of the esophagus. Most surgeons report fewer problems with the resection of tumors in the lower one-third. It appears likely that patients with upper-two-thirds tumors categorized as inoperable and thereafter referred for radiation therapy are less unfavorable in respect of tumor size and

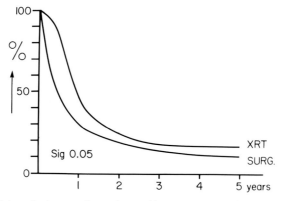

FIG. 7. Actuarial survival curves for patients with squamous esophageal cancer treated radically in Edinburgh from 1949 to 1969 show significantly higher survivals for irradiated patients at 1 and 5 years ($p = 0.05$), mainly because of the higher mortality in the first 2 months following surgery. (From Pearson, ref. 43, with permission.)

patient age than the surgical rejects from the lower third. This, rather than differences in radiocurability attributable specifically to the level in the esophagus, may be the reason for the relatively more favorable outcome following irradiation of upper-two-thirds tumors. The combined radiation therapy and surgical experience in Edinburgh is relevant (Fig. 4). Evaluation is complicated by the cross-linkages with sex, age, and method of treatment. Similar numbers have been irradiated in the upper, middle, and lower esophagus, but 281 at the lower end compared with only 25 at the upper end have been treated surgically. However, at all three levels the survival rates are higher following irradiation. The differences are statistically significant at the upper end (25% vs. 16%), in the middle (16% vs. 9%), and overall (17% vs. 11%), but imperceptible in the lower esophagus (12% vs. 11%). However, the comparability of the surgical and radiation groups is less well established than it would have been had there been a stratified and randomized trial. The 103 patients with lower-third tumors treated by irradiation included a higher proportion of older patients, but not a higher proportion of females, than the 281 surgically treated patients. There is no evidence that site, per se, is an important prognostic factor in this series, but because of the cross-linkages between site, sex, age, and method of treatment (because more patients with upper-end tumors are female, younger, and irradiated), upper-end tumors are associated with a better prognosis.

Age

The older the patient the more hazardous is radical treatment by radiation therapy or surgery, but age is less of a limitation for irradiation than for surgery.

Survival

No significant, prospective, randomized trial has yet been reported that compares surgery and radiation therapy in the management of any category of patients with esophageal cancer. There remains an element of conjecture in any provisional conclusions drawn from currently available material. The Edinburgh 1949 to 1969 series is of interest because it is the work of a team of radiation therapists and surgeons who together provided all the potentially curative treatment for this disease for a well-defined and stable population of 1.3 million persons. All patients with a diagnosis of esophageal cancer in the Regional Cancer Registry have been included. The surgical component of the material constitutes a notable record, as reported by Logan (25) and LeRoux (23). The radiation therapy component benefited greatly from the availability of a 4-MeV linear accelerator since 1955. Radiation therapists gained vital insight into the likely extent and anatomy of the tumor to be included in the irradiated volume by working closely with their surgical colleagues in the clinic, the operating room, and the autopsy room. Neither the surgery nor the radiation therapy of esophageal cancer can be optimal in the hands of occasional practitioners.

The Edinburgh experience is of disease apparently more extensive than that at the Linhsien County Hospital in China, but less extensive than that in Durban, Port

Elizabeth, Johannesburg, or Capetown. In the Edinburgh series there were as many females as males, which is a factor favoring longer survival not present to the same degree in most other series.

Figures 2, 4, and 7 may be examined together. The Edinburgh practice was to treat by surgery for thoracic esophageal cancer (followed occasionally by irradiation salvage) and by irradiation for cervical esophageal cancer from 1949 to 1956, by surgery for lower-half tumors and irradiation for upper-half tumors (and for old and frail patients with small tumors at any level) from 1957 to 1964, and by initial irradiation at all levels for squamous carcinoma and wider use of surgical salvage for irradiation failure from 1965 to 1969. Throughout, surgery has been preferred for adenocarcinoma (adenocarcinomas are excluded from Figs. 2, 4, and 7). During those 21 years the definitive treatment was irradiation for 401 patients, surgery for 405, and palliative measures for 549. Whatever view one takes of the causes of the effects observed over those 21 years, the increasing use of megavoltage irradiation has been attended by a striking increase in the overall 1-year survival and no decrease in the 5-year survival. A hundred patients have lived more than 5 years, and there is no hidden group of unfavorable patients not included in Fig. 2.

Functional Result

The long-term survivors following irradiation constitute a particularly fortunate group from the functional point of view. Most are euphagic, regain normal weight, and retain a normally functioning larynx, normal lungs, a normal cardia, and a normally functioning stomach.

COMBINATIONS OF RADIATION THERAPY AND SURGERY

Loco-regional or local treatment such as irradiation or surgery must fail to cure the 80% of patients who already have manifest or occult remote tumor spread when treated (43). However, some patients still free from remote spread suffer operative mortality, or primary recurrence within the irradiated volume, or recurrence at the margins of the irradiated or resected tissues. Many different combinations of irradiation and surgery have been tried in attempts to reduce these hazards. Robertson et al. (49) lucidly outlined the reasons for expecting benefit from preoperative irradiation. Akakura et al. (2) and Yamashita et al. (62) found that during a period when surgical technique altered little, the introduction of full preoperative irradiation to a dose of 5,000 to 6,000 rads in 4 to 6 weeks, followed 2 to 4 weeks later by resection, was associated with a striking improvement in resectability, reduction in the incidence of tumor at the margins of resection, and improvement in 5-year survival. Nakayama (32) and Nakayama and Kinoshita (33) reported that preoperative irradiation (four fractions of 500 rads) and three-stage esophagectomy and reconstruction have decreased operative mortality and increased survival. Parker and Gregorie (36), Rambo et al. (47), and Marks et al. (28) have had extensive experience with a preoperative dose of 4,500 rads in 18 fractions in 3.5 weeks, and they conclude that preoperative radiation offers a distinct advantage. Seymour and Pettit (51) and Nègre et al. (35) favor preoperative irradiation. The group at Fu Wai Hospital in Peking (13) and Doctor and Sirsat (9) have studied the effect of a range of doses used preoperatively. Werner et al. (58–60) have developed an impressive overall plan for the management of clearly categorized stages of esophageal cancer using preoperative methotrexate and irradiation or methotrexate and irradiation without surgery. Their early results are encouraging. Guernsey et al. (16) used doses of 6,600 rads in 7 weeks preoperatively and concluded that such a dose is too high. After a trial of three fractions of 800 rads preoperatively in 70 patients, Groves and Rodriguez-Antunez (15) have discontinued the practice.

Postoperative irradiation may be inferior to preoperative irradiation because the blood supply and oxygenation of residual tumor, and therefore its radiosensitivity, are believed to be reduced after surgery. However, in 39 patients who underwent curative resection of esophageal cancer and were found to have no demonstrable lymph node metastases, Kasai et al. (19) observed increased survival among those given postoperative irradiation, but there was no benefit from postoperative irradiation if lymph node metastases were present.

Thus there are indications that radiotherapy and surgery can usefully be combined, but because of lack of suitable controls, none of the evidence constitutes incontrovertible proof.

There are two ways of combining irradiation and surgery that occasionally have been attended by indisputable success. One is irradiation salvage following manifest local failure of surgery. The other is surgical salvage following manifest local failure of irradiation. Such successes are infrequent.

DISCUSSION

Reasons for Success and Failure

For most patients with esophageal carcinoma, radiation therapy fails to cure because of the great extent of the tumor (often occult metastases) by the time the diagnosis is established and treatment is started. Insidious onset, patient delay, and medical delay all contribute to this unfortunate situation (34). It is probably infrequent for esophageal carcinoma to cause its first symptom before the tumor is more than 2 cm long. Symptoms may be unremarkable until two-thirds of the circumference of the esophagus have been stiffened by tumor. The early symptoms appear trivial and may remit for several weeks. So poorly is the populace educated that a patient will tolerate dysphagia for an average of 4 months before medical advice is sought. In some communities, excessive intake of alcohol is a causative factor that also reduces patient awareness. Alcohol may reduce the patient's motivation and capacity to facilitate the procedures necessary for successful irradiation, and alcohol may reduce tissue and organ tolerance of full-dose irradiation. On the other hand, a patient who consults a physician early may have negative barium studies and endoscopy that lead to false reassurance. Brushings, washings, and cytology are not yet universally applied in the diagnosis of minimal dysphagia. It is clear from the experience in Linhsien County, Honan, as reported by Ackerman et al. (1) and Wu (61), that where esophageal cancer is so common as to be a public health problem, community education, medical education, and a screening program lead to early diagnosis and a high cure rate. There is no significant reported experience with radiation therapy for early esophageal cancer. Less than 1% of the Edinburgh series of 401 patients treated by radical irradiation had tumors of less than 3 cm demonstrable length. But experience with radiation therapy for lip cancer and early tongue cancer suggests that a 90% local eradication rate is a reasonable expectation following irradiation of squamous carcinomas less than 2 cm in diameter. The Linhsien experience suggests that such small tumors in the esophagus are not associated with a high incidence of occult distant metastases. To speculate, the Linhsien and Edinburgh experiences, taken together, suggest that both radiation therapy and surgery might benefit to similar degrees by earlier diagnosis of esophageal cancer, but the irradiated patients would suffer less treatment mortality and less morbidity and would end up with better function than similar patients treated surgically.

Nevertheless, it seems doubtful that the incidence of esophageal cancer is high enough in most communities in North America to justify a screening program.

Prospects for Improvement

1. Better education of the populace and medical profession, leading to improved interpretation of early symptoms.

2. Wider use of brushings, washings, and cytology.

3. Technical improvements in radiation therapy to reduce local failures and increase the volume of cancer that can be irradiated radically: (a) better dose, time, and fractionation factors; (b) an improved therapeutic ratio with selective hypoxic radiosensitizers; (c) improved localization of the deposition of radiation energy to the target volume and an improved therapeutic ratio within the target volume using neutrons, heavy ions, or pi-mesons (38); (d) the combination of radiation with hyperthermia or cytotoxic drugs in circumstances when the effects are more than additive (6).

4. More advantageous combinations of surgery with irradiation or with irradiation and chemotherapy (58,60).

5. Improved surgical salvage following irradiation failure by earlier and more certain diagnosis of local recurrence. Some patients die needlessly from operations carried out on suspicion of local irradiation failure when in fact irradiation has eradicated all tumor. Many more patients die because the fact of local failure of irradiation is not established until too late for salvage surgery to be practicable.

CONCLUSIONS

There are large variations among communities in the patterns of esophageal carcinoma, but with rare exceptions diagnosis and treatment come at a hopelessly late stage.

The seriousness of dysphagia is emphasized.

During the last 30 years there have been great improvements in local effectiveness for both radiation and surgical treatments of esophageal cancer, generally not matched by earlier diagnosis. The screening program in north China is an exceptional experience in a very high-incidence community that has led to the diagnosis of many early cancers which have been successfully treated by surgery. For lower-incidence areas, greater patient and physician awareness and the addition of brushings, washings, and cytology to improved barium studies and endoscopy for the investigation of persistent minimal dysphagia should contribute to earlier diagnosis.

There are no experimental data to prove that surgery is preferable to irradiation or that irradiation is preferable to surgery in the management of the various categories of esophageal cancer. However, close teamwork between the disciplines usually is fruitful. Neither irradiation nor the surgical treatment of esophageal cancer is optimal in the hands of the occasional practitioner. In communities where there are good and closely associated radiation therapy and surgical facilities, the greatest number of enjoyable years of life are likely to be obtained if patients with squamous carcinoma of the middle and upper thirds of the esophagus are treated initially by irradiation, with surgery held in reserve for local recurrences, and patients with squamous carcinoma of the lower third and all adenocarcinomas are treated surgically, unless medically unfit. For patients treated primarily by surgery, the addition of preoperative irradiation is likely to be beneficial.

Patients with more advanced disease usually can be helped by palliative irradiation, with intubation held in reserve until an adequate fluid diet can no longer be swallowed.

Prevention is conceivable and would be preferable.

REFERENCES

1. Ackerman, L. V., Weinstein, I. B., and Kaplan, H. S. (1978): Cancer of the esophagus. In: *Cancer in China*, edited by H. S. Kaplan and P. J. Tsuchitani, pp. 111–136. Liss, New York.
2. Akakura, I., Nakamura, Y., Kakegawa, T., Nakayama, R., Watanabe, H., and Yamashita, H. (1970): Surgery of carcinoma of the esophagus with preoperative radiation. *Chest*, 57:47–57.
3. Appelqvist, P. (1972): Carcinoma of the oesophagus and gastric cardia. *Acta Chir. Scand. [Suppl.]*, 430:3–92 (Major review article).
4. Baskind, A., and Marchand, P. E. (1978): Discussion of diagnosis in carcinoma of the oesophagus. In: *Carcinoma of the Oesophagus*, edited by W. Silber, pp. 211–216. A. A. Balkema, Capetown.
5. Beatty, J. D., DeBoer, G., and Rider, W. D. (1979): Carcinoma of the esophagus. *Cancer*, 43:2254–2267.
6. Cade, Sir S. (1978): Memorial symposium on the interaction of radiation and antitumor drugs. *Int. J. Rad. Oncol. Biol. Phys.*, 4:1–179.
7. Cox, R. (1957): The management of dysphagia due to malignant disease of the thoracic and abdominal oesophagus. *Ann. R. Coll. Surg.*, 21:133–176.
8. Deeley, T. J., and Francois, P. E. (1958): A technique for the irradiation of the upper oesophagus in megavoltage therapy. *Br. J. Radiol.*, 3:395–396.
9. Doctor, V. M., and Sirsat, M. V. (1967): A histopathological study of pre-operative radiated carcinoma of the esophagus. *Clin. Radiol.*, 18:422–427.
10. Elkon, D., Lee, M., and Hendrickson, F. R. (1978): Carcinoma of the esophagus: Sites of recurrence and palliative benefits after definitive radiotherapy. *Int. J. Rad. Oncol. Biol. Phys.*, 4:615–620.

11. Ellis, F. H., Jr., Jackson R. C., Kreuger, J. T., Moersch, H. J., Clagett, O. T., and Gage, R. P. (1959): Carcinoma of the esophagus and cardia. Results of treatment, 1946–1956. *N. Engl. J. Med.*, 260:351–358.
12. Flores, A. (1978): Personal communication.
13. Fu Wai Hospital and Institute for Oncology, Chinese Academy of Medical Sciences, Peking (1967): Combined preoperative irradiation and surgery for carcinoma of the esophagus. *China's Med.*, 6:473–478.
14. Garrett, M. J. (1971): Megavoltage technique for treatment of carcinoma of the post cricoid region. *Clin. Radiol.*, 22:136–138.
15. Groves, L. K., and Rodriguez-Antunez, A. (1973): Treatment of carcinoma of the esophagus and gastric cardia with concentrated preoperative radiation followed by early operation. *Ann. Thorac. Surg.*, 15:333–338.
16. Guernsey, J. M., Dogget, R. L. S., Mason, G. R., Kohatsu, S., and Oberhelman, H. A. (1969): Combined treatment of cancer of the esophagus. *Am. J. Surg.*, 117:157–161.
17. Gunnlaugsson, G. H., Wychulis, A. R., Roland, C., and Ellis, F. H. (1970): Analysis of the records of 1657 patients with carcinoma of the esophagus and cardia of the stomach. *Surg. Gynecol. Obstet.*, 130:997–1005.
18. Japanese Society for Esophgeal Diseases (1976): Guidelines for the clinical and pathological studies on carcinoma of the esophagus. *Jpn. J. Surg.*, 6:69–86.
19. Kasai, M., Mori, S., and Watanabe, T. (1978): Follow-up results after resection of thoracic esophageal carcinoma. *World J. Surg.*, 2:543–551.
20. Lachapèle, A. P., Lagarde, C., and Touchard, J. (1964): Bilan de sept ans d'expérience de cycloroentgenthérapie du cancer de l'oesophage. *J. Radiol. Electrol. Med. Nucl.*, 45:732–735.
21. Lane, F. W. (1976): The case for irradiation—Symposium on cancer of the esophagus. *Hospital Practice*, 11:68–73.
22. Leborgne, R., Leborgne, F., Jr., and Barlocci, L. (1963): Cancer of the oesophagus: Results of radiotherapy. *Br. J. Radiol.*, 36:806–811.
23. LeRoux, B. T. (1961): An analysis of seven hundred cases of carcinoma of the hypopharynx, the oesophagus and the proximal stomach. *Thorax*, 16:226–255.
24. Lewinsky, B. S., Annes, G. P., Mann, S. G., Green, J. P., Vaeth, J. M., Schroeder, A. F., and Cantril, S. T. (1975): Carcinoma of the esophagus. *Radiol. Clin.*, 44:192–204.
25. Logan, A. (1963): The surgical treatment of carcinoma of the oesophagus and cardia. *J. Thorac. Cardiovasc. Surg.*, 46:150–161.
26. Marcial, V. A., Tomé, J. M., Ubiñas, J., Bosch, A., and Correa, J. N. (1966): Role of radiation therapy in esophageal cancer. *Radiology*, 87:231–239.
27. Marchand, P. E. (1978): Diagnosis in carcinoma of the oesophagus. In: *Carcinoma of the Oesophagus*, edited by W. Silber, pp. 211–216. A. A. Balkema, Capetown.
28. Marks, R. D., Scruggs, H. J., and Wallace, K. M. (1976): Preoperative radiation therapy for carcinoma of the esophagus. *Cancer*, 38:84–89.
29. Martini, N., Goodner, J. T., D'Angio, G. J., and Beattie, E. J. (1970): Tracheoesophageal fistula due to cancer. *J. Thorac. Cardiovasc. Surg.*, 59:319–324.
30. Miller, C. (1962): Carcinoma of the thoracic esophagus and cardia: A review of 405 cases. *Br. J. Surg.*, 49:507–522.
31. Mustard, R. A., and Ibberson, O. (1956): Carcinoma of the esophagus. A review of 381 cases admitted to Toronto General Hospital 1937–1953 inclusive. *Ann. Surg.*, 144:927–940.
32. Nakayama, K. (1977): Experiences in the treatment of esophageal cancer of the upper and middle thoracic segment. *Surg. Annu.*, 9:125–132.
33. Nakayama, K., and Kinoshita, Y. (1974): Surgical treatment combined with preoperative concentrated radiation: Esophagus: Treatment: Cancer of the gastrointestinal tract. *J. Am. Med. Assoc.*, 227:178–181.
34. Nanson, E. M. (1976): Dysphagia: Caveat oesophagum. *N. Z. Med. J.*, 83:109–111.
35. Nègre, E., Pujol, H., Gary-Bobo, J., and Bordart, J. C. (1976): L'irradiation pré-opératoire dans le traitement des cancers di l'oesophage thoracique. *J. Chir. (Paris)*, 111:403–408.
36. Parker, E. F., and Gregorie, H. B. (1976): Carcinoma of the esophagus. Long term results. *J. Am. Med. Assoc.*, 235:1018–1020.
37. Parker, E. F., Gregorie, H. B., Arrants, J. E., and Ravenel, J. M. (1970): Carcinoma of the esophagus. *Ann. Surg.*, 171:746–751.

38. (1977): Particles and radiation therapy. Second international conference. *Int. J. Rad. Oncol. Biol. Phys.*, 3:1–424.

39. Pearson J. G. (1966): Radiotherapy of carcinoma of the oesophagus and post-cricoid region in south east Scotland. *Clin. Radiol.*, 17:242–257.

40. Pearson, J. G. (1969): The value of radiotherapy in the management of esophageal cancer. *Am. J. Roentgenol. Radium Ther. Nucl. Med.*, 105:500–513.

41. Pearson J. G. (1971): The value of radiotherapy in the management of squamous oesophageal cancer. *Br. J. Surg.*, 58:794–797.

42. Pearson, J. G. (1974): Carcinoma of the oesophagus—Operation or radiation. *Langenbecks Arch. Chir.*, 337:739–743.

43. Pearson, J. G. (1977): The present status and future potential of radiotherapy in the management of esophageal cancer. *Cancer*, 39:882–890.

44. Pearson, J. G., and LeRoux, B. T. (1974): Malignant tumors of the esophagus. In: *Diseases of the Esophagus*, edited by G. Vantrappen and J. Hellemans. In: *Handbuch der inneren Medizin*, dritter Band/erster Teil, fünfte Auflage, pp. 447–487. Springer-Verlag, Berlin.

45. Prager, G. R. (1973): Vertebral fixation of the oesophagus. A symptom in the posterior mediastinum. *Radiol. Clin. Biol.*, 42:174–175.

46. Proctor, D. S. C. (1968): Carcinoma of the oesophagus: A review of 523 cases. *S. Afr. J. Surg.*, 6:137–159.

47. Rambo, V. B., O'Brien, P. H., Miller, M. C., III., Stroud, M. R., and Parker, E. F. (1975): Carcinoma of the esophagus. *J. Surg. Oncol.*, 7:355–365.

48. Rider, W. D., and Mendoza, R. D. (1969): Some opinions on treatment of cancer of the esophagus. *Am. J. Roentgenol. Radium Ther. Nucl. Med.*, 105:514–517.

49. Robertson, R., Coy, P., and Mokkhavesa, S. (1967): The results of radical surgery compared with radical radiotherapy in the treatment of squamous carcinoma of the thoracic esophagus. The case for preoperative radiotherapy. *J. Thorac. Cardiovasc. Surg.*, 53:430–440.

50. Rubin, P. (1974): Comment: Pretreatment laparotomy: Esophagus: Treatment—Localized and advanced: Cancer of the gastrointestinal tract. *J. Am. Med. Assoc.*, 227:184–185.

51. Seymour, E. Q., and Pettit, H. S. (1973): An evaluation of long term survivors treated for cancer of the esophagus with preoperative x-ray therapy. *Radiology*, 106:423.

52. Shimkin, M. B. (1951): Duration of life in untreated cancer. *Cancer*, 4:1–8.

53. Stevens, K. R., Fry, R., and Stone, C. (1978): A new technique for irradiating thoracic inlet tumors. *Int. J. Rad. Oncol. Biol. Phys.*, 4:731–774.

54. Storey, C. F. (1962): *Acquired Surgical Lesions of the Esophagus*. Charles C Thomas, Springfield, Ill.

55. UICC (International Union against Cancer) (1978): *TNM Classification of Malignant Tumors*, ed. 3. UICC, Geneva.

56. Vaeth, J. M. (1978): Esophageal carcinoma. In: *Modern Radiation Oncology*, edited by H. A. Gilbert and A. R. Kagan, pp. 357–374. Harper & Row, New York.

57. Voutilainen, A., and Koulumies, M. (1965): Results of radiation therapy of cancer of the esophagus. *Ann. Chir. Gynaecol. Fenn.*, 54:40–51.

58. Werner, I. D. (1978): Pre and post-operative radical therapy for oesophageal carcinoma. In: *Carcinoma of the Oesophagus*, edited by W. Silber, pp. 340–345. A. A. Balkema, Capetown.

59. Werner, I. D. (1978): The palliative management of squamous carcinoma of the intra-thoracic and intra-abdominal oesophagus. In: *Carcinoma of the Oesophagus*, edited by W. Silber, pp. 445–448. A. A. Balkema, Capetown.

60. Werner, I. D., Silber, W., Madden P. C. W., Birkenstock, W. E., Perkin, H., and Stein, D. (1975): Carcinoma of the thoraco-abdominal oesophagus. *S. Afr. Med. J.*, 49:653–656.

61. Wu, Y. K., and Huang, K. C. (1979): Chinese experience in the surgical treatment of carcinoma of the esophagus. *Ann. Surg.*, 190:361–365.

62. Yamashita, H., Okura, J., Yoshioka, T., and Tanaka, Y. (1972): Preoperative irradiation in treatment of carcinoma of the oesophagus. *Australas Radiol.*, 16:250–257.

63. Younghusband, J. D., and Aluwihare, A. P. R. (1970): Carcinoma of the oesophagus: Factors influencing survival. *Br. J. Surg.*, 57:422–430.

Thoracic Oncology, edited by N. C. Choi and
H. C. Grillo. Raven Press, New York © 1983.

Mediastinal Tumors

J. Gordon Scannell

Department of Surgery, Massachusetts General Hospital, Boston, Massachusetts 02114

In the consideration of mediastinal tumors, one broad principle can be stated at the outset: Any diagnosis short of a histologic one is at best an educated guess, and in the case of certain teratomas this statement may even include histologic diagnoses. Given this uncertainty, it is generally agreed that except in unusual circumstances mediastinal tumors should be removed when technically possible, or at the very least an adequate biopsy should be obtained on which to base alternative forms of therapy.

There are numerous reasons for an aggressive approach. Space is at a premium in the mediastinum and thoracic inlet, where a space-taking lesion, should it grow, may seriously embarrass the airway, great vessels, or vital structures. Whether this increase is the result of continuing proliferation of cells, as in a neoplasm, or the result of hemorrhage, infarction, or infection in a benign cyst, the hazard is the same. The sudden increase in substernal goiter is a familiar example of this problem. Similarly, a bronchogenic cyst is susceptible to infection; it is easily removed if uninfected, but a source of disability and difficulty once infection has occurred.

In the past the diagnosis of mediastinal tumors has depended on conventional radiography, fluoroscopy, tomography, and at times special procedures to define the relationship of a mediastinal mass to adjacent structures (e.g., barium swallow, venography, arteriography). There is little question that in the foreseeable future further refinements in computerized tomography and ultrasound will add greatly to our prethoracotomy diagnostic acumen. Indeed, for purely cystic lesions, it may in some cases allow for simple aspiration as a substitute for limited thoracotomy.

The problem, of course, with needle aspiration biopsy of a mediastinal mass is the familiar one of obtaining inadequate or unrepresentative samples plus the theoretical possibility of implantation of tumor in areas not amenable to subsequent block excision. In the case of seeding of the pleural space, this includes contamination outside the usual field of radiation therapy. Certainly present techniques of fine-needle aspiration, as opposed to the older methods of large-needle "core" biopsies, have greatly reduced the likelihood of hemorrhage or tumor implantation, for which the evidence is largely anecdotal, although real. Cytologic differentiation of the biopsy, however, may tax even the most experienced of cytologists or pathologists. Therefore, an "excision" biopsy, or adequate incision biopsy if the tumor is clearly out of bounds in terms of its removal, is to be preferred. It is important to emphasize that if thoracotomy is to be freely advocated in order to establish the diagnosis of benign disease, it must not become synonymous with a painful or disfiguring incision. The surgical approach, particularly until the malignant or technically difficult nature of the lesion is established, should be designed with respect for the anatomic structure and function of the chest wall.

The mediastinum is conventionally divided into four compartments, although to a large degree the boundaries are arbitrary: anterior, superior, middle, and posterior. To some degree this dictates or at least suggests, optimal surgical access. Certainly, an anterior mediastinal mass is approached most directly by way of a median sternotomy unless it clearly extends posteriorly or to one side. A vertical midline incision may be used, or if cosmetic considerations are important, particularly in female patients a transverse submammary incision may be worth the extra effort and risk of superficial wound complications. A transverse bilateral anterior thoracotomy has limited application, except in children, for it can be an awkward incision to make, and exposure may be limited. In the case of an anterior mediastinal lesion that extends into the neck, median sternotomy can easily be extended for a cervicomediastinal exposure. Low anterior mediastinal lesions that lie clearly to one side may be approached by way of an anterolateral thoracotomy using a submammary incision to good cosmetic effect.

Direct access to superior mediastinal lesions, unless there is clearly significant posterior extension, is satisfactorily obtained by partial or total median sternotomy. The obvious exception, of course, is the substernal goiter, where the conventional collar incision is adequate, excellent access to the blood supply of the mass is provided, and extension by medial sternotomy is rarely required.

The usual approach to a posterior mediastinal lesion will be a standard posterolateral thoracotomy. If necessary, as in the case of a neurofibroma with intraspinal extension, this incision can be extended by a vertical limb over the dorsal spine to permit concomitant laminectomy and neurosurgical assistance. This will be discussed later.

For simple biopsy of an anterior mediastinal process, resection of one or more appropriate costal cartilages or in some cases merely a short anterior intercostal incision will be adequate, the so-called Chamberlain procedure or one of its many modifications. The principal hazards of this approach are two: hemorrhage from the internal mammary vessels, which must be carefully isolated and secured; opening of the pleura, with consequent pleural seeding.

Conventional mediastinoscopy, of course, has enormous utility in the biopsy of paratracheal and carinal lesions, particularly if tomography, conventional or computerized, suggests lymph node involvement. The indications for mediastinoscopy in the presence of a solitary lesion are a matter of individual judgment. For example, the transcervical approach for thymectomy in myasthenia gravis has its advocates, but in the presence of presumed thymoma the transcervical approach provides only limited access and introduces the likelihood of implantation should the tumor prove to be malignant.

The majority of benign mediastinal tumors are asymptomatic. The presence of symptoms, notably pain, dysphagia, dyspnea, or the finding of venous blockade of the superior vena caval system, enormously increases the likelihood of malignancy. Exceptions, of course, have been mentioned earlier: hemorrhage, infarction, or infection of a benign process leading to its rapid increase in size.

TUMORS OF THE ANTERIOR AND SUPERIOR MEDIASTINUM

The common tumors of the anterior and superior mediastinum are (a) teratogenous tumors, (b) tumors of thymic origin, (c) tumors or cysts of the thyroid or parathyroid, (d) isolated tumors of the lymphoma series, (e) neurogenic tumors (rarely), (f) tumors of blood vessel or lymphatic origin, (g) lipomata and miscellaneous tumors of mesodermal origin, and (h) processes simulating primary mediastinal tumors (e.g., aneurysm, pleuropericardial cysts, metastatic tumor, or giant lymph node hyperplasia). In all the preceding categories one finds a range from benign to highly malignant.

The common benign teratogenous tumor of the anterior and superior compartment is the dermoid cyst. Although this may occur at any age, the diagnosis usually is not made until adult life. The benign form presents as a smooth rounded mass, almost always an incidental radiologic finding unless infection has occurred. Demonstration of bone, teeth, and other differentiated structures by tomography, conventional or computerized, establishes a diagnosis preoperatively. The probability of gradual increase in size and the possibility of superimposed infection justify removal in the absence of serious systemic contraindications. Microscopically, dermoids are composed of predominantly ectodermal elements.

At the other end of the teratogenous spectrum are malignant teratomas. These are prone to invade or seriously compress adjacent structures, and they characteristically present as large, lobulated or irregular masses with a short or rapidly evolving history of mediastinal compression. Microscopically such tumors contain poorly differentiated tissues of entodermal, ectodermal, and mesodermal origin, of almost infinite variety in form and function including both exocrine and endocrine secretions. If one can demonstrate nonresectability by venography, barium swallow, or other clinical or radiologic evidence, open biopsy by anterior mediastinotomy should provide a reasonable basis for radiation therapy. Open biopsy is ordinarily preferable to needle biopsy by virtue of the sampling problem, except in extreme cases. Indeed, in patients with acute respiratory obstruction it may be prudent to proceed with emergency radiation therapy on clinical grounds, but this should be done only in most unusual circumstances.

Partial removal followed by radiation may be a workable compromise, particularly in the relatively small and manageable tumors when seemingly complete or nearly complete removal is possible. Not infrequently the bizarre histologic characteristics of a teratoma may be reflected in its clinical behavior, and a management plan of radiation followed by resection of the residual tumor mass can be justified.

THYMOMA

The Massachusetts General Hospital (MGH) experience with tumors of thymic origin has recently been reported by Wilkins and Castleman (1). As the authors point out, the patient population in this study had an unusually high proportion, 56 of 103 (54%), of thymoma patients with myasthenia gravis, 47 patients without. This unusually high incidence of myasthenia is due in large measure to the number of patients seen in the Myasthenia Gravis Clinic established at MGH in 1935 and for a long time a special interest of that institution.

The judgment whether a thymoma is benign or malignant is made on the basis of the gross characteristics of the tumor. Outright invasive growth into surrounding organs, intrathoracic or intrapleural metastases or both, is an indication of malignancy (stage III). Pericapsular growth into the mediastinal fat, adjacent pleura, or pericardium is also a criterion of malignancy, calling for a rating of stage II. A tumor is considered benign (stage I) when the capsule of the gland appears intact and growth occurs only within the capsule. Wilkins and Castleman agreed that the prognostic value of the histology of the tumor, spindle cell versus epithelial cell, is zero. Others have argued that spindle cell tumors are less frequently invasive than the epithelial form, but they agree that it is the invasive feature that is the determinant.

It is interesting to note that in the MGH series a relatively high proportion of thymomas with myasthenia gravis were otherwise asymptomatic, whereas in the nonmyasthenic group, chest pain, cough, fever, weakness, hoarseness, and dyspnea were relatively common. It is no surprise, then, that in the nonmyasthenic groups invasive tumors were twice as frequent as in the myasthenics.

The radiologic appearance of a thymoma is variable, but as a general rule the mass is anterior and extends frequently to fuse with the shadows of the pericardium and the pulmonary artery, particularly to the left. The recent use of computerized tomography in the diagnosis and evaluation of extent has contributed dramatically to the surgical management of this interesting group of tumors.

With few exceptions, median sternotomy, total thymectomy, and mediastinal dissection constitute the preferred operative approach. Preoperative needle aspiration biopsy, even if the lesion appears to be largely cystic, is rarely to be recommended and on theoretical grounds should be avoided if one accepts invasion of the capsule of the gland as a major criterion of malignancy.

Incomplete removal ordinarily is an indication for postoperative radiation therapy, and on an empirical basis postoperative irradiation appears to be reasonable in stage III and most stage II lesions, even if the tumor appears to be totally excised. Evidence for the value of irradiation in the latter two categories is inferential.

One conclusion emphatically brought out by the recent report from MGH is that improved methods of postoperative and long-term medical management of patients with thymoma and myasthenia gravis have reversed an earlier dictum by these same authors that the presence of myasthenia is an extremely ominous factor affecting survival. Quite clearly it is the invasive character of the tumor that is the most important predictor.

Long-term survival following removal of stage I thymoma has been encouraging, ranging in the MGH series from 92% among patients without myasthenia to 63%

among patients with myasthenia (this includes all patients in the series, which extends back to 1939, and the results are reported as cumulative survival).

Cumulative 5-year survival for all invasive stage II and stage III tumors was of the order of 55% (46% for those with myasthenia).

OTHER TUMORS OF THE ANTERIOR AND SUPERIOR MEDIASTINUM

Other tumors of the anterior and superior mediastinum include adenomatous enlargement of both the thyroid and parathyroids. Intimately related embryologically to the pharyngeal pouches and the embryologic anlage of the thymus, which normally descends through the thoracic inlet, it is not surprising to find colloid adenomata of the thyroid (not a true neoplasm) and less commonly parathyroid adenoma adjacent to or involved in thymic tissue.

There are many well-known clues to the diagnosis of substernal goiter, notably upward motion on swallowing, the position of the mass within the thoracic inlet, positive isotope scans for ectopic functioning thyroid tissue. Only a few additional remarks are needed. Substernal goiters commonly produce venous obstruction, but in this instance without the usual grim clinical implications of a superior vena caval syndrome. Simple venography may be reassuring in this regard. Laryngeal nerve paralysis may occur but it is rare. Compression of the trachea by its lateral displacement may be radiologically dramatic without corresponding clinical airway obstruction, quite distinct from the airway encroachment that occurs with invasive anaplastic carcinoma, which usually occurs at a cervical level.

Of particular interest is the substernal goiter that descends posterior to the great vessels and presents as a posterior superior mediastinal mass. As with any thyroid mass, the blood supply will descend from the neck, and the surgical approach is primarily cervical, with sternotomy extension if necessary. Posterior mediastinal goiters may be associated with unusual variations in the course of the recurrent nerve.

Neurogenic tumors may present in the anterior or superior mediastinum, but they are rare enough to qualify for single case reports, often with a review of the literature appended. Their biological behavior differs little from that of neurogenic tumors in the posterior mediastinum. Tumors of the lymphoma series, including Hodgkin's disease, may present as solitary lesions in the anterior mediastinum, although more commonly they are found in the middle mediastinum. If the tumor is actually solitary at the time of exploration, removal can be justified if it can be accomplished without hazard to adjacent vital structures. This opportunity rarely arises. Although lymphoma and Hodgkin's disease may be found in the anterior mediastinum, as indicated above, they are generally middle mediastinal, paratracheal, and hilar tumors, and the predominant differential diagnosis will be sarcoid or giant lymph node hyperplasia. The diagnosis usually is made at mediastinoscopy. The treatment is irradiation or chemotherapy or both.

TUMORS OF THE MIDDLE MEDIASTINUM

In addition to being the site for lymphoma, the middle mediastinum is a common habitat for bronchogenic and enterogenous cysts, not true neoplasms, to be sure, but frequently masquerading as such. The diagnosis may require astute radiologic observation, once again tremendously aided by computerized tomography. Because bronchogenic and enterogenous cysts are in close proximity or in actual communication with the airway and upper gastrointestinal tract, superimposed infection is common. In the absence of specific contraindications, local removal at a time of election is indicated.

It is always a source of some surprise to encounter a large, apparently solitary mediastinal mass that proves to be a metastatic node. An occult carcinoma of the lung and an unsuspected renal carcinoma are the two most likely sources. Removal of a solitary mediastinal metastasis requires no apology, particularly because the diagnosis is generally made after the fact.

The bête noire of the middle mediastinum is, of course, the unsuspected aneurysm. The diagnosis of thoracic aortic aneurysm should be, but is not always, straightforward, and with the techniques of arteriography and computerized tomography it can be made with great accuracy. Diagnostic oversight, however, seems to be part of the human condition.

Pericardiocoelomic cysts commonly masquerade as mediastinal tumors. Their location and radiologic characteristics, particularly with the sophisticated techniques now available, should allow an accurate prethoracotomy diagnosis. Under these circumstances one can justify aspiration of "spring-water" cysts, a procedure much discussed, though probably rarely performed by thoracic surgeons of those early times when even the simplest thoracotomy was an event.

NEUROGENIC TUMORS AND THE POSTERIOR MEDIASTINUM

The posterior mediastinum is the primary breeding area and habitat for a long list of neurogenic tumors, each with its benign and malignant counterparts. The final classification (neurilemoma, neurofibroma, ganglioneuroma, paraganglioma, etc.) provides an indication of the point of origin of the tumor in question. Usually slow-growing, they may undergo "malignant degeneration" if incompletely removed, and, of course, some are malignant and invasive at the outset. Pheochromocytoma, a functioning tumor of neural crest origin, may present as an intrathoracic lesion but so rarely as merely to warrant mentioning en passant. So also neuroblastoma, a highly malignant tumor of childhood that requires an extensive surgical excision, irradiation, and chemotherapy.

Of major clinical importance is the relationship of a posterior mediastinal mass to the intercostal foramen, with possible intraspinal extension, the aptly named dumbbell neurofibroma. Ganglioneuroma and paraganglioma, which take origin from cells of the autonomic chain and its ganglia, rarely extend into the spinal foramen. However, such tumors may be highly vascular, and their removal may require adequate exposure through a posterolateral approach. Whereas ganglioneuromas and other tumors that take origin in the sympathetic system tend to remain exclusively intrathoracic, neurofibromata and neurilemomas, the latter derived from cells forming the sheath of Schwann, hence the name Schwannoma, are commonly involved with intercostal nerves at their entrance into the chest through the intervertebral foramen. The radiologic clue to this point of origin is distortion of this foramen and widening of the corresponding intercostal space. Carefully focused tomography and computerized tomographic scanning can be most helpful. Involvement of the nerve at the level of the intervertebral foramen imposes two major surgical problems: (a) possible intraspinal extension of the tumor, usually without evidence of neurologic deficit; (b) difficulty in control of the blood supply to the tumor, requiring maneuvers such as undue traction and tamponade that can lead to serious intraspinal damage at a high or midthoracic level.

Certainly, the unexpected finding of an extension of the tumor through the spinal foramen complicates the thoracic procedure. Hemorrhage may be difficult to control, and under these circumstances the surgeon may settle for partial removal, transecting the tumor at the foramen and leaving the intraspinal removal for a later date. Although the dual location of the neurofibroma is uncommon, the problem is of sufficient importance that it should be defined preoperatively by polytome roentgenograms and myelography if the former are positive, or by careful computerized tomography. Forearmed with knowledge that the tumor has an intraspinal extension, we advocate a combined procedure using an incision that permits both standard posterolateral thoracotomy and laminectomy. Operation is carried out in the usual lateral thoracotomy position. An appropriate interspace is chosen, and the intrathoracic portion of the tumor is completely mobilized so that only its intraforamenal isthmus remains attached. If total mobilization is impossible from within, laminectomy is carried out through a vertical posterior midline extension of the standard thoracotomy incision. We have used this approach successfully in three patients. A similar concept, that is, a one-stage combined operation, has been advocated by the group at the Mayo Clinic, who have described a curved paraspinal incision and a laminectomy, with resection of the posterior portion of an appropriate rib.

Partial excision of neurofibromata is to be avoided if at all possible, although wide en bloc resection is unnecessary. Recurrence is rare, but growth of residual tumor can be most troublesome. The majority of single neurofibromata and other neurogenic tumors are slowly growing, but their removal is indicated to establish their true nature and to avoid future difficulties should they advance to an awkward size. Obviously, should the tumor be responsible for unwanted hormonal abnormalities, particularly in the case of paragangliomas, removal is clearly indicated. Multiple neurofibromata as part of von Recklinghausen's disease may be treated expectantly, unless under observation a given tumor shows significant increase.

MISCELLANEOUS TUMORS AND PSEUDOTUMORS

At the outset of this chapter it was implied that the mediastinum is the site of an enormous variety of tumors and processes that have the appearance of neoplasms.

In addition to the common lesions already discussed, meaningful differential diagnosis should include the following: (a) lipoma and liposarcoma; (b) fibroma and fibrosarcoma; (c) hemangioma and malignant tumors of vascular origin; (d) lymphangioma, notably cystic hygroma; (e) intrathoracic meningocele; (f) giant lymph node hyperplasia (Castleman's disease).

Lipomata, at times unusually discrete well-formed mediastinal fat tabs, are not uncommon. Even conventional tomography may be sufficiently convincing to permit continuing observation of such lesions, and sophisticated tomography and sonography offer promise of even greater diagnostic assurance. The incidence of malignant change presumably is low, the indications for removal are diagnostic uncertainty or the possibility of infarction and sudden increase in size in tumors of threatening proportions.

The protean nature of mediastinal fat is well illustrated by the clinical entity of pericardial fat necrosis (2). Eight such cases are on record. The characteristic clinical picture is that of rapid onset of anterior chest pain or repeated attacks of pain that may mimic myocardial or pulmonary infarction followed by the appearance of a juxtacardiac mass in the chest roentgenogram. Similar in clinical course and pathologic appearance to infarction of an epiploic appendage, their pathogenesis is obscure, because torsion of mediastinal fat is mechanically unlikely and has not been encountered in the reported cases.

In the differential diagnosis of solid mediastinal masses, fibroma and its malignant variant fibrosarcoma must be considered. Without entering into the argument regarding the origin of such tumors, suffice it to say that preoperative diagnosis is beyond the bounds of reasonable certainty, and the operative indications and management will be an individualized affair. The relationship to solitary benign fibrous mesothelioma will be considered in another chapter.

Hemangiomata, hemangiosarcoma, and its many variants and vascular abnormalities simulating blood vessel neoplasms must always be considered in poorly defined mediastinal masses. Usually asymptomatic, a clue to their diagnosis may be the presence of a bruit or unusual vascular patterns in adjacent tissue. Where doubt exists and technical difficulties can be predicted, preoperative angiography is of great value.

Comparable to and closely allied to blood vessel tumors are neoplasms and abnormalities of lymphatic origin. Usually in the superior mediastinum, these may or may not be related to the thoracic duct. The most striking example, of course, is the large cystic hygroma, predominantly a pediatric problem, usually cervical in presentation but commonly with mediastinal extension. Occasionally it may be confined to the mediastinum.

A most unusual but important posterior mediastinal lesion, indistinguishable at first glance from neurofibroma with intraspinal extension, is intrathoracic meningocele. The lesion is characteristically associated with widening of the intervertebral foramen, erosion of rib and adjacent vertebrae, and even, at times, diffuse neurofibromatosis. Preoperative diagnostic evaluation will parallel that for neurofibroma with bony spinal changes. If the process is enlarging or is causing symptoms, excision may be indicated at the discretion of the neurosurgeon.

No discussion of miscellaneous or unusual mediastinal masses would be complete without mention of giant lymph node hyperplasia, variously described as lymph-nodal hamartoma, benign giant lymphoma, angiofollicular mediastinal lymph-node hyperplasia, etc. It is also referred to by the eponym Castleman's disease, at least at MGH, to recognize his original description of the entity in 1956. In the course of studying tumors of the thymus gland, he encountered 13 cases in which enlarged mediastinal lymph nodes resembled thymic tumors grossly, radiologically, and even microscopically and had been so reported. On careful study, however, it became apparent that although numerous lymph follicles were present, the lesions had two distinct histologic patterns (hyaline vascular and plasma cell types) and were of lymph node origin. First reported in 1956, the subject was reviewed in 1972, with a total of 81 cases from the AFIP and MGH. Seventy of the 81 presented as solitary mediastinal tumors, 25 in the anterior superior mediastinum. The masses varied from 1.5 to 16 cm in greatest diameter. The majority of the mediastinal masses, 74 of 81, were of the hyaline vascular type. Of these patients, 13 had symptoms of tracheobronchial compression, respiratory tract infections, cough, dyspnea, hemoptysis, and pain. Hematologic abnormalities, notably anemia and hyperglobinemia, were for the most part related to the plasma cell variety. In all cases, surgical excision, preferably total, was considered to be the treatment of choice, with almost certain prospect of cure. Apparently radiation therapy was not effective.

SUMMARY AND CONCLUSIONS

Tumors of the mediastinum and processes resembling tumors continue to pose fascinating challenges in differential diagnosis, settled in the final analysis by surgical exploration. It is safe to predict that increasingly sophisticated radiographic and related techniques will greatly improve our diagnostic acumen and therefore our preoperative planning. Conventional ground rules have proved reasonable and sound. However, the respective roles of surgical therapy, radiation therapy, and chemotherapy, the latter used as primary treatment or adjunctively, will require further definition on a cooperative basis.

REFERENCES

1. Wilkins, E. W., Jr., and Castleman, B. (1979): Thymoma: A continuing survey at the Massachusetts General Hospital. *Am. Thor. Surg.*, 28:252–256.
2. Behrendt, D. M., and Scannell, J. G. (1968): Pericardial fat necrosis. *N. Engl. J. Med.*, 275:448–449.
3. Byron, F. X., Alling, E. E., and Samson, P. C. (1949): Intrathoracic meningocele. *J. Thorac. Surg.*, 18:294–303.
4. Keller, A. R., Hochholzer, L., and Castleman, B. (1972): Hyaline-vascular and plasma-cell types of giant lymph node hyperplasia of the mediastinum and other locations. *Cancer*, 29:3.

Thoracic Oncology, edited by N. C. Choi and
H. C. Grillo. Raven Press, New York © 1983.

Pathology of Pleural Neoplasms

Eugene J. Mark

Department of Pathology, Massachusetts General Hospital, Boston, Massachusetts 02114

The pleura is composed of layers of three different tissues (3), each responsible for different types of neoplasm. The surface mesothelial layer gives rise to diffuse mesothelioma (Fig. 1); the submesothelial fibrous layer gives rise to localized mesothelioma; and the interstitial layer, with its rich supply of capillaries and lymphatics, hosts metastases, lymphoma, and leukemia. Visceral pleura contains two layers of elastica, the inner serving as the anatomic boundary between pleura and lung. Parietal pleura has a structure similar to visceral pleura but less regular in organization. The characteristic elastic layers serve as guideposts in histologically locating the pleura (a feature that is always helpful when infection or neoplasm or fibrous tissue has obliterated the pleural space) and thereby distinguishing visceral pleura from lung and parietal pleura from chest wall. Elastic tissue is seen to best advantage with special stains.

Primary neoplasms of the pleura were virtually unknown in the first part of the twentieth century. As late as the 1950's some authors doubted their very existence and considered all malignant pleural neoplasms to be metastases. However, as the incidence of diffuse malignant pleural tumors has increased continuously since 1940, and continues to increase (16,29), the histologic characteristics which serve to define a primary pleural mesothelioma have become recognized, just as the characteristics of an infectious agent often first become apparent during an epidemic. Metastatic carcinoma remains the most common neoplasm which involves the pleura. Diffuse malignant mesothelioma remains the greatest challenge in diagnosis. The classification of pleural neoplasms used here is given in Table 1.

TABLE 1. *Pleural neoplasms*

Diffuse malignant mesothelioma
Localized fibrous mesothelioma
Metastases
Carcinoma
Sarcoma
Lymphoma
Leukemia

DIFFUSE MALIGNANT MESOTHELIOMA

Mesothelial cells derive from the mesoderm but also line a space in the body and thus have both mesenchymal and epithelial aspects. Diffuse malignant mesothelioma, reflecting this binary potential, exhibits pathological features of both a sarcoma and a carcinoma. Until fairly recently, conservative pathologists maintained that a diagnosis of malignant mesothelioma could be made with assurance only at autopsy. Gradually the diagnosis came to be made at full exploratory thoracotomy, and now a diagnosis is sought on small biopsy obtained at limited thoracotomy or even on needle biopsy of the pleura.

Grossly, malignant mesothelioma usually has spread diffusely over the pleural surface of one hemithorax by the time of diagnosis. Occasionally, at open thoracotomy early in the disease, the tumor may seem to be confined to one area, more often on the parietal than visceral pleura. Extensive growth involves both parietal and visceral pleura, obliterates the pleural space, encases and compresses the lung, invades outward into chest wall, and invades inward along the interlobular septa to the hilum of the lung. Involvement of the contralateral pleura, pericardium, or peritoneum occurs in approximately one-third of cases (22,30). Blood vessel invasion is common, as is direct extension through the diaphragm into the abdominal cavity. Mediastinal lymph node invasion occurs more commonly by direct extension than by lymphatic invasion, a feature characteristic of sarcomas. Distant metastases appear, in order of decreasing frequency, in liver, lung, bone, spleen and adrenal.

Histologically, the essential feature is a mixture of malignant stromal-like cells and malignant epithelial-like cells, thus resulting in both sarcomatous and carcinomatous patterns. The sarcomatous areas may have anaplastic spindle cells with numerous mitoses, but in early lesions the cells may be spaced far apart, the nuclei may be rather uniform and deceptively innocuous, and the histology may mimic reative fibrous proliferation. Malignant cartilage and bone and dystrophic calcification sometimes appear (9,21). The carcinomatous areas may have tubular, alveolar or slit-like spaces (Fig. 1). The epithelial-like cells may form papillary structures and psammoma bodies (20). Advanced lesions usually exhibit anaplastic and pleomorphic epithelial-like cells, but early lesions characteristically have cells with relatively regular, oval, normochromatic nuclei and abundant cytoplasm (Fig. 2). The proportion of sarcomatous versus carcinomatous pattern has no prognostic value. If either pattern appears alone, as might be anticipated if the sample of tissue is small, diagnosis on pure histologic grounds might have to be presumptive. Additional methods which can be utilized in the biopsy diagnosis of diffuse malignant mesothelioma are histochemistry (13), quantitation of hyaluronic acid in tissue (2), transmission electron microscopy (27,31), scanning electron microscopy (8), electrophoresis of tissue glycosaminoglycans extracted from the tumor (32), immunopathologic analysis, and antisera for human mesothelial cells in an indirect immunofluorescent assay (25). Three important facts about the histochemistry of mesothelioma follow: (i) diastase-resistant, periodic-acid-Schiff-positive, intracellular globules of neutral mucopolysaccharide are not found in mesothelioma and

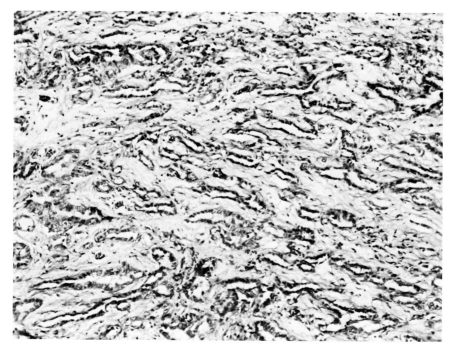

FIG. 1. Diffuse malignant mesothelioma (×160). Tubuloalveolar pattern results from clefts of variable size and shape lined by cuboidal cells with epithelial features. Loose fibrous stroma separates the clefts.

suggest carcinoma; (ii) hyaluronidase-sensitive, colloidal-iron-positive, intracellular globules of acid mucopolysaccharide are not found in carcinoma and suggest mesothelioma; (iii) mucicarmine-positive, intracellular globules of mucin can be found in either mesothelioma or carcinoma.

Exposure to asbestos is responsible for the great majority of cases of diffuse malignant mesothelioma of the pleura and for two other pleural abnormalities, hyaline plaques and recurrent pleural effusions (12). The hyaline plaque consists of firm, discrete, hypocellular fibrosis which typically appears grossly as candle-drippings on the parietal or visceral pleura of basal segments, calcifies, and serves as a radiologic and pathologic marker of probable inhalation of asbestos. The recurrent pleural effusions are often associated with atypical mesothelial hyperplasia, which probably represents a precursor lesion of diffuse malignant mesothelioma. Asbestos also causes interstitial fibrosis of the lung (asbestosis) and an increase in incidence of bronchopulmonary carcinomas.

LOCALIZED FIBROUS MESOTHELIOMA

Localized fibrous mesothelioma is a slowly growing mesenchymal neoplasm which occupies the thoracic cavity by compressing or indenting the lung. It occurs at all ages above 12 years and is slightly more common in women than men.

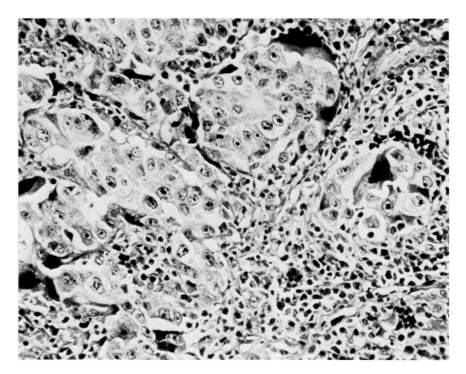

FIG. 2. Diffuse malignant mesothelioma (×400). Solid nests of cells with epithelial features have pleomorphic nuclei with large nucleoli. An occasional, giant, hyperchromatic nucleus is present. Lymphocytes separate the tumor cells.

Approximately 40% of patients are asymptomatic when the lesion is first discovered. Among patients with symptoms, cough, chest pain, dyspnea and/or pulmonary osteoarthropathy are each found in at least one-third of cases (4). Other signs and symptoms include hemoptysis, fever, night sweats, pleural effusion, palpitations, weight loss, hypoglycemia, and a heavy or rolling sensation in chest. The proportion of patients who are asymptomatic at time of diagnosis has increased in recent years, which probably reflects earlier diagnosis by increased use of chest radiographs in asymptomatic populations (4,24).

Three-fourths of fibrous mesotheliomas arise from the visceral pleura and one-fourth from the parietal pleura. The essential pathologic features are a partial or complete capsule surrounding the neoplasm, cells producing collagen, and nuclei which are spindle-shaped and for the most part lack atypicality (Fig. 3). Other pathologic features depend in part on the size of the tumor. Those less than 10 cm in greatest diameter are typically nodular, embedded subpleurally within the lung beneath a smooth pleural surface, solid and hyalinized, poorly vascular, and composed of cells without pleomorphism or mitoses (Fig. 4). Those more than 10 cm in greatest diameter are typically pedunculated, within the pleural cavity, covered by pleural adhesions, edematous and hemorrhagic, highly vascular, and may have foci of cellular pleomorphism and rare mitoses (4). Myxoid areas may predominate

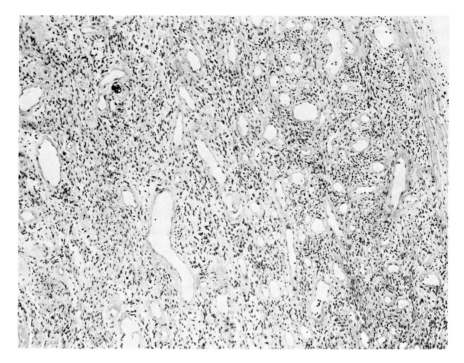

FIG. 3. Localized fibrous mesothelioma (×100). Spindle-shaped nuclei and fibrillar stroma are perforated by numerous, thin-walled, ectatic, blood vessels. Smooth intact pleura *(upper right)* encompasses the tumor.

(19). Although both small and large fibrous mesotheliomas are mostly encapsulated, strands of cells may infiltrate for a short distance into adjacent lung, diaphragm, or chest wall. Ultrastructurally, the cells may have features of either mesothelial cells or fibroblasts. Under some conditions mesothelial cells derive from fibroblasts. The cell of origin of fibrous mesothelioma is probably the submesothelial fibroblast, a cellular constituent of normal pleura (1).

Localized fibrous mesothelioma of the pleural behaves in a benign fasion in 90% of cases. In the other 10% the tumor is directly responsible for the patient's death because of massive intrathoracic growth, due either to recurrence or to late diagnosis. No single pathologic feature indicates malignancy, but large and cellular tumors with more than 10 mitoses per 10 high power fields are more likely to behave badly (7). Localized fibrous tumors of the pleura virtually never metastasize. Thus, they differ from the rarer primary pleural fibrosarcoma (15), which lacks a capsule, has generalized nuclear atypicality and extensive mitotic activity, and metastasizes.

METASTASES IN THE PLEURA

Carcinoma

Pleural carcinomatosis represents metastasis in and/or on the pleura. Biopsy of the visceral or parietal pleura is necessary for diagnosis if malignant cells are

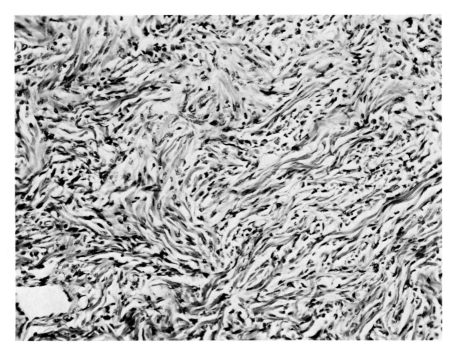

FIG. 4. Localized fibrous mesothelioma (×256). Dark spindle-shaped nuclei and wavy collagen fibers are arranged in fascicles. Nuclear pleomorphism and mitoses are not present.

confined to pleural lymphatics and/or pleural tissue and have not yet migrated to the pleural surface or shed into an effusion. Metastatic carcinoma to the pleura involves visceral pleura only in one-third of cases, and closed needle biopsy of the parietal pleura only will miss these cases. Positive cytology of a pleural effusion means that malignant cells cover the serosal surface and have seeded into the pleural cavity. Positive pleural cytology is the first manifestation of carcinoma in almost one-half of the cases of malignant pleural effusion.

Most common sites of the primary tumor responsible for pleural carcinomatosis are lung, breast, ovary and stomach. Among the lung carcinomas the most common histologic types, in order of decreasing frequency, are adenocarcinoma, squamous cell carcinoma, small cell carcinoma, and large cell carcinoma. If a carcinomatous effusion is clinically unilateral, the primary carcinoma will be ipsilateral in over 90% of the cases if the primary exists in the lung, breast or ovary. Bilateral pleural involvement by carcinoma of the lung suggests tertiary spread from hepatic metastases and bilateral parenchymal metastases (6).

Pseudomesotheliomatous carcinoma is a variant of peripheral adenocarcinoma of the lung which grows primarily into and through the pleura, spreads along the pleural surface, and encases the lung. The primary tumor is small, subpleural, and difficult to find radiologically or grossly (11). The mimicry of pseudomesotheliomatous carcinoma to diffuse malignant mesothelioma is the crucial problem for a definitive biopsy diagnosis of mesothelioma when carcinomatous but no sarcomatous areas are found histologically, regardless of the gross finding of encasement of lung by pleural tumor.

Sarcoma

Pleural sarcomatosis occurs infrequently late in the course of disease of a known primary sarcoma or very rarely as the initial manifestation of an occult primary sarcoma (23). In the latter event it can be mistaken as the sarcomatous phase of a diffuse malignant mesothelioma. Sarcomas classically embolize via blood vessels, so when the metastases reach the subpleural region of the lung or the pleura they may thrombose and destroy blood vessels and cause infection, parenchymal or pleural hemorrhage, and hemothorax. Angiosarcomas arising in large vessels of both the systemic and pulmonary circulation show a particular tendency to metastasize to the pleura (23).

LYMPHOMA

Pulmonary lymphoma may involve interstitium, airspaces or vessels. Since the interstitium of the pleura is continuous with that of the pulmonary parenchyma, lymphoma within the periphery of the lung will usually extend into the pleura (Fig. 5). Malignant cells may then shed into a pleural effusion, and a cytologic diagnosis of malignant lymphoma can be made from the pleural fluid (33). However, most pleural effusions associated with either pulmonary or generalized lymphoma are due not to pleural lymphoma but rather to mediastinal nodal lymphoma, obstruction of lymphatic return, and lymphedema of the pleural cavity. In a large clinical series 7% of all patients with lymphoma including Hodgkin's disease had pleural effusions, but less than one-fifth of these 7% had a positive cytology (33). In another clinical series of Hodgkin's lymphoma in particular, 11% of patients had pleural effusions (17). The relative frequency of histopathologic types of lymphoma in those patients with pleural effusion is not different from those patients without effusion (33).

Multiple myeloma differs from lymphoma, as pleural effusion occurs in only 1 to 2% of patients. Nodal enlargement in multiple myeloma is unusual, and the effusion is due to actual infiltration of the pleura by malignant plasma cells (14).

Angioimmunoblastic lymphadenopathy may infiltrate the lung and pleura and cause exudative pleural effusion (18).

LEUKEMIA

Pleural infiltration by leukemic cells is found at autopsy in approximately 15% of cases of leukemia. Parenchymal infiltration, by comparison, occurs twice as commonly. Half of the cases with pleural leukemia have associated parenchymal leukemia. The other half have pleural leukemia as the major thoracic manifestation of the disease unassociated with parenchymal disease (10). If a pleural effusion is present, it will contain leukemic cells. The pleura may be massively thickened by

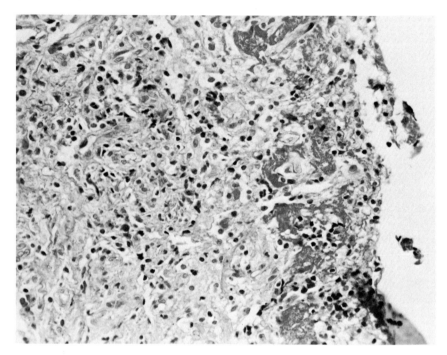

FIG. 5. Lymphoma of small cell type (×400). Thickened fibrous pleura *(left)* is diffusely infiltrated by small, dark, round cells of the lymphoma. Darker staining fibrin on pleural surface *(right)* also contains lymphoma cells.

the leukemic cells. Selectively pleural involvement occurs particularly in chronic lymphocytic leukemia and in chronic myelocytic leukemia with acute blastic transformation (5,10). Rarely, pleural leukemia will presage an accelerated phase of chronic myelogenous leukemia or a relapse of acute myelogenous leukemia in a patient whose disease is in remission in the bone marrow (5,34).

REFERENCES

1. Alvarez-Fernandez, E., and Diez-Nau, M. D. (1979): *Cancer*, 43:1658–1663.
2. Arai, H., Kang, K. Y., Sato, H., Satoh, K., Nagai, H., Motomiya, M., and Konno, K. (1979): *Am. Rev. Respir. Dis.*, 120:529–532.
3. Barrett, N. R. (1970): *Thorax*, 25:515–524.
4. Briselli, M., Mark, E. J., and Dickersin, G. R. (1981): *Cancer*, 47:2678–2689.
5. Carey, R. W., Galdabini, J. J. (1976): *N. Engl. J. Med.*, 294:1333–1338.
6. Chernow, B., and Sahn, S. A. (1977): *Am. J. Med.*, 63:695–702.
7. Dalton, W. T., Zolliker, A. S., McCaughey, W. T. E., Jacques, J., and Kannerstein, M. (1979): *Cancer*, 44:1465–1475.
8. Dionne, G. P., and Wang, N. (1977): *Cancer*, 40:707–715.
9. Goldstein, B. (1979): *Thorax*, 34:375–379.
10. Green, R. A., and Nichols, N. J. (1959): *Am. Rev. Respir. Dis.*, 80:833–844.
11. Harwood, T. R., Gracey, D. R., and Yokoo, H. (1976): *Am. J. Clin. Pathol.*, 65:159–167.
12. Hasan, F. M., Nash, G., and Kazemi, H. (1978): *Am. J. Med.*, 65:649–654.

13. Kannerstein, M., Churg, J., and Magner, D. (1973): *Ann. Clin. Lab. Sci.*, 3:207–211.
14. Kapadia, S. B. (1977): *Arch. Pathol. Lab. Med.*, 101:534–536.
15. Klima, M., and Gyorkey, F. (1977): *Virchows Arch. A. Path. Anat. and Histol.*, 376:181–193.
16. Legha, S. S., and Muggia, F. M. (1977): *Ann. Intern. Med.*, 87:613–621.
17. MacDonald, J. B. (1977): *Thorax*, 32:664–667.
18. Myers, T. J., Cole, S. R., and Pastuszak, W. T. (1978): *Cancer*, 40:266–271.
19. Nwafo, D. C., and Adi, F. C. (1978): *Thorax*, 33:520–523.
20. Oels, H. C., Harrison, E. G., Jr., Carr, D. T., and Bernatz, P. E. (1971): *Chest*, 60:564–570.
21. Persaud, V., Bateson, E. M., and Bankay, C. D. (1970): *Cancer*, 26:920–928.
22. Ratzer, E. R., Pool, J. L., and Melamed, M. R. (1967): *Am. J. Roent.*, 99:863–880.
23. Scannell, J. G., and Mark, E. J. (1979): *N. Engl. J. Med.*, 300:1477–1482.
24. Scharifker, D., and Kaneko, M. (1979): *Cancer*, 43:627–635.
25. Singh, G., Whiteside, T. L., and Dekker, A. (1979): *Cancer*, 43:2288–2296.
26. Sladden, R. A. (1964): *J. Clin. Pathol.*, 17:602–607.
27. Suzuki, Y., Churg, J., and Kannerstein, M. (1976): *Am. J. Path.*, 85:241–262.
28. Tang, C. K., Gray, G. F., and Keuhnelian, J. G. (1976): *Cancer*, 37:1887–1890.
29. Taryle, D. A., Lakshminarayan, S., and Sahn, S. A. (1976): *Medicine*, 55:153–162.
30. Wanebo, H. J., Martini, N., Melamed, M. R., Hilaris, B., and Beattie, E. J., Jr. (1976): *Cancer*, 38:2481–2488.
31. Wang, N. (1973): *Cancer*, 38:2481–2488.
32. Waxler, B., Eisenstein, R., and Battifora, H. (1979): *Cancer*, 44:221–227.
33. Weick, J. K., Kiely, J. M., Harrison, E. G., Jr., Carr, D. T., and Scanlon, P. W. (1973): *Cancer*, 31:848–853.
34. Wu, K. K., and Burns, C. P. (1974): *Cancer*, 33:1179–1182.

Thoracic Oncology, edited by N. C. Choi and H. C. Grillo. Raven Press, New York © 1983.

Mesothelioma

J. Gordon Scannell

Department of Surgery, Massachusetts General Hospital, Boston, Massachusetts 02114

The appropriate treatment of pleural mesothelioma may not occupy absolute center stage, but it is a matter of great interest and debate in the theater of thoracic oncology. This is more particularly true of the diffuse malignant form of the disease than of the localized, usually benign form of fibrous mesothelioma that at times exhibits a malignant potential.

As Chahinian and Holland (1) suggest in their excellent review of the diffuse malignant form, epidemiologic studies have predicted an increasing incidence of this disease in the next decade, in large measure because neoplasms associated with current levels of industrial exposure to asbestos will not be evident until the 1990s, so great is the lag phase of the malign agent in asbestos that has been given such great visibility by Selikoff (2). Certainly the experience at Mt. Sinai, together with reports from Memorial Sloan-Kettering (3), the Mayo Clinic (4), and the group at Newcastle-upon-Tyne (5), is in accord with the gathering storm we have encountered at the Massachusetts General Hospital (MGH). At the latter institution, proximity to shipyards has been in part responsible for a steady increase in asbestosis and asbestos-related neoplasms. The massive building projects of World War II led to unusually high asbestos exposure, the result of insulating pipes under conditions of poor ventilation. This experience at a large urban hospital in the past 20 years has been reported by Hasan, Nash, and Kazemi (6). Similar conditions were reported by the group at Newcastle-upon-Tyne. By way of contrast, reports from the Mayo Clinic (7) of a large series of localized mesotheliomas, benign and malignant, indicate no discernible relationship to asbestos exposure.

It is quite apparent that localized and diffuse mesotheliomas are distinct entities and should be so regarded in any discussion of modes of treatment and results thereof.

LOCALIZED FIBROUS MESOTHELIOMA OF THE PLEURA

Localized mesotheliomas of the pleura, both benign and malignant variants, have been recently reviewed by Okike, Bernatz, and Woolner of the Mayo Clinic (7). Of 60 patients with localized pleural mesotheliomas, 52 had tumors that were histologically and clinically benign. Each patient's normal life expectancy was unaltered or almost certainly improved by successful removal of the tumor. Seven of 8 patients in whom a diagnosis of malignant (though localized) mesothelioma was made on the basis of histologic characteristics died of recurrent disease, usually

347

within 2 years of operation. There was one notable survival at 9 years. The remaining patient in the group died of carcinoma of the pancreas within 5.5 months of the initial operation, thereby raising some question about the initial diagnosis. In none of the localized malignant lesions was there evidence of asbestosis, either in the histologic section of adjacent lung or in the clinical history of the patient.

In the Mayo Clinic series, 28 of 52 patients with benign disease were asymptomatic. Ten patients, however, presented with hypertrophic pulmonary osteoarthropathy and clubbing, an interesting association described some 30 years ago by Clagett et al. (8) from the same institution. The explanation for the extrathoracic manifestations is not forthcoming, although the same dramatic relief of symptoms followed resection of the localized benign mesothelioma that would be expected following resection of a peripheral carcinoma of the lung with similar extrapulmonary manifestations.

A review of 8 cases of solitary fibrous tumors of the pleura encountered at MGH in the two years 1977–1978 was published in 1981 (9). Five of the 8 patients were asymptomatic; 2 patients complained of chest pain, and 1 patient complained of dyspnea and cough. None had osteoarthropathy. None had the bizarre endocrine abnormalities that have been reported with similar tumors, including recurrent hypoglycemia. None had clinical or histologic evidence of asbestosis. Presumably the cell of origin was the mesenchymal cell present in the areolar tissues subjacent to the mesothelial lining.

This agrees with the series reported from Mt. Sinai in 1979. The latter represents a carefully studied group of 18 patients over a period of 17 years. These patients had solid fibrous tumors of the visceral pleura and had undergone successful total resection. Total excision was curative. The majority of the tumors were well encapsulated, took origin from the visceral pleura, and were composed predominantly of spindle cells with more or less hyalinized stroma. No relationship to environmental pollutants was established.

The relative incidence of benign localized mesothelioma versus the diffuse malignant variety may well be the product of referral patterns. For example, at the Memorial Sloan-Kettering Cancer Center, where the emphasis is on malignant disease, only 10 of 76 patients with pleural mesothelioma seen in the years 1939 to 1972 had the localized benign form.

Although the terms *localized* and *benign* imply a rather straightforward and relatively easy surgical approach, it must be noted that many of these localized tumors achieve great size and often are quite vascular. Their total removal can be a taxing surgical exercise.

DIFFUSE MALIGNANT MESOTHELIOMA

Traditionally the prognosis and clinical course of diffuse malignant mesothelioma have been so dismally catastrophic that surgical radiologic and chemotherapeutic attempts to help the unfortunate patients with this disease remind one of Bruce Bainsfeather's dictum of World War I: "If you know a better 'ole, go to it."

An example of this philosophy is the experience of the thoracic surgeons at Newcastle-upon-Tyne, Butchart, Barnsley, and Holden (5). Ashcroft was their pathologist. Asbestos exposure on Tyneside occurs in many industries, notably shipbuilding. Faced with a relatively large series of patients with diffuse malignant mesothelioma, these authors challenged traditional conservative approaches. As a result, they reported 29 patients who underwent pleuropneumonectomy between the years 1959 and 1972. The interval between onset of symptoms (characteristically chest pain) and operation ranged from 2 months to 4 years. During the same period, 17 patients received combinations of medical treatment; although they were similar, by no means can they be considered matched controls. Of the 29 surgical patients, 28 had epithelial tumors or mixed epithelial-mesenchymal tumors.

A radical surgical approach was used. Pleuropneumonectomy, together with removal of adjacent pericardium, diaphragm, and mediastinal contents, was required in 24 patients; in 5 patients minimal diaphragmatic involvement obviated the need for diaphragmatic resection and prosthetic reconstruction.

In view of the magnitude of the procedure, it is not surprising that the operative mortality was 31% (50% in the 8 patients aged 60 to 69). Major complications occurred in 45% of the patients. Two of the 29 survived more than 2 years; both were classified stage I; that is, tumor was confined to the ipsilateral pleura, lung, and pericardium.

Undaunted by past failures, the authors suggest a positive approach, namely, pleuropneumonectomy in patients under age 60 who are fit, without evidence of lymph node involvement by mediastinoscopy, and without peritoneal or contralateral spread, and where the tumor is primarily helpful. Certainly these are reasonable limits with respect to the local extent of tumor and its extension. Computerized body tomography can be enormously helpful. This we have found true in our own experience.

The surgical results reported by Butchart et al. have been matched by those of Delaria, Jensik, Faber, and Kittle of Chicago (11). They reported a series of 18 patients in whom the diagnosis of malignant mesothelioma was made. Eleven underwent extrapleural pneumonectomy, without an operative death. Of the 11, one patient aged 59 remains disease-free at 48 months. This patient had an epithelial tumor and was given cyclophosphamide adjunctively. One of the 11 patients is reported "disease-free" at 4 months(!). The remainder were either dead or living with disease at the time of the report (1978).

Similarly discouraging patient salvage following pleurectomy and in two cases pneumonectomy has been reported from Memorial Sloan-Kettering. Isolated long-term survivals suggest that in the unusual case an apparently diffuse malignant mesothelioma is, indeed, a variant of the localized disease. Unfortunately, in all the series reported, the quality of survival remains an undisclosed item.

Perhaps the most balanced review of the subject of diffuse malignant mesothelioma now available is that of Chahinian and Holland (1), previously referred to. These authors point out quite correctly that statements in the literature vary considerably with regard to life expectancy in this disease and that there has been no published series in which matched groups of patients have been subjected to a variety of treatments in a prospective study.

Palliative procedures in a poorly defined group of patients suffering from a highly lethal and usually painful disease of variable duration and progression are notably difficult to evaluate. This, of course, does not invalidate the attempt to palliate but makes its evaluation extremely difficult. Curative resection has already been discussed, and, indeed, the experience of Butchart and his colleagues is the most enlightening. Unfortunately, conventional radiotherapy and chemotherapy have had limited success. Adriamycin, DTIC (dimethyltriazonimidazol carboximide), vinblastine, cyclophosphamide, methotrexate, etc., alone or in combination, with or without adjuvant radiation therapy, with and without partial surgical extirpation, are all in the protocol stage. Unfortunately, at the present time the clinical prospect is not encouraging.

Certainly the experience at MGH is consonant with the foregoing reports and reviews. Diffuse malignant mesothelioma remains a tremendous therapeutic challenge. The relationship to asbestos exposure appears well established, though not an essential condition. Pain, notably pain that is disproportionate to the radiologic findings of pleural thickening, is a clue to the early diagnosis, particularly of the diffuse mesenchymal type. Pleural effusion and multiple pleural masses are the commonly encountered radiologic findings. Needle biopsy of the pleura has been generally equivocal, and therefore open biopsy usually is recommended. Even a liberal open biopsy may leave room for doubt. For many years the epithelial nature of most malignant mesotheliomas was interpreted variously as "endothelioma" (12) or, in the case of MGH in the days of Tracy Mallory, as extension of an unusual adenocarcinoma from the subjacent lung, and the diagnosis of mesothelioma was not made.

The availability of computerized axial tomography should greatly improve our assessment of the extent of tumor with respect to contralateral or extrathoracic spread, particularly when surgical intervention is contemplated. When extrathoracic extension has occurred, heroic attempts to extirpate the bulk of tumor appear to be ill-advised.

Attempts at radical excision have been sporadic and rarely successful. Partial excision and pleurectomy in an effort to produce pleurodesis is rarely feasible. Pleurodesis by tube thoracotomy and the instillation of tetracycline or other sclerosing agents have met with varying degrees of temporary success. Conventional radiotherapy usually has little to offer, although in a few fortunate patients it has provided some relief of pain. Chemotherapy is on an entirely empiric basis.

The problem of diffuse malignant mesothelioma is far from resolved. For that matter, the natural history of the disease is still poorly defined. That the incidence of the disease is increasing seems evident. It is hoped that further refinements of histologic and electron microscopic techniques may help define the nature of this challenging problem (13).

REFERENCES

1. Chahinian, A. P., and Holland, J. F. (1978): Treatment of diffuse malignant mesothelioma: A review. *Mt. Sinai J. Med.*, 45:54–67.
2. Selikoff, I. J. (1976): Lung cancer and mesothelioma during prospective surveillance of 1249 asbestos insulation workers, 1963–1974. *Ann. N.Y. Acad. Sci.*, 271:448–456.
3. Wanebo, H. J., Martini, N., Melamed, M. R., Hilaris, B., and Beattie, E. J., Jr. (1976): Pleural mesothelioma. *Cancer*, 38:2481–2488.
4. Oels, H., Harrison, E. G., Jr., Carr, D. T., and Bernatz, P. E. (1971): Diffuse malignant mesothelioma of the pleura: A review of 37 cases. *Chest*, 60:564–570.
5. Butchart, E. G., Ashcroft, T., Barnsley, W. C., and Holden, M. P. (1976): Pleuropneumonectomy in the management of diffuse malignant mesothelioma of the pleura. *Thorax*, 31:15–24.
6. Hasan, F. M., Nash, G., and Kazemi, H. (1978): Asbestos exposure and related neoplasia. The 28 year experience of a major urban hospital. *Am. J. Med.*, 65:649–654.
7. Okike, H., Bernatz, P. E., and Woolner, L. B. (1978): Localized mesothelioma of the pleura. Benign and malignant varieties. *J. Thorac. Cardiovasc. Surg.*, 75:363–372.
8. Clagett, O. T., McDonald, J. R., and Schmidt, H. W. (1952): Localized pleural mesothelioma. *J. Thorac. Surg.*, 24:213–230.
9. Briselli, M., Mark, G. J., and Dickersin, G. R. (1981): Solitary fibrous tumors of the pleura. *Cancer*, 47:2678–2689.
10. Scharifker, D., and Kaneko, M. (1979): Localized fibrous mesothelioma of pleura (submesothelial fibroma). *Cancer*, 43:627–635.
11. Delaria, G. A., Jensik, R., Faber, L. P., and Kittle, C. F. (1978): Surgical management of malignant mesothelioma. *Ann. Thorac. Surg.*, 26:375–382.
12. Robertson, H. E. (1924): "Endothelioma" of the pleura. *J. Cancer Res.*, 8:317–375.
13. Scannell, J. G. (1981): Mesothelioma: What the options offer. *Your Patient and Cancer*, 1:53–60.

Thoracic Oncology, edited by N. C. Choi and
H. C. Grillo. Raven Press, New York © 1983.

Treatment of Malignant Pleural Effusion

John M. Head

*Veterans Administration Medical and Regional Office Center,
White River Junction, Vermont 05001*

Pleural effusion is a common and distressing complication of neoplastic disease, especially carcinoma of the breast. Although malignant effusions sometimes respond to systemic therapy directed against the underlying disease, they often become persistent and progressive. Multiple thoracentesis is required for relief of ventilatory restriction and discomfort that often are augmented by chest wall, mediastinal, or pulmonary involvement. Unfortunately, removal of large volumes of proteinaceous pleural fluid can cause severe nutritional (protein) depletion in patients whose homeostatic mechanisms are already weakened. The pleural effusion itself often becomes the major problem confronting the patient during the months before the terminal state is reached.

The ideal treatment of malignant effusions should be simple, quick, flexible, effective, and free of side effects; the end result should be full expansion of the lung and permanent control of the effusion. Of course, no such perfect solution exists, despite a long search. Methods employed have included multiple thoracentesis, tube thoracostomy, irradiation of the hemithorax, instillation of a variety of radioactive, chemotherapeutic and sclerosing agents, and pleurectomy. All have been effective to some extent, but all have undesirable side effects, and some are more flexible than others.

In the search for an effective agent that could be instilled into body cavities to inhibit fluid formation, attention was focused (over 25 years ago) on antineoplastic agents such as radioactive gold, thio-TEPA, and nitrogen mustard. These were followed by quinacrine, which appeared to have tumoricidal properties *in vitro*. When it was found to be effective, flexible, and almost nontoxic, quinacrine became the agent of choice for many physicians in spite of the fact that its cancericidal activity was found to be negligible. This demonstrated that irritating substances were effective in effusion control, regardless of the course of the underlying tumor. The earlier observations that irritating solutions (such as silver nitrate, talc, or sucrose) would produce a reliable pleurodesis were confirmed. The use of radioactive materials declined owing to their inherent logistical problems and variable results. Indeed, any agent, to be effective, must be irritating, whether or not it has an antitumor action. Nitrogen mustard is a prime example.

After quinacrine became unavailable for intracavitary use, several agents such as tetracycline, erythromycin, and bleomycin were advocated. All have enjoyed some measure of success. Recent experience with Corynebacterium parvum has shown that certain malignant effusions, especially those caused by mesothelioma, can be controlled by this agent (1).

A current Veterans Administration cooperative study is attempting to determine whether simple chest tube placement or Tetracycline instillation through a chest tube is the most effective form of treatment. Unfortunately, a limited dose of Tetracycline is specified, so no profound answers will be obtained. From data not yet published, it is evident that effusions caused by certain tumors (i.e., breast) are easily controlled by low dose Tetracycline, whereas effusions caused by tumors such as lung cancer are relatively incorrigible (3). In the author's experience, the latter can be controlled if a sufficient (large) dose of sclerosing agent is used. Several factors influence the choice of agent and dosage: (a) the ability to obtain full expansion of the lung prior to chemical pleurodesis; (b) the rapidity of fluid formation; (c) size of the thorax; (d) patient condition and age; (e) reactivity of the pleura (some patients show very little response to a given dose of a given agent and require much larger total doses than others, by a factor of five or six; other patients demonstrate intense obliterative pleuritis after a single modest dose); (f) known allergy; (g) toxicity. Therefore, a successful program must begin with the art of medicine and end with the administration of an effective medicine. The latter should be chosen to fit the problem. Skill and judgment still exert a greater effect on outcome in the management of malignant effusions than does science.

CLINICAL PROCEDURE

Indications for Pleurodesis

Pleurodesis is indicated when (a) there is persistent, progressive, or recurring pleural effusion of moderate to large size that does not respond to specific treatment of the underlying tumor, (b) the effusion causes symptoms, (c) estimated longevity is more than a month or two, (d) a satisfactory degree of lung expansion can be obtained, and (e) the condition of the patient is good enough to withstand the treatment.

Evaluation

Patient evaluation is relatively simple, although considerable judgment on the part of the physician who is to perform the pleurodesis is necessary. First, it should be determined that the effusion is the result of malignant disease and not of congestive heart failure or other unrelated conditions. This may be difficult if patients have no history of cardiac, renal, or hepatic disease but have impaired organ function caused by tumor or its treatment. Thoracentesis and analysis of the fluid usually will give the answer. Malignant effusions generally have the high protein content of an exudate, frequently contain red blood cells, and usually show malignant cells if a sufficient volume is studied by cytologic and cell block techniques. All available fluid should be removed by thoracentesis and a large sample of it scrutinized for malignant cells.

Following thoracentesis, five important bits of information can be gained.

1. The degree of relief of symptoms can be judged. (If there is little relief, pleurodesis will be disappointing.)

2. The ability of the lung to reexpand can be evaluated.

3. The rate of reaccumulation can be measured. (It is obvious that treatment of an effusion that accumulates at a rate of 600–700 ml per day is much more pressing than treatment of one with a daily rate of 30 ml.)

4. The underlying lung and pleura can be assessed more accurately radiographically.

5. Pulmonary function can be measured more accurately. This is an important consideration, because all methods of effusion control produce some degree of respiratory impairment for at least 1 or 2 weeks. If there is severe impairment of pulmonary function, the treatment may be lethal; i.e., when there is extensive lymphangitic intrapulmonary tumor spread, an effusion may be virtually untreatable. By the same token, bilateral effusions should never be treated simultaneously.

Compromises must be made in the selection of patients for pleurodesis. For example, it is fairly common to find that good reexpansion of the lung cannot be obtained owing to pleural thickening and rigidity that occur when effusions have been present for months. In this event, chemical pleurodesis can be attempted, with the realization that the degree of collapse will be permanent and that a fluid-filled space may remain. However, it is possible to stop the progression of effusion fairly regularly in this circumstance, and thus it may be worthwhile. Because pleural rigidity and loculations tend to develop eventually, the decision to perform chemical pleurodesis should be made as early as possible.

Specific Methods of Treatment

Surgery

Pleurectomy is effective therapy for malignant effusions, perhaps the most reliable of all. Surgery is appropriate for the occasional patient who is very well and unusually stable and whose slow-growing tumor has done little but provoke a pesky effusion. It is especially suited to treatment of multiloculated effusions that cannot be drained by a chest tube. Unfortunately, most patients who have malignant effusions have 6 months or less to live and will not easily withstand thoracotomy. Adequate postoperative suction drainage must be obtained in order to achieve rapid and permanent reexpansion of the lung.

Chemical Pleurodesis

The general peocedure is the same regardless of the agent used. Full expansion of the lung should be obtained if possible; the degree obtained will be permanent. Usually a low axillary or posterolateral intercostal tube (preferably Silastic or polyethylene) is inserted, under local anesthesia. Large effusions should be evacuated slowly in order to avoid marked mediastinal shift with its attendant discomfort and vasovagal reflexes. Usually the tube is placed on gentle suction overnight, and a chest X-ray is obtained in the morning to assess completeness of drainage and reexpansion of the underlying lung. If the appearance is satisfactory, chemical pleurodesis is begun by instilling the chosen agent, diluted in 50 to 100 ml of sterile normal saline or water, through the chest tube. Sterile precautions should be used. The chest tube is clamped for 4 to 6 hr; during this time the patient should be rotated through prone, supine, and both lateral positions for a few minutes each with the bed flat. Usually this routine is repeated two or three times to ensure distribution of the agent throughout the pleural space. The tube is placed back on suction again overnight.

Although several single-dose regimens have been advocated, our experience indicates that the best results are obtained by fractionating the dose into three to five daily doses. For example, 300 mg of tetracycline is given the first day. If there is brisk pleural reaction (manifested by pain and fever), the same dose is repeated the following day. In the case of a small fragile patient whose fluid accumulates at a modest rate, the total dose of 600 mg may suffice; drainage will slow, and the chest tube can be removed 24 to 48 hr later. However, when there is little evidence of reaction, or when there is rapid accumulation in a large chest, the daily dose should be increased to 500 mg, and administration should be continued until drainage slows appreciably (preferably to 75 ml per day or less) before the chest tube is withdrawn. Sometimes it is necessary to deliver as much as 3,000 mg over 5 to 6 days in order to gain control of the effusion.

Very often fluid drainage becomes more copious and thin after the first dose. Also, some patients experience immediate and severe pain on instillation of the sclerosing solution. This can be controlled by including 75 to 100 mg of lidocaine in the solution.

Chest radiographs often become very difficult to interpret during the 2 to 4 weeks following chemical pleurodesis, owing to pleural thickening and locule formation (1). Physical examination provides the most accurate information about lung expansion and aeration during this period. After pleural swelling subsides, most of the density obscuring radiologic detail disappears, usually leaving a visible pleural thickening of 1 to 5 mm.

Side effects. All effective sclerosing agents produce pleuritis and hence some degree of pain, fever, malaise, and temporary ventilatory restriction. Should side effects be lacking completely, it is doubtful that enough reaction is being produced to accomplish permanent pleural symphysis. However, there is some difference in the degrees of severity of side effects of different specific agents. Of the drugs in common use during the past 15 years, nitrogen mustard usually causes the most violent side effects (especially pain, vomiting, and fever), which tend to be of relatively short duration. Quinacrine, while it was in use, seemed to occupy an intermediate position. Tetracycline and erythromycin usually cause low-grade fever, moderate discomfort, and malaise of longer duration.

Selection of specific sclerosing agent. Quinacrine was the prototype of an effective, flexible agent with little specific toxicity. Tetracycline and erythromycin also satisfy these criteria, although allergic reaction occurs occasionally. They also have the theoretical advantage of preventing infection in the pleural space. They can be used during chemotherapy or radiation therapy and do not usually augment bone-marrow depression. They are nontoxic within the required dosage range and are the preferred agents for use today.

Nitrogen mustard is an effective sclerosing agent, and it has specific cancericidal properties. It is ideal for the treatment of lymphomatous effusions *when the patient is not receiving any other form of therapy.* It has been stated that intracavitary mustard is not absorbed. On the contrary, its absorption is capricious, and we have seen fatal bone-marrow depression following intracavitary administration of nitrogen mustard in patients who had received recent chemotherapy or radiation therapy. Therefore, it should not be combined with such treatment, and the intracavitary dose (usually in two or three divided daily doses) should not exceed that normally given intravenously. Flexibility is therefore limited. If satisfactory pleurodesis is not produced by the total dose of 0.4 mg/kg, another agent should be used to "top it off." Also, it is not necessary to clamp the chest tube for 4 to 6 hr, because the cellular effect of mustard is very rapid. Rotation of the patient, in order to distribute the drug, should be done immediately after instillation.

Radiation Therapy

On occasion, intractable pleural effusion accompanies a malignancy in the homolateral hemithorax. When this occurs, radiation therapy of the hemithorax is the treatment of choice, usually with a modest dose to the entire field followed by a step-up dose restricted to the visible tumor mass. Radiation therapy has the same limitation as nitrogen mustard: When a tolerable total dose is not effective in controlling the effusion, another agent must be used to finish the job.

Results

Successful control of malignant pleural effusion can be achieved most of the time (60%–80% in various reports). In our own experience, 63% of those who survived 6 months or more were free of fluid (2). Several patients whose lung reexpansion was incomplete had persistent fluid pockets but required no further treatment (another 13%). Frank early failures were uncommon, but later recurrences did develop approximately 15% of the time.

It is difficult to judge the effect on mortality of pleurodesis in patients who are already quite ill with malignancy. Respiratory failure will occur when pulmonary function is severely impaired before pleurodesis, and it can be expected if bilateral effusions are treated simultaneously. Clear-cut complications are uncommon. Empyema is one such, and should be anticipated. It has occurred in 6% of our patients, becoming manifest 2 to 6 weeks after removal of the chest tube. Owing to the dense pleural adhesions that generally follow therapy, empyema cavities usually will be small and localized and therefore responsive to relatively conservative drainage methods.

Occasionally, allergy to the instilled drug will become a problem.

Because of the setting in which chemical and radiotherapeutic pleurodesis is used, little is known about long-range effects. As a rule, they are overshadowed by the progress of the primary disease.

CONCLUSIONS

The management of distressing malignant pleural effusions requires imagination, flexibility, sensitivity, and compassion. Massive effusions should be controlled early if serious debility is to be avoided. The result is related more to the skill of the physician than to the choice of method, but methods specific to the causative neoplasm should be employed whenever possible. Although side effects of pleurodesis are common, serious complications are not. It is important to recognize the typical radiographic changes that follow chemopleurodesis, because they may be quite confusing for several weeks. Simultaneous bilateral pleurodesis is hazardous and should be avoided.

REFERENCES

1. Felletti, R. and Ravazzoni, C. (1983): *Thorax*, 38:22.
2. McLoud, T. C., Isler, R., and Head, J. M. (1980): The radiologic appearance of chemical pleurodesis. *Radiology*, 135:313–317.
3. O'Donnell, J. (1983): *personal communication.*

Thoracic Oncology, edited by N. C. Choi and
H. C. Grillo. Raven Press, New York © 1983.

Surgery of Pulmonary Metastases

John M. Head

*Veterans Administration Medical and Regional Office Center,
White River Junction, Vermont 05001*

Although it was known by 1900 that removal of tumor metastases was attended by prolonged remission on occasion, planned excision of distant metastases was not done until the late 1920s. In 1927, Diviš reported the planned removal of a metastatic sarcoma from the lung (2). In this country, Barney and Churchill recorded successful lobectomy for metastatic renal carcinoma in 1933 (1). It was only a matter of time before metastases from other primary sites engaged surgical interest. As experience grew, it became possible to define ground rules for case selection, which are still changing as the efficacy of adjuvant therapy improves. For example, sporadic attempts were made to excise multiple metastases from the breast (seldom with success) until chemotherapy became the more effective treatment. Removal of metastatic deposits in organs such as the brain, liver, etc., followed, again with varying degrees of success. Owing to the ease of both detection and removal of metastases in the lung, the lung is still the most common target for excisional therapy.

Based on surgical experience during the 20 years after the Churchill-Barney report, fairly rigid criteria were adopted to govern case selection, and attempts to broaden these were consistently thwarted. These criteria remain valid today:

1. The primary neoplasm should be controlled. This usually implies a long interval between excision of the primary tumor and treatment of metastasis, preferably with a long disease-free interval.

2. Metastatic disease should be "solitary," not part of a metastatic "shower."

3. There should be no other metastases evident.

4. Because little was known about the tendency of metastases themselves to spread to regional nodes at the lung root, and because subsequent solitary metastases might dictate resection, conservative operations were advised. Fortunately, limited resections have low morbidity and mortality rates.

It was found that a reasonable number of patients with pulmonary metastases from the kidney, colon, and uterus met these criteria and that 30% to 35% of them survived without evidence of tumor for 5 years after pulmonary resection. A few soft-tissue sarcomas were also favorable. In general, patients with metastases from breast, upper GI tract, bone, lung, and melanoma did poorly.

By 1965, most interested physicians were aware that the criteria for case selection were, in reality, a crude statement of tumor biologic behavior and that leisurely cohesive tumors were favorable, whereas tumors with rapid growth and spreading factors were not. Joseph, Morton, and Atkins (4) added to this statement with the demonstration that the doubling times of metastatic tumors also provided a useful estimate of longevity and outcome. According to their data, metastases need not be solitary to warrant excision, but they do need to be leisurely. (On the other hand, it would be ludicrous to suggest that 20 metastases in both lungs might be of the same gravity as a single nodule showing a similar growth rate.) Today, surgeons operate on patients whose lungs harbor several nodules, usually with multiple wedge excisions, in an attempt to remove all visible disease. It is too soon to assess the results accurately, but there has been some measure of success. Improved diagnostic techniques have altered the picture further and have sharpened case selection. Conventional tomography reveals small multiple metastases that were missed in the past. Now computerized tomography is revolutionizing the detection of metastases throughout the body and obviates fruitless attempts to excise disease that is not surgical in scope.

The final word on the treatment of metastases is but a dream of the perfect "silver bullet" that will make surgery unnecessary. Until that day arrives, judgment, careful study, and compassionate aggression are the keys to the surgical treatment of pulmonary metastases.

The concept of tumor "debulking" has become popular in recent years and is not without logic. However, as Moore (6) has well stated, the success of debulking followed by chemotherapy depends on the availability of really effective immune or chemical therapy, not on surgical enthusiasm. The mechanisms of metastatic tumor implantation in the lung are somewhat obscure. Logically, pulmonary metastases should occur much more commonly than they do. Many factors are involved, including capillary network diameter, immune responses, lysosomal enzymes, spreading factors, tissue factor-thromboplastin-platelet interactions, and fibrin deposition or lysis. Wilkins (9) summarizes much of this knowledge. To date, therapeutic manipulation of these basic factors has not been effective except in the case of certain tumors (i.e., small cell carcinoma of lung) whose spread has been influenced by anticoagulation (13).

CURRENT EXPERIENCE

Indications for Resection of Pulmonary Metastases

As discussed in the previous section, the ideal patient for cure of metastatic disease has a single metastasis that appeared several years after curative resection of the primary (with no evidence of local recurrence) and that is enlarging slowly in the lung; nothing more than lobectomy should be required; cardiopulmonary function should be adequate to permit safe resection; the surgical approach should be the best form of therapy available.

By focusing on the concept of biologic behavior of the tumor, a moderate number of patients who do not meet all these criteria can be included, i.e., those with several small, slowly growing nodules from the colon. Others who meet most of the criteria can be excluded, i.e., those whose apparently solitary metastases from melanoma of the eye appear years after primary operation but then show a very short doubling time.

With the advent of more effective chemotherapy, a potential area is being developed for the excision of visible metastases from specific tumors to set the stage for medicinal treatment of remaining (reduced) cell populations. For example, Giritsky et al. (3) have reported favorable results of combined surgical-medical therapy of metastatic sarcomas of bone in children. Extension of this approach to the management of similar tumors in adults may not be as useful in improving longevity; more experience is needed in order to be certain.

The discussion to this point has been keyed to the cure of patients with metastatic disease. Palliative surgery should be considered also. In a few cases, resection of metastases is necessary to relieve bronchial obstruction or to stop bleeding if other forms of therapy have failed to do so. This is not a common problem, because only 10% to 12% of patients with limited or moderate metastatic disease have involvement of a major bronchus. Peculiarly, bronchial involvement reduces the cure rate for patients who seem to fit the criteria for curative resection. As is true of palliative surgery in general, pulmonary resection in the face of known residual disease must truly relieve a real problem and improve the patient's well-being if postoperative disaster is to be avoided. Healing may be poor, and resistance to infection nil. Therefore, major surgery for palliation must be performed expertly after good preparation.

Methods of Evaluation

Radiologic techniques yield much useful information about pulmonary metastases, most of which are first noted on standard chest X-rays performed periodically during routine tumor follow-up visits. When a possible abnormality is detected, the examination customarily is repeated 2 or 3 weeks later to rule out evanescent small zones of pneumonitis, artifacts, etc. At this point, a complete workup is indicated to rule out the presence of metastases to liver, brain, bone, etc., and should always include full-lung tomography to obtain a realistic estimate of the number and location of pulmonary lesions. At this juncture, at least 4 weeks will have elapsed since the original detection. Measurements of metastases are made on standard chest films, and diameters are plotted on semilog paper (4) to give a growth slope from which volumetric doubling time can be calculated. Should the doubling time be less than 20 days, it is unlikely that pulmonary resection will be successful. When doubling time is prolonged (more than 40 days), resection usually is indicated. The midrange group must be evaluated carefully. It should be remembered that patients who have one cancer may harbor other synchronous or metachronous primaries. Indeed, 10% of patients with a history of cancer who develop new pulmonary lesions are found to have bronchogenic carcinoma. Thus, three to five cytologic examinations of the sputum are in order. Bronchoscopy should be performed unless the disease is small and peripheral. Bronchial brushing and/or needle aspiration may be needed in questionable or poor-risk cases. Because most metastases are parenchymal, the yield from sputum cytologic examination will be low. The indications for surgical staging by mediastinoscopy or mediastinotomy are not clear. Pulmonary metastases do spread to hilar and mediastinal lymph nodes, but less commonly and more slowly than do most lung cancers (8,10,11). Mediastinal exploration, or at least radionuclide scanning, should be done prior to resection if a pulmonary metastasis is large, is central in location, or is of long duration. Secondary metastases will be found in about 25% of such patients.

The usual preoperative assessment of cardiopulmonary function should be done, and the possibility and scope of pulmonary resection should be matched to the patient's physiologic tolerances. Preparation using chest physiotherapy, postural drainage, bronchodilators, and antibiotic therapy for established sepsis is the same as that before any thoracotomy.

Occasionally it is desirable to give a course of preoperative radiation therapy in an attempt to shrink a large central metastasis so that resection may be safe and perhaps more limited.

Surgical Approach

Surgery for pulmonary metastases should be conservative. Pneumonectomy is justified only when necessary for the removal of a large, slowly growing, solitary, centrally located metastasis. Local lymph nodes should be assessed and dissected if involved.

Lobectomy is indicated for the removal of metastatic disease located in a single lobe or for a solitary nodule lying deep within the parenchyma. Again, regional nodes deserve attention. Simple wedge excisions, occasionally segmental resections, are preferred in the treatment of small subpleural metastases, especially when multiple. Mediastinal nodes are not often involved in this setting, but should be checked. A definite margin of normal lung must be removed. The "shelling out" of metastases often is followed by local recurrence.

A reasonable approach to bilateral pulmonary metastasis requires careful thought. When the lesions are small and amenable to wedge excisions, median sternotomy and simultaneous bilateral resection, as popularized by Urschel and others, are satisfactory. The task is accomplished in one session, and the wound is more comfortable than that following posterolateral thoracotomy. However, if one or more of the metastases require a formal resection such as lobectomy, most surgeons will find staged posterolateral thoracotomies more to their liking. Also, left lower lobe lesions are difficult to reach through an anterior midline incision.

Results

At the Massachusetts General Hospital (MGH) and the White River Junction Veterans Hospital, 205 patients have had 244 operations for removal of pulmonary metastases. Only 2 patients have died because of operation, and complications have been relatively infrequent (12). The primary sites of the original tumors are shown in Table 1. The overall 5-year survival has been just under 32%, similar to the salvage of resectable primary carcinoma of the lung (Fig. 1).

Certain specific tumors are worthy of mention. To date we have no long-term survivors following resection of metastatic melanoma or osteogenic sarcoma. Several recent adult patients who were managed by surgical debulking plus chemotherapy for metastatic bone sarcoma are not included in this series, but there is no evidence as yet that their outcome will be as favorable as that reported in children (3).

By contrast, the prognosis for patients with pulmonary metastasis from colon, kidney, fibrosarcoma, testis, and uterus is reasonable, with the expectation that one in three will survive 5 years or longer if the patients are correctly chosen. Patients with metastatic breast cancer do well after pulmonary resection if the case selection is very careful (Table 2).

Tumor doubling times were not calculated in the majority of patients reported here. The technique is useful and should be employed more widely than it is. Doubling times are indispensable in selecting those patients with several metastases who are suitable for operation. Occasionally the method also will point out changes in the behavior of a tumor. For example, we have treated 4 patients known to have apparently solitary pulmonary metastases that had been observed for prolonged

TABLE 1. *Primary sites of original tumors[a]*

Colon	46
Kidney, bladder	42
Sarcomas	42
Testis	17
Breast	16
Uterus, ovary	14
Melonoma	13
Miscellaneous	15
	205

[a]244 operations

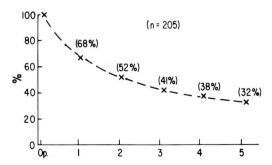

FIG. 1. Survival following excision of pulmonary metastases, all types.

TABLE 2. *5-year cumulative survival*

	N	Survival (%)
Breast	(16)	60
Testis	(17)	50
Kidney-bladder	(44)	46
Uterus-ovary	(14)	34
Colon-rectum	(46)	21
Sarcoma	(42)	18
Melanoma	(13)	0

[a]Entire series = 205; overall cumulative survival = 32%.

periods of time. During initial observation, doubling times were very long (favorable), until sudden growth occurred, and doubling times were recalculated to be within the span of 18 to 30 days (unfavorable). In each case there was rapid spread, with the appearance of additional nodules, signifying a poor prognosis from the surgical point of view. Whether or not earlier resection would have prevented this dissemination is unknown, as is the cause of the change in growth rate. Unfortunately, immunologic competence was not tested in these patients before and after the change in growth rate, which would have been necessary in order to assess the role of competence in tumor behavior.

Personal observations also corroborate the statements of Joseph et al. (5) and Plesnicar et al. (7) that there may be variations in growth rates of simultaneous pulmonary metastases in the same individual. We have no data to support their (probably correct) conclusion that the prognosis is related to the fastest-growing nodule.

CONCLUSIONS

Experience has shown that, in some cases, the course of a patient who develops pulmonary metastases is markedly improved by pulmonary resection. The key is the biologic behavior of the individual tumor, both with and without adjuvant chemotherapy and/or radiation therapy. In other words, case selection versus therapy selection is paramount.

The most significant factors governing prognosis are (a) control of the primary, (b) absence of extrapulmonary metastases, (c) growth rate of metastases in the lung, (d) disease-free interval, and (e) cell type.

Other less significant factors are (a) number of metastases, (b) size and location of metastases (i.e., the prognosis tends to be poor if pneumonectomy is required), and (c) availability of effective chemotherapy.

Although few studies of immunocompetence have been reported in patients with pulmonary metastases, immune mechanisms probably play an important role in determining outcome.

From these thoughts, a therapeutic algorithm may be developed (Fig. 2).

Careful judgment is required in borderline cases showing intermediate growth rates, short disease-free intervals, and multiple metastases. If no effective alternative

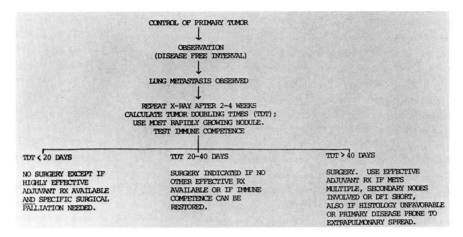

FIG. 2. Therapeutic algorithm for pulmonary metastases.

treatment is available, excision of pulmonary metastases may well be the treatment of choice. However, when all known criteria are favorable, an aggressive surgical attack on pulmonary metastases is both justifiable and rewarding.

REFERENCES

1. Barney, J. D., and Churchill, E. D. (1938): Adenocarcinoma of the kidney with metastases to the lung cancer cured by nephrectomy and lobectomy. *Trans. Am. Assoc. Genitourin. Surg.*, p. 71.
2. Diviš, G. (1927): *Acta. Chir. Scand.*, 62:329.
3. Giritsky, A. S., Etcubanas, E. and Mark, J. B. D. (1978): Pulmonary resection in children with metastatic osteogenic sarcoma. *J. Thorac. Cardiovasc. Surg.*, 75:354–362.
4. Joseph, W. L., Morton, D. L., and Adkins, P. C. (1971): Prognostic significance of tumor doubling time in evaluation operability in pulmonary metastatic disease. *J. Thorac. Cardiovasc. Surg.*, 61:23.
5. Joseph, W. L., Morton, D. L., and Adkins, P. C. (1971): Variation in tumor doubling time in patients with pulmonary metastatic disease. *J. Surg. Oncol.*, 3:143–149.
6. Moore, G. E. (1980): Debunking debulking. *Surg. Gynecol. Onc.*, 150:395–396.
7. Plesnicar, S., Klanjscek, G., and Modic, S. (1978): Actual doubling time values of pulmonary metastases from malignant melanoma. *Aust. N.Z. J. Surg.*, 48:23–25.
8. Sugarbaker, E. V., Cohen, A. M., and Ketcham, A. S. (1971): *Ann. Surg.*, 174:161.
9. Wilkins, E. W., Jr. (1983): In: *Thoracic and Cardiovascular Surgery*, edited by Glenn, Baue, Geha, et al., p. 448. Appleton-Century-Crofts, Norwalk, Connecticut.
10. Wilkins, Jr., E. W., Burke, J. F., and Head, J. M. (1961): The surgical management of metastatic neoplasms in the lung. *J. Thorac. Cardiovasc. Surg.*, 42:298.
11. Wilkins, Jr., E. W., and Head, J. M. (1965): Pulmonary neoplasms: Surgical experience at Massachusetts General Hospital, 1930–1963. *Postgrad. Med.*, 37:584.
12. Wilkins, Jr., E. W., Head, J. M., and Burke, J. F. (1978): Pulmonary resection for metastatic neoplasms in the lung. Experience at the Massachusetts General Hosptial. *Am. J. Surg.*, 135:480.
13. Zacharski. L. R., Henderson, W. G., Pickles, F. R., et al.: (1981): *J.A.M.A.*, 245:831.

Subject Index